Clinical Value of Hybrid PET/MRI

Editors

MINERVA BECKER
VALENTINA GARIBOTTO

MAGNETIC RESONANCE IMAGING CLINICS OF NORTH AMERICA

www.mri.theclinics.com

Consulting Editors
SURESH K. MUKHERJI
LYNNE S. STEINBACH

November 2023 • Volume 31 • Number 4

ELSEVIER

1600 John F. Kennedy Boulevard • Suite 1800 • Philadelphia, Pennsylvania, 19103-2899

http://www.mri.theclinics.com

MAGNETIC RESONANCE IMAGING CLINICS OF NORTH AMERICA Volume 31, Number 4
November 2023 ISSN 1064-9689, ISBN 13: 978-0-443-18272-3

Editor: John Vassallo (j.vassallo@elsevier.com)
Developmental Editor: Shivank Joshi

Magnetic Resonance Imaging Clinics of North America (ISSN 1064-9689) is published quarterly by Elsevier Inc., 360 Park Avenue South, New York, NY 10010-1710. Months of issue are February, May, August, and November. Business and Editorial Offices: 1600 John F. Kennedy Blvd., Ste. 1800, Philadelphia, PA 19103-2899. Customer Service Office: 3251 Riverport Lane, Maryland Heights, MO 63043. Periodicals postage paid at New York, NY and additional mailing offices. Subscription prices are $408.00 per year (domestic individuals), $783.00 per year (domestic institutions), $100.00 per year (domestic students/residents), $455.00 per year (Canadian individuals), $1021.00 per year (Canadian institutions), $573.00 per year (international individuals), $1021.00 per year (international institutions), $100.00 per year (Canadian students/residents), and $275.00 per year (international students/residents). International air speed delivery is included in all *Clinics* subscription prices. All prices are subject to change without notice. **POSTMASTER:** Send address changes to *Magnetic Resonance Imaging Clinics*, Elsevier Health Sciences Division, Subscription Customer Service, 3251 Riverport Lane, Maryland Heights, MO 63043. Customer Service (orders, claims, online, change of address): Elsevier Health Sciences Division, Subscription **Customer Service, 3251 Riverport Lane, Maryland Heights, MO 63043. Tel:1-800-654-2452 (U.S. and Canada); 314-447-8871 (outside U.S. and Canada). Fax: 314-447-8029. E-mail: journalscustomerservice-usa@elsevier.com (for print support); journalsonlinesupport-usa@elsevier.com (for online support).**

Reprints. For copies of 100 or more of articles in this publication, please contact the Commercial Reprints Department, Elsevier Inc., 360 Park Avenue South, New York, NY 10010-1710. Tel.: 212-633-3874; Fax: 212-633-3820; E-mail: reprints@elsevier.com.

Magnetic Resonance Imaging Clinics of North America is covered in the *RSNA Index of Imaging Literature, MEDLINE/PubMed (Index Medicus),* and *EMBASE/Excerpta Medica.*

Contributors

CONSULTING EDITORS

SURESH K. MUKHERJI, MD, MBA, FACR
Clinical Professor of Radiology and Radiation
Oncology, University of Louisville, Peoria,
Illinois, USA; Robert Wood Johnson Medical
School, Rutgers University, New Brunswick,
New Jersey, USA; Faculty, Otolaryngology
Head Neck Surgery, Michigan State University,
Farmington Hills, Michigan, USA; National
Director of Head and Neck Radiology, ProScan
Imaging, Carmel, Indiana, USA

LYNNE S. STEINBACH, MD, FACR
University of California, San Francisco, San
Francisco, California, USA

EDITORS

MINERVA BECKER, MD, EBiHNR
Professor of Radiology, Chair, Unit of Head and
Neck and Maxillofacial Radiology, Division of
Radiology, Diagnostic Department, University
Hospitals of Geneva; Department of Radiology
and Medical Informatics, Geneva University,
Geneva, Switzerland

VALENTINA GARIBOTTO, MD
Associate Professor of Nuclear Medicine, Chair
Division of Nuclear Medicine and Molecular
Imaging, Diagnostic Department, University
Hospitals of Geneva; Chair Department of
Radiology and Medical Informatics, Geneva
University; CIBM Center for Biomedical
Imaging, Geneva, Switzerland

AUTHORS

DIONYSIOS ADAMOPOULOS, PhD
Department of Medical Specialties,
Cardiology, Geneva University Hospital,
Geneva, Switzerland

ABASS ALAVI, MD
Professor, Department of Radiology, Hospital
of the University of Pennsylvania, Philadelphia,
Pennsylvania, USA

HOSSEIN ARABI, PhD
Division of Nuclear Medicine and Molecular
Imaging, Geneva University Hospital, Geneva,
Switzerland

MINERVA BECKER, MD, EBiHNR
Professor of Radiology, Chair, Unit of Head and
Neck and Maxillofacial Radiology, Division of
Radiology, Diagnostic Department, University

Hospitals of Geneva; Department of Radiology
and Medical Informatics, Geneva University,
Geneva, Switzerland

CAROLINA BEZZI, MSc
Vita-Salute San Raffaele University, Nuclear
Medicine Department, IRCCS San Raffaele
Scientific Institute, Milan, Italy

DIOMIDIS BOTSIKAS, MD
Department of Radiology, Geneva University
Hospitals, Geneva, Switzerland

SILVIA CARRARO, MD
Medical Doctor, Specialist in Pediatrics, Unit of
Pediatric Allergy and Respiratory Medicine,
Women's and Children's Health Department,
Associate Professor of Pediatrics, University-
Hospital of Padova, Padova, Italy

FRANCESCO CASTRONOVO, MD
Radiation Oncology Clinic, Oncology Institute of Southern Switzerland, Ente Ospedaliero Cantonale, Bellinzona, Switzerland

ONOFRIO A. CATALANO, MD
Associate Professor, Department of Radiology, Massachusetts General Hospital, Harvard Medical School, Boston, Massachusetts, USA; Athinoula A. Martinos Center for Biomedical Imaging, Harvard Medical School, Charlestown, Massachusetts, USA

DIEGO CECCHIN, MD
Medical Doctor, Specialist in Nuclear Medicine, Associate Professor of Nuclear Medicine at the University of Padova, Department of Medicine, Director of the Postgraduate School of Nuclear Medicine of Padova, Director, Complex Unit of Nuclear Medicine, Department of Medicine (DIMED), University-Hospital of Padova, Padova, Italy

MICHELLE CHEN, BA
Department of Radiology, Keck School of Medicine of University of Southern California, Health Science Campus, Los Angeles, California, USA

ARTURO CHITI, MD
Vita-Salute San Raffaele University, Nuclear Medicine Department, IRCCS San Raffaele Scientific Institute, Milan, Italy

CLAUDIO DE VITO, MD
Diagnostic Department, Division of Clinical Pathology, Geneva University Hospitals, Geneva, Switzerland

LETIZIA DEANTONIO, MD
Radiation Oncology Clinic, Oncology Institute of Southern Switzerland, Ente Ospedaliero Cantonale, Bellinzona, Switzerland; Faculty of Biomedical Sciences, Università della Svizzera italiana, Lugano, Switzerland

JEAN-FRANÇOIS DEUX, MD, PhD
Professor, Diagnostics Department, Radiology, Geneva University Hospitals, Geneva, Switzerland

NICOLAS DULGUEROV, MD
Department of Clinical Neurosciences, Clinic of Otorhinolaryngology, Head and Neck Surgery, Unit of Cervicofacial Surgery, Geneva University Hospitals, Geneva, Switzerland

FELIPE S. FURTADO, MD
Department of Radiology, Massachusetts General Hospital, Harvard Medical School, Boston, Massachusetts, USA; Athinoula A. Martinos Center for Biomedical Imaging, Harvard Medical School, Charlestown, Massachusetts, USA

VALENTINA GARIBOTTO, MD
Associate Professor of Nuclear Medicine, Chair Division of Nuclear Medicine and Molecular Imaging, Diagnostic Department, University Hospitals of Geneva; Chair Department of Radiology and Medical Informatics, Geneva University; CIBM Center for Biomedical Imaging, Geneva, Switzerland

SAMUELE GHEZZO, MSc
Vita-Salute San Raffaele University, Nuclear Medicine Department, IRCCS San Raffaele Scientific Institute, Milan, Italy

ALI GHOLAMREZANEZHAD, MD
Associate Professor, Department of Radiology, Keck School of Medicine of University of Southern California, Health Science Campus, Los Angeles, California, USA

CHIARA GIRAUDO, MD
Medical Doctor, Specialist in Radiology, Complex Unit of Nuclear Medicine of Padova, Department of Medicine (DIMED), Researcher, University-Hospital of Padova, Padova, Italy

CARL GLESSGEN, MD
Diagnostics Department, Radiology, Geneva University Hospitals, Geneva, Switzerland

REECE J. GOIFFON, MD, PhD
Department of Radiology, Massachusetts General Hospital, Harvard Medical School, Boston, Massachusetts, USA

ELSA HERVIER, MD
Diagnostics Department, Nuclear Medicine and Molecular Imaging, Geneva University Hospital, Geneva, Switzerland

AURÉLIE KAS, MD, PhD
Department of Nuclear Medicine, Pitié-Salpêtrière Hospital, APHP Sorbonne Université; Sorbonne Université, INSERM, CNRS, Laboratoire d'Imagerie Biomédicale, LIB, Paris, France

SANAZ KATAL, MD, MPH
Medical Imaging Department of St. Vincent's
Hospital, Melbourne, Victoria, Australia

UMAR MAHMOOD, MD
Professor, Department of Radiology,
Massachusetts General Hospital, Harvard
Medical School, Boston, Massachusetts, USA

ISMINI C. MAINTA, MD
Department of Nuclear Medicine and
Molecular Imaging, Geneva University
Hospitals, Geneva, Switzerland

PAOLA MAPELLI, MD, PhD
Vita-Salute San Raffaele University, Nuclear
Medicine Department, IRCCS San Raffaele
Scientific Institute, Milan, Italy

RENÉ NKOULOU, MD
Diagnostics Department, Nuclear Medicine
and Molecular Imaging, Geneva University
Hospitals, Geneva, Switzerland

GAETANO PAONE, MD
Faculty of Biomedical Sciences, Università
della Svizzera italiana, Lugano, Switzerland;
Clinic for Nuclear Medicine and Molecular
Imaging, Imaging Institute of Southern
Switzerland, Ente Ospedaliero Cantonale,
Bellinzona, Switzerland

MARIA PICCHIO, MD
Vita-Salute San Raffaele University, Nuclear
Medicine Department, IRCCS San Raffaele
Scientific Institute, Milan, Italy

NADYA PYATIGORSKAYA, MD, PhD
Neuroradiology Department, Pitié-Salpêtrière
Hospital, APHP Sorbonne Université;
Sorbonne Université, Institut du Cerveau,
Paris, France

ÁLVARO BADENES ROMERO, MD
Department of Radiology, Massachusetts
General Hospital, Harvard Medical School,
Boston, Massachusetts, USA; Athinoula A.
Martinos Center for Biomedical Imaging,
Harvard Medical School, Charlestown,
Massachusetts, USA; Department of Nuclear
Medicine, Joan XXIII Hospital, Tarragona, Spain

LAURA ROZENBLUM, MD
Department of Nuclear Medicine, Pitié-
Salpêtrière Hospital, APHP Sorbonne
Université; Sorbonne Université, INSERM,

CNRS, Laboratoire d'Imagerie Biomédicale,
LIB, Paris, France

PANIZ SABEGHI, MD
Department of Radiology, Keck School of
Medicine of University of Southern California,
Health Science Campus, Los Angeles,
California, USA

BABAK SABOURY, MD, MPH
Department of Radiology, Hospital of the
University of Pennsylvania, Philadelphia,
Pennsylvania, USA; Department of Radiology
and Imaging Sciences, Clinical Center,
National Institutes of Health, Bethesda,
Maryland, USA

ANA MARIA SAMANES GAJATE, MD
Nuclear Medicine Department, IRCCS San
Raffaele Scientific Institute, Milan, Italy

MADALEINE SERTIC, MD
Department of Radiology, Massachusetts
General Hospital, Harvard Medical School,
Boston, Massachusetts, USA

ILEKTRA SFAKIANAKI, MD
Department of Radiology, Geneva University
Hospitals, Geneva, Switzerland

ISAAC SHIRI, PhD
Department of Nuclear Medicine and
Molecular Imaging, Geneva University
Hospitals, Geneva, Switzerland

ALESSANDRO SPATARO, MD
Department of Biomedical and Dental
Sciences and of Morpho-Functional Imaging,
Nuclear Medicine Unit, University of Messina,
Messina, Italy

FARZANEH TARAVAT, MD
Department of Radiology, Keck School of
Medicine of University of Southern California,
Health Science Campus, Los Angeles,
California, USA

GIORGIO TREGLIA, MD
Faculty of Biomedical Sciences, Università
della Svizzera italiana, Lugano, Switzerland;
Clinic for Nuclear Medicine and Molecular
Imaging, Imaging Institute of Southern
Switzerland, Ente Ospedaliero Cantonale,
Bellinzona, Switzerland; Faculty of Biology and
Medicine, University of Lausanne, Lausanne,
Switzerland

JEAN-PAUL VALLEE, MD, PhD
Professor, Diagnostics Department,
Radiology, Geneva University Hospitals,
Geneva, Switzerland

THOMAS J. WERNER, MS
Department of Radiology, Hospital of the
University of Pennsylvania, Philadelphia,
Pennsylvania, USA

HABIB ZAIDI, PhD
Professor of Medical Physics, Diagnostic
Department, Division of Nuclear Medicine and
Molecular Imaging, Geneva University
Hospitals, University of Geneva, Geneva
University Neurocenter, University of Geneva,
Geneva, Switzerland; Department of Nuclear
Medicine and Molecular Imaging, University of
Groningen, University Medical Center

Groningen, Groningen, Netherlands;
Department of Nuclear Medicine, University of
Southern Denmark, Odense, Denmark

THOMAS ZILLI, MD
Chief, Radiation Oncology Clinic, Oncology
Institute of Southern Switzerland, Ente
Ospedaliero Cantonale, Bellinzona,
Switzerland; Faculty of Biomedical Sciences,
Università della Svizzera italiana, Lugano,
Switzerland; Faculty of Medicine, University of
Geneva, Geneva, Switzerland

PIETRO ZUCCHETTA, MD
Medical Doctor, Specialist in Nuclear
Medicine, Vice-Director, Complex Unit of
Nuclear Medicine, Department of Medicine
(DIMED), University-Hospital of Padova,
Padova, Italy

Contents

More than a decade has passed since the clinical deployment of the first commercial whole-body hybrid PET/MR scanner in the clinic. The major advantages and limitations of this technology have been investigated from technical and medical perspectives. Despite the remarkable advantages associated with hybrid PET/MR imaging, such as reduced radiation dose and fully simultaneous functional and structural imaging, this technology faced major challenges in terms of mutual interference between MRI and PET components, in addition to the complexity of achieving quantitative imaging owing to the intricate MRI-guided attenuation correction in PET/MRI. In this review, the latest technical developments in PET/MRI technology as well as the state-of-the-art solutions to the major challenges of quantitative PET/MR imaging are discussed.

Hybrid PET/MRI is highly valuable, having made significant strides in overcoming technical challenges and offering unique advantages such as reduced radiation, precise data coregistration, and motion correction. Growing evidence highlights the value of PET/MRI in broad clinical aspects, including inflammatory and oncological imaging in adults, pregnant women, and pediatrics, potentially surpassing PET/CT. This newly integrated solution may be preferred over PET/CT in many clinical conditions. However, further technological advancements are required to facilitate its broader adoption as a routine diagnostic modality.

Head and neck squamous cell carcinoma (HNSCC) can either be examined with hybrid PET/MR imaging systems or sequentially, using PET/CT and MR imaging. Regardless of the acquisition technique, the superiority of MR imaging compared to CT lies in its potential to interrogate tumor and surrounding tissues with different sequences, including perfusion and diffusion. For this reason, PET/MR imaging is preferable for the detection and assessment of locoregional residual/recurrent HNSCC after therapy. In addition, MR imaging interpretation is facilitated when combined with PET. Nevertheless, distant metastases and distant second primary tumors are detected equally well with PET/MR imaging and PET/CT.

Dedicated MR imaging is highly performant for the evaluation of the primary lesion and should regularly be added to whole-body PET/MR imaging for the initial staging. PET/MR imaging is highly sensitive for the detection of nodal involvement and could be combined with the high specificity of axillary second look ultrasound for the confirmation of the N staging. For M staging, with the exception of lung lesions, PET/MR imaging is superior to PET/computed tomography, at half the radiation dose. The predictive value of multiparametric imaging with PET/MR imaging holds promise to improve through radiomics and artificial intelligence.

Hybrid positron emission tomography (PET)/magnetic resonance imaging (MRI) is highly suited for abdominal pathologies. A precise co-registration of anatomic and metabolic data is possible thanks to the simultaneous acquisition, leading to accurate imaging. The literature shows that PET/MRI is at least as good as PET/CT and even superior for some indications, such as primary hepatic tumors, distant metastasis evaluation, and inflammatory bowel disease. PET/MRI allows whole-body staging in a single session, improving health care efficiency and patient comfort.

Hybrid PET/MR imaging offers a unique opportunity to acquire MR imaging and PET information during a single imaging session. PET/MR imaging has numerous advantages, including enhanced diagnostic accuracy, improved disease characterization, and better treatment planning and monitoring. It enables the immediate integration of anatomic, functional, and metabolic imaging information, allowing for personalized characterization and monitoring of neurologic diseases. This review presents recent advances in PET/MR imaging and highlights advantages in clinical practice for neuro-oncology, epilepsy, and neurodegenerative disorders. PET/MR imaging provides valuable information about brain tumor metabolism, perfusion, and anatomic features, aiding in accurate delineation, treatment response assessment, and prognostication.

The present systematic review and meta-analysis are focused on the diagnostic accuracy of PSMA PET/MRI in primary prostate cancer assessment. A literature search was conducted on the PubMed database using the terms "PSMA" AND "prostate cancer" or "prostate" AND "PET/MRI" or "PET MRI" or "PET-MRI" or "PET-MR" AND "primary" or "staging." Ten articles were eligible for analysis after applying the exclusion criteria. PET/MRI showed better diagnostic accuracy in detecting primary PCa compared to multiparametric (mp) MRI and PET alone. The pooled sensitivity and specificity of 68Ga-PSMA PET/MRI at the per-patient level were 0.976 (CI: 0.943–0.991) and 0.739 (CI: 0.437–0.912); respectively. PSMA PET/MRI has good sensitivity in detecting primary PCa, especially in patients with PIRADS 3 PCa.

In the last few years, technological advances in MR imaging, PET detectors, and attenuation correction algorithms have allowed the creation of truly integrated PET/MR imaging systems, for both clinical and research applications. These machines allow a comprehensive investigation of cardiovascular diseases, by offering a wide variety of detailed anatomical and functional data in combination. Despite significant pathophysiologic mechanisms being clarified by this new data, its clinical relevance and prognostic significance have not been demonstrated yet.

PET/MR imaging is a one-stop shop technique for pediatric diseases allowing not only an accurate clinical assessment of tumors at staging and restaging but also the diagnosis of neurologic, inflammatory, and infectious diseases in complex cases. Moreover, applying PET kinetic analyses and sequences such as diffusion-weighted imaging as well as quantitative analysis investigating the relationship between disease metabolic activity and cellularity can be applied. Complex radiomics analysis can also be performed.

The use of hybrid PET/MR imaging for radiotherapy treatment planning has the potential to reduce tumor and organ displacements caused by different scan times and setup changes. Although with mixed results mainly due to single-center studies with small sample size, PET/MR imaging could provide better target delineation, especially by reducing coregistration discrepancies on computed tomography simulation scan and offering better soft tissue contrast. The main limitation to drive stronger conclusions is due to the relatively low availability of hybrid PET/MR imaging systems, mainly limited to large academic centers.

MAGNETIC RESONANCE IMAGING CLINICS OF NORTH AMERICA

SERIES OF RELATED INTEREST

Advances in Clinical Radiology
www.advancesinclinicalradiology.com
Neuroimaging Clinics
www.neuroimaging.theclinics.com
PET Clinics
www.pet.theclinics.com
Radiologic Clinics
www.radiologic.theclinics.com

VISIT THE CLINICS ONLINE!
Access your subscription at:
www.theclinics.com

PROGRAM OBJECTIVE

The goal of *Magnetic Resonance Imaging Clinics of North America* is to keep practicing physicians up to date with current clinical practice by providing timely articles reviewing the state of the art in patient care.

TARGET AUDIENCE

All practicing physicians and healthcare professionals who provide patient care utilizing findings from Magnetic Resonance Imaging.

LEARNING OBJECTIVES

Upon completion of this activity, participants will be able to:
1. Review the diagnostic accuracy of PET (Positron Emission Tomography) and MRI (Magnetic Resonance Imaging).
2. Discuss PET/MRI specificity in the detection, classification, staging, and treatment response evaluation of malignant lesions.
3. Recognize the central role imaging plays in the diagnosis and management of various cancers.

ACCREDITATION

The Elsevier Office of Continuing Medical Education (EOCME) is accredited by the Accreditation Council for Continuing Medical Education (ACCME) to provide continuing medical education for physicians.

The EOCME designates this journal-based CME activity enduring material for a maximum of 10 *AMA PRA Category 1 Credit*(s)™. Physicians should claim only the credit commensurate with the extent of their participation in the activity.

All other healthcare professionals requesting continuing education credit for this enduring material will be issued a certificate of participation.

DISCLOSURE OF CONFLICTS OF INTEREST

The EOCME assesses conflict of interest with its instructors, faculty, planners, and other individuals who are in a position to control the content of CME activities. All relevant conflicts of interest that are identified are thoroughly vetted by EOCME for fair balance, scientific objectivity, and patient care recommendations. EOCME is committed to providing its learners with CME activities that promote improvements or quality in healthcare and not a specific proprietary business or a commercial interest.

The planning committee, staff, authors, and editors listed below have identified no financial relationships or relationships to products or devices they or their spouse/life partner have with commercial interest related to the content of this CME activity:
Dionysios Adamopoulos, MD, PhD; Abass Alavi, MD; Hossein Arabi, PhD; Minerva Becker, MD; Carolina Bezzi, MSc; Diomidis Botsikas, MD; Silvia Carraro, MD; Francesco Castronovo, MD; Onofrio A. Catalano, MD; Michelle Chen; Arturo Chiti, MD; Claudio de Vito, MD; Letizia Deantonio, MD; Cecchin Diego, MD; Nicolas Dulguerov, MD; Felipe S. Furtado, MD; Valentina Garibotto, MD; Samuele Ghezzo, MSc; Ali Gholamrezanezhad, MD; Chiara Giraudo, MD; Reece J. Goiffon, MD, PhD; Elsa Hervier, MD; Aurélie Kas, MD, PhD; Sanaz Katal, MD-MPH; Kothainayaki Kulanthaivelu, BCA, MBA; Michelle Littlejohn; Umar Mahmood, MD; Ismini C. Mainta, MD; Paola Mapelli, MD, PhD; René Nkoulou, MD; Gaetano Paone, MD; Maria Picchio, MD; Nadya Pyatigorskaya, MD, PhD; Álvaro Badenes Romero, MD; Laura Rozenblum, MD; Paniz Sabeghi, MD; Babak Saboury, MD, MPH; Ana Maria Samanes Gajate, MD; Madaleine Sertic, MD; Ilektra Sfakianaki, MD; Isaac Shiri, PhD; Alessandro Spataro, MD; Farzaneh Taravat, MD; Giorgio Treglia, MD; Jean-Paul Vallee, MD, PhD; Thomas J. Werner, MSE; Habib Zaidi, PhD; Thomas Zilli, MD; Pietro Zucchetta, MD

UNAPPROVED/OFF-LABEL USE DISCLOSURE

The EOCME requires CME faculty to disclose to the participants:
1. When products or procedures being discussed are off-label, unlabelled, experimental, and/or investigational (not US Food and Drug Administration [FDA] approved); and
2. Any limitations on the information presented, such as data that are preliminary or that represent ongoing research, interim analyses, and/or unsupported opinions. Faculty may discuss information about pharmaceutical agents that is outside of FDA-approved labelling. This information is intended solely for CME and is not intended to promote off-label use of these medications. If you have any questions, contact the medical affairs department of the manufacturer for the most recent prescribing information.

TO ENROLL

To enroll in the *Magnetic Resonance Imaging Clinics of North America* Continuing Medical Education program, call customer service at 1-800-654-2452 or sign up online at http://www.theclinics.com/home/cme. The CME program is available to subscribers for an additional annual fee of USD 270.00.

METHOD OF PARTICIPATION

In order to claim credit, participants must complete the following:
1. Complete enrolment as indicated above.
2. Read the activity.

3. Complete the CME Test and Evaluation. Participants must achieve a score of 70% on the test. All CME Tests and Evaluations must be completed online.

CME INQUIRIES/SPECIAL NEEDS

For all CME inquiries or special needs, please contact elsevierCME@elsevier.com.

Foreword

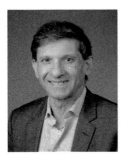 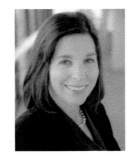

Suresh K. Mukherji, MD, MBA   Lynne S. Steinbach, MD, FACR
Consulting Editors

I was very impressed and somewhat surprised by Drs Minerva Becker and Valentina Garibotto's candor regarding the evolution of PET-MR imaging in their preface. Instead of touting PET/MR imaging as a "wonder modality," they give an elegant and accurate description of the history of PET-MR imaging using the analogy of the Gartner "Hype Cycle." The initial excitement of high expectations was followed by the realities of trying to demonstrate the tangible benefits of combining two important modalities into an hybrid modality to justify the high costs to hospital administrators, payors, and patients.

We have entered the "reality" phase of the lifecycle of PET-MR imaging, which is why we decided to devote this issue to the clinical applications of PET-MR imaging. There are practical articles devoted to the current role of PET-MR imaging for evaluating various disorders of the head and neck, brain, breast, abdomen, and cardiac. There are also more advanced articles devoted to prostate specific membrane antigen (PSMA) PET/MR imaging for intraprostatic tumor assessment and metabolic imaging for radiation therapy treatment planning.

A very special debt of gratitude to Drs Becker and Garibotto and all the article authors. The articles beautifully illustrate state-of-the-art reviews by recognized experts. I also want to thank Drs Becker and Garibotto for their willingness to take on such a challenging and timely topic.

On a personal note, I have known my friend Minerva Becker for many years and congratulate her on her recent election as second Vice-President of the European Society of Radiology (ESR). Minerva will ascend to the Presidency of the ESR in 2025 and President of the European College of Radiology in 2026. The future of European Radiology is incredibly bright with such a talented person at its helm!

Suresh K. Mukherji, MD, MBA, FACR
University of Louisville, ProScan Imaging
Carmel, IN 46032, USA

Lynne S. Steinbach, MD, FACR
University of California San Francisco
505 Parnassus Avenue
San Francisco, CA 94143-0628, USA

E-mail addresses:
sureshmukherji@hotmail.com (S.K. Mukherji)
lynne.steinbach@ucsf.edu (L.S. Steinbach)

Magn Reson Imaging Clin N Am 31 (2023) xiii
https://doi.org/10.1016/j.mric.2023.08.003
1064-9689/23/© 2023 Published by Elsevier Inc.

Preface
PET/MR Imaging in Clinical Practice: After Expectations and (Some) Disillusion, a Slope of Enlightenment

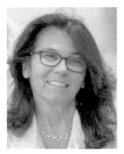 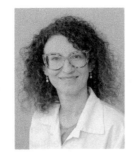

Minerva Becker, MD, EBiHNR   Valentina Garibotto, MD
Editors

Like many other technical innovations, PET/MR hybrid imaging has followed Gartner's hype cycle theory that the innovation trigger leads to a peak of inflated expectations, followed by a dip of disillusionment, and finally, a slope of enlightenment leading to a plateau of productivity. Since its introduction in the clinical field in 2010, the method has raised very high expectations across almost all clinical applications. The previous issue of the *Magnetic Resonance Imaging Clinics of North America* about this topic published in 2017 was still influenced by the initial enthusiasm.

In the current issue, we invited experts to share their view on PET/MR imaging based on the evidence that has been collected over a decade of clinical use. The presentation of the main technological progresses focuses on quantitative approaches that are of particular interest in an academic environment, given that PET/MR imaging has a place not only in clinical routine but also in research. Unsurprisingly, the typical clinical indications for PET/MR imaging occurred in those clinical domains in which both PET and MR imaging were already routinely used as complementary modalities before the advent of combined PET/MR imaging acquisition. Key examples include advanced oncologic imaging in different organ systems and metabolic imaging in order to assess the viability of tissue of the brain and heart. Particular clinical interest has also been given to pediatric imaging, head and neck cancer, and radiation therapy planning.

The most important advantages of combining the information of PET and MR imaging enable radiologists and nuclear physicians together (1) to interrogate tissue by evaluating many different biomarkers, adding metabolic information to perfusion, diffusion, and other signal behaviors; (2) to localize changes with regard to anatomic structures that can be visualized only with MR imaging; (3) to facilitate image interpretation in complex situations (eg, after surgery of radiation therapy); and (4) to obtain information for both specific anatomic regions (eg, for local tumor staging) and large body regions (eg, for M staging).

Magn Reson Imaging Clin N Am 31 (2023) xv–xvi
https://doi.org/10.1016/j.mric.2023.08.002
1064-9689/23/© 2023 Published by Elsevier Inc.

Despite all these advantages, the impact of combined PET/MR imaging on patient care still remains difficult to measure and depends on clinical situations. In clinical practice, the added value that combined acquisition of PET and MR imaging can bring to patient care must be weighed against the relatively high cost and examination time involved in this technique as opposed to separate acquisitions of each modality. Finally, although the use of multiple biomarkers often facilitates the diagnosis, this may also be quite challenging, as the different parameters may be contradictory.

The initial hype is over, and the community of PET/MR imaging users is now on the path of enlightenment, adequately discussing the pros and cons about this fascinating diagnostic approach in an informed and critical way and with evidence-based methodologies. We invite the reader to discover the key clinical aspects of this combined modality in this issue of *Magnetic Resonance Imaging Clinics of North America*.

Minerva Becker, MD, EBiHNR
Division of Radiology
Diagnostic Department
University Hospitals of Geneva
Rue Gabrielle Perret Gentil 14
CH 1211 Geneva, Switzerland

Valentina Garibotto, MD
Division of Nuclear Medicine and Molecular Imaging
Diagnostic Department
University Hospitals of Geneva
Rue Gabrielle Perret Gentil 14
CH 1211 Geneva, Switzerland

E-mail addresses:
Minerva.Becker@hcuge.ch (M. Becker)
Valentina.Garibotto@hcuge.ch (V. Garibotto)

Recent Advances in Positron Emission Tomography/Magnetic Resonance Imaging Technology

Hossein Arabi, PhD[a], Habib Zaidi, PhD[a,b,c,d],*

KEYWORDS

• PET/MRI • Multimodality imaging • Instrumentation • Quantitative imaging • Attenuation correction

KEY POINTS

- Contrary to the widespread adoption of hybrid PET/CT scanners in clinical setting, PET/MR imaging bears only a small fraction of the total PET market.
- PET/MR imaging is challenged by MRI-guided attenuation correction of PET data, mutual MR-PET components interferences, body truncation, and metal artifacts.
- The trend is toward developing compact PET inserts for existing MRI scanners, providing high spatial resolution and reasonable cost.
- Deep learning-guided approaches will be predominately employed to address the major challenges of quantitative PET/MR imaging.

INTRODUCTION

Over a decade has passed since the introduction of PET/MR hybrid systems in the clinic, wherein the main advantages and drawbacks of PET/MR imaging from a medical, technical, and logistics/workflow perspective have been investigated.[1,2] In contrast to the widespread adoption of hybrid PET/CT scanners in the clinical setting, PET/MR imaging couldn't reach many sites and may bear only 5% of the total PET market.[3] This trend could be attributed to the high cost and new paradigms introduced by this technology, workflow, and logistics issues, and the challenges associated with quantitative PET/MR imaging. Since the introduction of PET/MRI systems, substantial efforts have been made to find/establish the key clinical applications of this modality in order to justify/promote its utilization.

Though PET/MR systems are not as popular as PET/CT scanners, they cause reduced patient radiation exposure, which is critical in childbearing women, pediatric patients, and patients undergoing sequential response to therapy and recurrence monitoring.[4,5] Moreover, superior soft-tissue contrast and visualization in MR images (compared to CT images) would lead to enhanced lesion detectability and diagnostic accuracy in addition to complementary functional information that could be provided by MR imaging.[6,7] Furthermore, simultaneous PET and MR imaging would enable motion correction to PET data to compensate for respiratory and cardiac motions as well as patient movement due to pain and anxiety during PET imaging.[8] Reduced positron range and improved PET image quality (higher spatial resolution) are expected for high-energy positron-emitting PET radiotracers due to the presence of the MR magnetic

[a] Division of Nuclear Medicine and Molecular Imaging, Geneva University Hospital, Geneva 4 CH-1211, Switzerland; [b] Geneva University Neurocenter, Geneva University, Geneva CH-1205, Switzerland; [c] Department of Nuclear Medicine and Molecular Imaging, University of Groningen, University Medical Center Groningen, Groningen 9700 RB, Netherlands; [d] Department of Nuclear Medicine, University of Southern Denmark, Odense 500, Denmark
* Corresponding author. Division of Nuclear Medicine and Molecular Imaging, Geneva University Hospital, Geneva 4 CH-1211, Switzerland.
E-mail address: habib.zaidi@hcuge.ch

Magn Reson Imaging Clin N Am 31 (2023) 503–515
https://doi.org/10.1016/j.mric.2023.06.002
1064-9689/23/© 2023 Elsevier Inc. All rights reserved.

field in simultaneous PET MR imaging at high magnetic field strength.[9] Moreover, co-registered MR data (in simultaneous PET/MR imaging) could be employed for MRI-guided PET image reconstruction and partial volume correction to enhance the overall quality and quantitative accuracy of PET images.[10,11]

Despite the advantages associated with simultaneous PET/MR imaging, this technology yet faces major challenges regarding attenuation correction for PET data, mutual MR-PET components interferences, body truncation due to the limited transaxial MR field-of-view, and artifacts in MR images due to the metal implants.[12]

In this review, the latest technical developments in PET/MR systems design and technological developements as well as the state-of-the-art solutions to the major challenges of quantitative PET/MR imaging are discussed.

ADVANCES IN POSITRON EMISSION TOMOGRAPHY/MAGNETIC RESONANCE IMAGING INSTRUMENTATION

The major challenge to developing simultaneous PET/MR devices is to minimize/nullify the interference between the magnetic field of MR imaging and the readout electronics of PET detectors.[13] In this regard, PET photomultiplier tubes (PMT) were replaced by semiconductor components in PET detectors. The very first simultaneous PET/MRI system (for small-animal imaging) exploited avalanche photodiodes (APD) coupled to lutetium oxyorthosilicate (LSO) crystals in a 7T MR scanner.[14,15] Using the same technology, Siemens Healthcare (Erlangen, Germany) built a prototype PET insert for simultaneous brain imaging in a 3T MR scanner with a 36 cm inner diameter.[16] PET detectors were shielded in copper cassettes to minimize magnetic field interferences. No noticeable interferences were reported between PET and MR components, such as PET signal distortion, eddy currents in PET shields, and inhomogeneities of the magnetic field (B0).[17]

The first whole-body PET/MR scanner (Ingenuity TF PET/MRI) was installed by Philips Healthcare in 2010. To avoid the interferences between PET and MR components, sequential hybrid imaging was adopted in this scanner, wherein the time of flight (TOF)-PET component of the Philips Gemini PET/CT was combined with Philips Achieva 3T MRI scanner (using a turntable-based mechanism). Owing to the sequential acquisition, no novel instrumental development was considered in the PET component, and still, PMTs (together with LYSO crystals) were employed in the PET detectors with minor modifications.[18,19] The Biograph mMR

(hybrid whole-body PET/MR, Siemens) was the first commercial whole-body scanner allowing for simultaneous MR imaging and PET data acquisition.[20] To reduce the sensitivity of the PET detectors to the 3T magnetic field, APDs were employed as readout electronics of photon detectors (LSO) with a crystal size of $4 \times 4 \times 20$ mm^3, leading to a spatial resolution of 4.3 mm (FWHM). Due to the slower temporal performance of ADPs compared to PMTs, the PET device does not benefit from TOF capability. Even though the PET component was fully integrated within the MR scanner, no significant distortion was observed in the RF field (B1) and magnetic field (B0) homogeneity as well as interferences of MR signals with the PET electronics.[20] 4-channels coils were later introduced in this system for dedicated MR imaging (breast scans) which caused 11% reduction in the PET statistical counts (photon attenuation).[21] Simultaneous PET and MR (3T) imaging SIGNA system was introduced by GE Healthcare in 2014 using Lutetium-based scintillator (LBS) crystal and Light Tight RF Shield with copper coating. The PMTs or ADPs were replaced with Silicon Photomultipliers (SiPMs) in this scanner providing a similar gain of 10^6 for PMTs (compared to 10^2 provided by ADPs) and 400 ps temporal resolution compared to 1 ns for PMTs.[22] These commercial PET/MR scanners have a large MR bore size of 70 cm to accommodate the PET component, however, the bore size of PET devices would be 60 cm in diameter, which may cause claustrophobia issues and limit the choice of subjects in terms of body size. The most recently released simultaneous uPMR790 PET/MRI scanner (United Imaging Healthcare Co. Ltd., Shanghai, China) has shown reliable performance with its 60 cm transverse field-of-view (FOV) of and 32 cm FOV.[23]

APDs are highly sensitive photodiodes that convert light into electricity based on the photoelectric effect. In the early PET/MR systems, APDs gained popularity owing to their very low sensitivity to the magnetic field, though they provide remarkably lower amplification gain compared to PMTs (10^2 vs 10^6).[24] SiPMs addressed the shortcomings of APDs through providing similar amplification gains to PMTs while requiring a low supply voltage (eg, 40 v vs 400 v for APDs). SiPMs are the dominant photodetectors in PET technology, however, the trend is toward using fully digital SiPMs wherein the photons are counted/detected in a digital format which renders the sensor less susceptible to electronic noise, magnetic field interferences, and temperature variations.[25]

Owing to the efficient performance of SiPMs in strong magnetic fields, brain PET inserts gained momentum and were designed and built for 7T

MR imaging using this technology. In this regard, Cubresa BrainPET, a PET insert for MR scanners (compatible with major MR scanners), was designed to provide simultaneous PET and 3T MR imaging capability comparable or superior to commercial competitors.[26] As a PET insert, the Cubresa BrainPET is conveniently lifted and mounted on the bed of MR scanners. The BrainPET technology relies on the preclinical Cubresa NuPET family (animal PET inserts for 7T MR scanners) with LYSO detectors coupled to SiPM modules.[27] The Cubresa NuPET inserts are compatible with commercial MR scanners operating at 1.5 to 9.4 T MR field strengths.[28] The Cubresa NuPET inserts (different versions) provide transaxial FOV of 59 mm to 250 mm and spatial resolution of 0.9 mm to 1.7 mm.[28] The major PET performance parameters, such as spatial resolution, SNR, and quantitative accuracy were altered when PET inserts were operating at 7T magnetic field, while MR parameters (Bruker 7T MRI scanner, Biospin, Billerica, MA) were not affected by the presence of the PET inserts.[28,29]

The MINDView PET brain imager was designed to function as an insert into 3T mMR scanner benefiting from monolithic LYSO detectors. The effective FOV of the scanner is 24 cm in diameter and 15.4 cm in axially. This PET scanner provided spatial resolution of less than 2 mm and exhibited no remarkable performance deviation when MR sequences such as MPrage and ultrashort time echo were simultaneously acquired.[30]

To perform brain PET scanning in a single bed position, a brain PET insert based on LSO and SiPM modules was designed and built for the 7T Magnetom (Siemens Healthineers) MRI scanner.[31] This PET insert is equipped with depth of interaction (DOI) capability and provides axial and transaxial FOVs of 16.7 and 25.6 cm, respectively. Though this scanner offers a peak sensitivity of 18.9 kcps/MBq and a spatial resolution of 2.5 mm (according to the NEMA NU 2 standard), its performance within simultaneous MR imaging should be improved. **Fig. 1** depicts this brain PET insert prototype together with PET images of the hot-rod and 3D Hoffman phantoms.

In an effort to build a flexible PET scanner to be attached/linked to existing MR scanners, fxPET scanner was developed using a dual arc-shape spinning detector covering 135°. The ring diameter and axial extent of this scanner are 77 and 15 cm, respectively, which enables whole-body sequential PET/MR imaging.[32] In the context of simultaneous data acquisition, the approach adopted by the TRIMAGE consortium should be considered, where simultaneous electroencephalography (EEG)/PET/MR scans are performed for a comprehensive study of basic mechanisms in the brain.[33] The PET component has an inner diameter and axial FOV of 26 and 16 cm, respectively, inserted into a 1.5 T MR scanner.

PRECLINICAL POSITRON EMISSION TOMOGRAPHY/MAGNETIC RESONANCE IMAGING SYSTEMS

The majority of preclinical PET/MRI scanners employ LYSO crystals readout by SiPMs owing to their high resolution and compact design. One such example is the hybrid SimPET scanner (Brightonix Imaging Inc., Seoul, South Korea). This PET/MR scanner benefits from a permanent 1T magnet and a PET ring which is capable to work within a 7T magnetic field with an inner bore diameter of 6.0 cm. SimPET-X PET insert was later introduced for total-body mouse PET/MR scanning (using LSO crystals) with 11 cm axial FOV and remarkably superior sensitivity compared to SimPET.[34]

Bruker BioSpin (Ettlingen, Germany), as one of the major vendors in the preclinical field, offered a dedicated PET insert to operate in a 9.4 T magnetic field followed by the release of a sequential PET system for MR scanners up to 15.2 T.[35] NuPET (Cubresa, Winnipeg, MB, Canada) and HALO (Inviscan Imaging Systems, Strasbourg, France) PET inserts were designed to fit into most commercially available MR scanners. Mediso Medical Imaging Systems (Budapest, Hungary) and MR Solutions (Guildford, Surrey, United Kingdom) companies produced preclinical PET/MR and PET inserts which could operate in standalone or sequential modes.[36]

SAFIR-I, a preclinical PET insert for 7T MRI scanners, was built for high-rate kinetic examination of rats and mice using injected activity up to 500 MBq. This scanner, with an axial FOV of 54.2 mm and an inner diameter of 114 mm, allows for time frames of a few seconds with an acceptable signal-to-noise ratio and spatial resolution of about 2 mm (at the center of the FOV).[37] Representative PET images of the rat brain obtained from the SAFIR-I PET scanner at 5 s time frame are presented in **Fig. 2**.

A recent survey on the Cubresa NuPET insert (Cubresa, Inc., Winnipeg, MB) inserted in a Bruker 7T MRI scanner (Bruker Biospin, Billerica, MA) revealed that some key characteristics of PET imaging, such as quantitative accuracy, signal-to-noise ratio (SNR), and spatial resolution, as well as MRI SNR, were adversely affected in the presence of both PET and MR components.[28] PET images of the Derenzo phantom filled with ^{18}F-FDG and ^{68}Ga are shown in **Fig. 3** when the PET

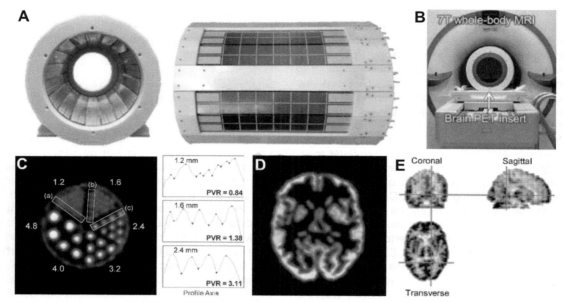

Fig. 1. (*A*) Prototype brain PET insert built by Won and colleagues,[31], (*B*) Brain PET scanner inserted in a 7T MR scanner, (*C*) PET image of the hot-rod phantom along with line profiles through the 1.2 mm, 1.6 mm, and 2.4 mm hot rods. PVR refers to the peak valley ratio. (*D*) PET image of 3D Hoffman brain phantom. (Adapted with permission from[31] under a Creative Commons License.)

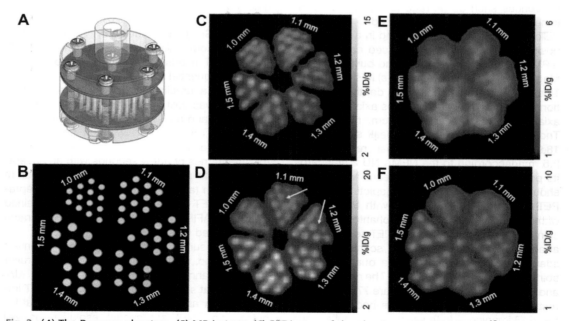

Fig. 2. (*A*) The Derenzo phantom, (*B*) MR images, (*C*) PET image of the phantom with 3.7 MBq of ^{18}F-FDG at the center of the FOV, (*D*) PET image of the phantom when the PET component[28] was inserted into the MRI scanner, (*E*) PET image of the phantom with 3.7 MBq ^{68}Ga at the center of the FOV, and (*F*) PET image of the phantom (with ^{68}Ga) when the PET component was inserted into the MRI scanner. (Reprinted with permission from Springer Nature[28] under a Creative Commons License.)

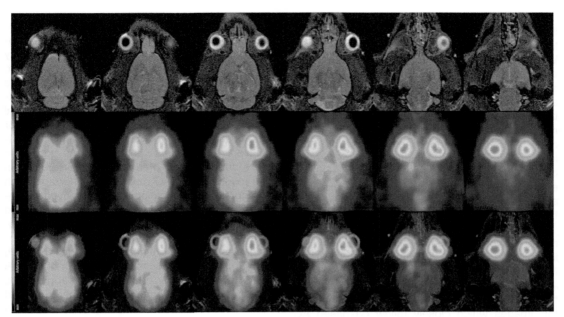

Fig. 3. (Top row) MR images (coronal views) of a rat brain obtained with a T2-TurboRARE sequence, (Middle row), Corresponding PET images at high activity (>300 MBq) in a single 5-s time frame, (Bottom row) Fused PET and MR images acquired on the scanner described in.[37] (Reprinted from[37] under a Creative Commons License.)

component was outside and within the MRI scanner. A similar study on the MR Solutions PET insert (model I-402, Guildford, UK) installed in a 3T MRI scanner demonstrated no significant interference between PET and MR components when they were operating in a stand-alone or simultaneous PET and MR acquisition mode.[38]

PROGRESS IN MAGNETIC RESONANCE IMAGING-GUIDED ATTENUATION CORRECTION IN HYBRID POSITRON EMISSION TOMOGRAPHY/MAGNETIC RESONANCE IMAGING

The major challenge impacting quantitative PET/MR imaging is the correction for attenuated photons within the body and other devices in the PET FOV. Since MR signals indicate tissue proton density and relaxation times and are not correlated with electron density, photon attenuation coefficients of materials cannot be directly estimated from MR images.[39] In addition to estimating linear attenuation coefficients from MR signals, quantitative PET/MR imaging faces the challenges of image artifacts due to metallic implants, body truncation in MRI-derived attenuation correction maps (AC maps), MRI hardware inside the PET FOV, and mismatches between MR and PET images.[40] A number of reports demonstrated that MRI Gadolinium-based contrast agents do not have a significant impact on PET quantification.[41]

In early PET/MRI systems, simple segmentation/classification of major tissue classes from T1-weighted and Dixon MR sequences was conducted to generate AC maps for PET data.[18,42] Due to the extremely short T1 relaxation time of cortical bone, bony structures were missing in the segmentation-based AC maps and they only included air, lung, soft-tissue, and fat tissue types.[43,44] The omission of bony structures from PET AC maps led to noticeable bias in the estimation of tracer uptake within/close to bones.[45] To address this issue, ultrashort, and zero echo time sequences were employed for bone visualization and inclusion in MRI-derived PET AC maps.[46,47] However, due to long acquisition times and misclassification of adjacent bone and air, these sequences were not feasible in head and neck imaging.[48]

An alternative approach to include bony structures in MRI-derived AC maps is to employ an offline bone template (consisting of major bone structures such as skull, hip, femur, and spine) that is to be aligned/registered to the MR image of the patient (referred to as atlas-based methods).[49] The SIGNA (GE Healthcare) and mMR (Siemens Healthineers) hybrid PET/MR scanners are equipped with short echo time MR sequences or atlas-based methods to include bony structures in brain AC maps.[43] Mixed feedback was received from the clinical implementation of the atlas-based method concerning inaccurate bone alignment and gross misregistration errors.[50]

Anatomic abnormalities would not be taken into account in atlas-based approaches, thus leading to remarkable patient-wise errors.[51] With respect to the fact that raw PET data inherently bear information about both emission and attenuation, maximum likelihood attention and activity reconstruction (MLAA) approaches could be employed to generate patient-specific PET AC maps and/or PET attenuation-corrected images.[52] Though this approach suffers from high levels of noise and uncertainties in the estimation of the attenuation coefficients, the quantitative errors due to metallic implants (metal artifacts) and body truncation could be diminished by this approach.[53,54]

The remarkable performance of convolutional neural networks is about to bring a paradigm shift in multimodality medical imaging, including PET/MRI technology.[55,56] Promising results have been achieved using deep learning approaches in synthetic CT generation or PET map estimation from MR images which closely follow CT-based AC maps.[57] Moreover, deep learning approaches have enabled novel approaches to address the challenge of AC in PET/MR imaging such as directly applying attenuation and scatter correction on non-AC PET images in the image domain,[58] estimation of attenuation correction factors in the sinogram domain,[59] estimation of accurate PET AC maps from the outcome of MLAA approaches,[60] and synthetic CT generation from non-AC PET images.[61] Overall, these approaches have reported quantitative bias of less than 10% for the recovery of activity concentration compared to ground truth CT-based AC of PET data, which is considered as clinically tolerable errors. A comparison of segmentation-based, atlas-based, and deep learning-based synthetic CT generation from MR images are depicted in Fig. 4.

Hardware-based Attenuation Correction

In addition to photon attenuation within the patient's body, MR equipments (eg, MR coils, patient positioning devices, and so forth) inside the PET FOV cause significant photon attenuation which should be taken into account for quantitative PET imaging.[62] Rigid MR hardware could be easily modeled within PET image reconstruction using a predetermined attenuation map. However, flexible MR hardware (eg, carotid coils and headphones) require localization, including markers, ultra-short echo time sequences, and depth cameras, before applying AC.[63,64] In addition, novel MR hardware has been designed to have a lightweight and low density in order to reduce photons attenuation within PET imaging.[65,66]

Strategies for Dealing with Body Truncation

Oncological PET/MR imaging suffers from inhomogeneity of the magnetic field and nonlinearity of the gradient field which leads to geometric distortion and truncation in the transverse plane (patients' arms are normally truncated), considering that the MR FOV is smaller than the typical 60 cm PET FOV. This geometric distortion or body truncation would be reflected in MRI-derived AC maps, wherein MLAA algorithms were suggested to predict the missing areas in the resulting PET AC maps. The other approach to address the truncation issue (employed in clinical routine) is magnetic field harmonization based on gradient enhancement (HUGE), which compensates for the gradient and magnetic field inhomogeneities through optimizing readouts for each arm and the entire slices at the margin of the MR FOV.[67] In addition, deep learning approaches have enabled the completion of the truncated MR-derived AC maps relying only on the truncated MR images,[68] or applying direct attenuation and scatter correction in the image domain.[69] Representative PET images reconstructed using HUGE plus Dixon and Dixon plus MLAA are shown in Fig. 5.

Metal Artefact Reduction Techniques

Due to the susceptibility of MR magnetic fields to metallic objects, the presence of dental fillings, endoprostheses, and surgical devices would result in voids and/or distorted areas in MR images which would adversely impact the MRI-derived PET AC maps, and consequently PET quantification and lesion detectability.[70,71] To address the issue of metallic artifacts in PET/MR imaging, dedicated MR sequences have been developed to show no or less susceptibility to metal implants. This includes the MAVRIC sequence, which works on the basis of multispectral 3D data acquisition with low sensitivity to metal implants.[71] However, due to the very long acquisition time, its clinical application for MRI-guided AC was not practically feasible.[72] MLAA algorithms are alternative approaches to estimate and/or correct PET AC maps from raw PET data.[73] Atlas-based AC map generation and impainting methods are also capable of diminishing the adverse impact of metal artifacts in PET AC maps.[51] Similar to body truncation, deep learning approaches could be employed to compensate for metal artifacts in the PET AC map,[68] or directly apply attenuation and scatter correction in the image domain to avoid the negative impact of metal artifacts.[74] Nevertheless, none of the proposed metal artifact reduction methods have provided reliable and

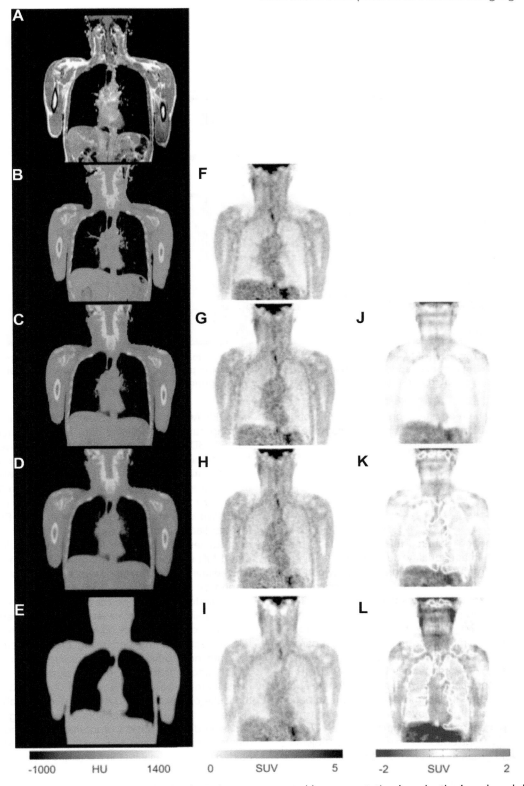

Fig. 4. Representative synthetic or pseudo-CT images generated by segmentation-based, atlas-based, and deep learning-based methods along with the corresponding PET images and the bias maps with respect to the reference CT-based PET AC. (*A*) MR images, (*B*) Reference CT, (*C*) Deep learning-based AC map, (*D*) Atlas-based AC map, (*E*) Segmentation-based AC map, (*F*) PET-CT, (*G*) PET-deep, (*H*) PET-atlas, (*I*) PET-segmentation, and (*J*), (*K*), and (*L*) shows their corresponding bias map with respect to the reference PET-CT, respectively. (Reprinted under a Creative Commons License.[51])

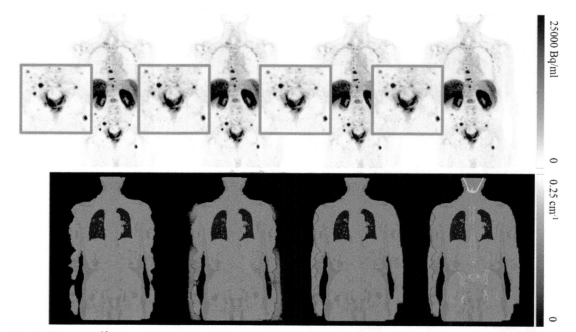

25000 Bq/ml

0

0.25 cm⁻¹

0

Fig. 5. (Top row) ¹⁸F-PSMA PET images reconstructed with four different AC approaches, (Bottom row) corresponding AC maps obtained from standard Dixon, MLAA with Dixon prior, HUGE with Dixon, HUGE with Dixon, and bones. (Reprinted under a Creative Commons License from Springer Nature.[50])

robust image reconstruction in the context of clinical PET/MR imaging, and as such, this issue warrants further investigation.[3]

MAGNETIC RESONANCE IMAGING-GUIDED MOTION CORRECTION IN POSITRON EMISSION TOMOGRAPHY/MAGNETIC RESONANCE IMAGING

Patient motion during PET imaging is a major source of image quality degradation leading to blurred structures, misalignment between PET and MR images (or AC map), and quantification errors.[75] An advantage of simultaneous PET/MR imaging (compared to PET/CT) could be the capability of MR imaging to provide the required information for motion correction, wherein cardiac, respiratory, and gross patient motions could be detected by MR sequences. Cardiac PET/MR imaging, in contrast to PET/CT, requires longer acquisition time and thus is more susceptible to patient and internal organ movements, wherein a mean misalignment error of 7 ± 4 mm between PET and AC images was observed in 90% of the subjects.[76] To avoid gross motion errors, strict quality control of MRI-guided AC is required in cardiac PET imaging, where multiple AC sequences could be acquired (no issues with radiation dose) to select the most appropriate one for PET AC. MRI-guided motion estimation is an efficient approach for artifact-

free PET AC owing to the absence of exposure to ionizing radiation, wherein fast MR sequences, such as 3D multi-echo could be triggered several times by control devices such as EEG electrodes or respiratory belts.[77] MR sequences that allow for the direct estimation of motion vectors in MR space are attractive options for AC of PET data and have shown promising results in FDG PET/MR cardiac imaging.[78,79] A disadvantage of these approaches would be the time needed for dedicated MR sequences and the navigation capabilities within PET imaging which may confine diagnostic MR imaging.

Respiratory motion correction could be conducted using only the emission data; however, since these methods rely on regions with high uptake to estimate the underlying motion vectors, they are not applicable to radiotracers with low target tracer uptake.[80] MLAA algorithms and deep learning-based AC solutions could address the issue of emission and AC image mismatches. However, they are not capable of correcting the emission data for patient or internal organ movements within PET imaging. In this regard, MRI-guided approaches with the capability of providing real-time motion assessment would be the optimal solution for applying motion correction to PET data as well as corresponding AC maps.

In brain PET imaging, due to head bulk motion, motion-corrected image reconstruction (MCIR) could be conducted, wherein motion information is extracted from MR imaging (magnetization-prepared rapid gradient echo) within PET acquisition (gated PET image reconstructions are transformed to a common gate a posteriori).[81] An example of MRI-guided PET motion correction is presented in Fig. 6.

Deep learning approaches have been successfully applied to estimate motion information from navigator MR sequences (using generative adversarial neural networks), where improved quantitative accuracy, as well as superior visualization quality, was reported compared to the reconstruct-transform average approach.[8,82,83] Radial schemes of MRI acquisitions were employed to estimate and model organ motion in abdominal PET/MR imaging and conducting PET and MR MCIR. Using this strategy, both PET and structural MR images will be corrected for internal organ motion (sharper organ boundaries), thus offering improved diagnostic accuracy.[84]

MAGNETIC RESONANCE IMAGING-GUIDED PARTIAL VOLUME CORRECTION IN HYBRID POSITRON EMISSION TOMOGRAPHY/ MAGNETIC RESONANCE IMAGING

A distinct advantage of simultaneous PET/MR imaging is the possibility of using prior knowledge extracted from MR images to enhance the quality of PET image reconstructions (MRI-guided PET reconstruction).[85] Statistical priors, extracted from the anatomic MRI data, could be employed within PET image reconstruction (modeled in the system matrix) to improve image reconstruction convergence, suppress noise, enhance the quantitative accuracy, and perform partial volume correction.[86,87]

Partial volume correction (PVC), which leads to enhanced quantitative accuracy as well as improved visual quality of PET images, could greatly benefit from high-contrast structural MR images perfectly aligned to the PET signals in simultaneous PET/MR imaging.[87] PVC approaches relying solely on MR signals to perform PVC, would cause factitious signals in case of mismatches between emission and structural information.[88] Moreover, these approaches tend to suppress signals present only in PET images with no counter structure in MR images. To address this issue, synergistic PET and multiparametric MR priors are employed to diminish the sensitivity to signal mismatches between PET and MRI data and preserve the unique structures in PET images, such as lesions with no equivalent edges/signals on MR images.[85] Nevertheless, these approaches may show high sensitivity to the high noise levels in PET images since strong noise signals would be regarded as genuine structures.[10]

To match the resolutions of PET and MR images, MR images are commonly down-sampled to PET images since increased noise levels and Gibbs artifacts are observed when PET data are upsampled. In this regard, a smooth Lange prior was considered in MRI-guided PET image reconstruction (maximum a posteriori) to perform PVC at a high spatial resolution on PET images.[87]

Recently, deep learning solutions have been proposed to apply post-reconstruction PVC either with or without using MRI support.[89,90] The aim of these approaches was to apply fast PVC without the need for co-registered structural MR information. An example of this approach is presented in Fig. 7. The bulk of research in MRI-guided PET image reconstruction and post-reconstruction PVC

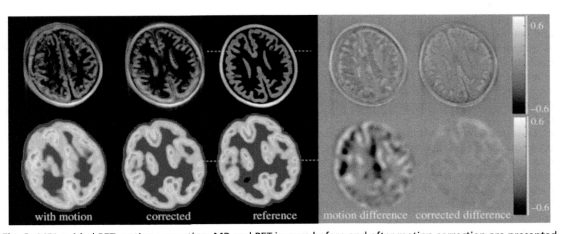

Fig. 6. MRI-guided PET motion correction. MR and PET images before and after motion correction are presented together with the difference maps before and after motion correction. (P M Johnson et al 2019. Rigid-body motion correction in hybrid PET/MRI using spherical navigator echoes, Physics in Medicine & Biology, 64 (8), NT03. DOI 10.1088/1361-6560/ab10b2.[83])

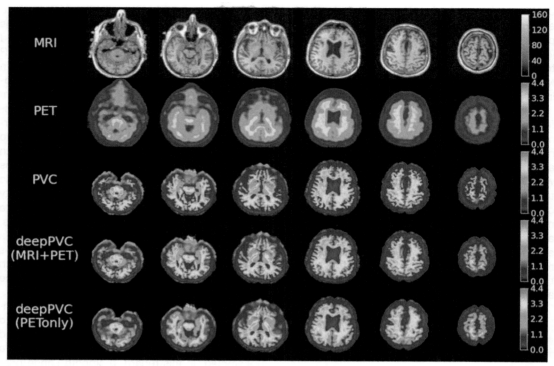

Fig. 7. Deep learning-based partial volume correction of PET data with and without using anatomic MRI information. (Reprinted with permission from Springer Nature.[90])

has been conducted in brain PET/MR imaging, which is less vulnerable to misalignment errors. The feasibility of MRI-guided PET PVC in other body regions and whole-body imaging warrants further research and development efforts.[91]

SUMMARY AND FUTURE PERSPECTIVES

Over a decade has passed since the introduction of hybrid PET/MRI scanners into clinical practice and yet this technology has yet to found its niche in clinical setting. This could be attributed to the lack of key applications or irreplaceable features of this modality compared to hybrid PET/CT imaging, rather than its technical challenges/limitations, including attenuation correction for PET data. Owing to the continuous advances in detectors and electronic readouts, the trend is toward developing compact PET inserts for existing MRI scanners providing high spatial resolution and reasonable cost. This technology is attracting much attention in research environment owing to the fact that simultaneous PET/MR imaging would enable accurate motion correction of PET data, partial volume correction, MRI-assisted PET image reconstruction or low-dose PET imaging, and MRI-based cardiac or respiratory gated imaging.

Owing to the extraordinary performance of artificial intelligence or deep learning approaches, algorithms belonging to this category are predominately employed to address the major challenges in PET/MR imaging, such as AC synthetic CT estimation from MR images, body truncation, attenuation and scatter correction of PET data, noise and metal artifact reduction.

DISCLOSURE

The authors have no potential conflicts of interest to disclose.

ACKNOWLEDGMENTS

This work was supported by the Swiss National Science Foundation under grant SNRF 320030_176052 and the Private Foundation of Geneva University Hospitals under grant RC-06 to 01.

REFERENCES

1. Zaidi H, Del Guerra A. An outlook on future design of hybrid PET/MRI systems. Med Phys 2011;38(10): 5667–89.
2. Zaidi H, Becker M. The Promise of hybrid PET/MRI: Technical advances and clinical applications. IEEE Sign Proc Mag 2016;33(3):67–85.

3. Bogdanovic B, Solari EL, Villagran Asiares A, et al. PET/MR Technology: Advancement and Challenges. Semin Nucl Med 2022;52(3):340–55.

4. Currie GM, Leon JL, Nevo E, et al. PET/MR Part 4: Clinical Applications of PET/MRI. J Nucl Med Technol 2021. https://doi.org/10.2967/jnmt.121.263288.

5. Torigian DA, Zaidi H, Kwee TC, et al. PET/MR Imaging: Technical aspects and potential clinical applications. Radiology 2013;267(1):26–44.

6. Mannheim JG, Schmid AM, Schwenck J, et al. PET/MRI Hybrid Systems. Semin Nucl Med 2018;48(4):332–47.

7. Becker M, Zaidi H. Imaging in head and neck squamous cell carcinoma: the potential role of PET/MRI. Br J Radiol 2014;87(1036):20130677.

8. Chen S, Fraum TJ, Eldeniz C, et al. MR-assisted PET respiratory motion correction using deep-learning based short-scan motion fields. Magn Reson Med 2022;88(2):676–90.

9. Meng X, Liu H, Li H, et al. Evaluating the impact of different positron emitters on the performance of a clinical PET/MR system. Med Phys 2022;49(4):2642–51.

10. Bland J, Mehranian A, Belzunce MA, et al. Intercomparison of MR-informed PET image reconstruction methods. Med Phys 2019;46(11):5055–74.

11. Gao Y, Zhu Y, Bilgel M, et al. Voxel-based partial volume correction of PET images via subtle MRI guided non-local means regularization. Phys Med 2021;89:129–39.

12. Afaq A, Faul D, Chebrolu VV, et al. Pitfalls on PET/MRI. Semin Nucl Med 2021;51(5):529–39.

13. Herzog H, Lerche C. Advances in clinical PET/MRI instrumentation. Pet Clin 2016;11(2):95–103.

14. Catana C, Wu Y, Judenhofer MS, et al. Simultaneous acquisition of multislice PET and MR images: initial results with a MR-compatible PET scanner. J Nucl Med 2006;47(12):1968–76.

15. Judenhofer MS, Catana C, Swann BK, et al. PET/MR images acquired with a compact MR-compatible PET detector in a 7-T magnet. Radiology 2007;244(3):807–14.

16. Schmand M, Burbar Z, Corbeil J, et al. BrainPET: First human tomograph for simultaneous (functional) PET and MR imaging. Soc Nuclear Med 2007;45.

17. Kolb A, Wehrl HF, Hofmann M, et al. Technical performance evaluation of a human brain PET/MRI system. Eur Radiol 2012;22(8):1776–88.

18. Zaidi H, Ojha N, Morich M, et al. Design and performance evaluation of a whole-body Ingenuity TF PET-MRI system. Phys Med Biol 2011;56(10):3091–106.

19. Kalemis A, Delattre BM, Heinzer S. Sequential whole-body PET/MR scanner: concept, clinical use, and optimisation after two years in the clinic. The manufacturer's perspective. Magma 2013;26(1):5–23.

20. Delso G, Fürst S, Jakoby B, et al. Performance measurements of the Siemens mMR integrated whole-body PET/MR scanner. J Nucl Med 2011;52(12):1914–22.

21. Aklan B, Paulus DH, Wenkel E, et al. Toward simultaneous PET/MR breast imaging: systematic evaluation and integration of a radiofrequency breast coil. Med Phys 2013;40(2):024301.

22. Roncali E, Cherry SR. Application of silicon photomultipliers to positron emission tomography. Ann Biomed Eng 2011;39(4):1358–77.

23. Chen S, Gu Y, Yu H, et al. NEMA NU2-2012 performance measurements of the United Imaging uPMR790: an integrated PET/MR system. Eur J Nucl Med Mol Imaging 2021;48(6):1726–35.

24. Renker D. Geiger-mode avalanche photodiodes, history, properties and problems. Nucl Instrum Methods Phys Res 2006;567(1):48–56.

25. Gundacker S, Heering A. The silicon photomultiplier: fundamentals and applications of a modern solid-state photon detector. Phys Med Biol 2020;65(17):17tr01.

26. Lundin A. Barrow Neurological Institute Adds PET Imaging System for Research Activities. AXIS Imaging News 2022.

27. CUBRESA NuPET™ System. https ://www.cubre sa.-com/nupet/. Accessed 2023.

28. Pollard AC, de la Cerda J, Schuler FW, et al. Evaluations of the performances of PET and MRI in a simultaneous PET/MRI instrument for pre-clinical imaging. EJNMMI physics 2022;9(1):1–14.

29. Lerche C, Lenz M, Bi W, et al. Design and simulation of a high-resolution and high-sensitivity BrainPET insert for 7T MRI. Nuklearmedizin-Nucl Med. 2020;59(02):V96.

30. Gonzalez AJ, Gonzalez-Montoro A, Vidal LF, et al. Initial results of the MINDView PET insert inside the 3T mMR. IEEE Trans Radiat Plasma Med Sci 2018;3(3):343–51.

31. Won JY, Park H, Lee S, et al. Development and Initial Results of a Brain PET Insert for Simultaneous 7-Tesla PET/MRI Using an FPGA-Only Signal Digitization Method. IEEE Trans Med Imaging 2021;40(6):1579–90.

32. Watanabe M, Kawai-Miyake K, Fushimi Y, et al. Application of a Flexible PET Scanner Combined with 3 T MRI Using Non-local Means Reconstruction: Qualitative and Quantitative Comparison with Whole-Body PET/CT. Mol Imaging Biol 2022;24(1):167–76.

33. Del Guerra A, Ahmad S, Avram M, et al. TRIMAGE: A dedicated trimodality (PET/MR/EEG) imaging tool for schizophrenia. Eur Psychiatry 2018;50:7–20.

34. Kim KY, Son JW, Kim K, et al. Performance Evaluation of SimPET-X, a PET Insert for Simultaneous Mouse Total-Body PET/MR Imaging. Mol Imaging Biol 2021;23(5):703–13.

35. Doss KKM, Mion PE, Kao Y-CJ, et al. Performance evaluation of a PET of 7T bruker micro-PET/MR

based on NEMA NU 4-2008 standards. Electronics 2022;11(14):2194.

36. Miyaoka RS, Lehnert AL. Small animal PET: a review of what we have done and where we are going [published online ahead of print 2020/05/02]. Phys Med Biol 2020;65(24).

37. Bebié P, Becker R, Commichau V, et al. SAFIR-I: Design and Performance of a High-Rate Preclinical PET Insert for MRI. Sensors 2021;21(21) [published online ahead of print 2021/11/14].

38. Emvalomenos G, Trajanovska S, Pham BTT, et al. Performance evaluation of a PET insert for preclinical MRI in stand-alone PET and simultaneous PET-MRI modes. EJNMMI Phys 2021;8(1):68.

39. Mehranian A, Arabi H, Zaidi H. Vision 20/20: Magnetic resonance imaging-guided attenuation correction in PET/MRI: Challenges, solutions, and opportunities. Med Phys 2016;43(3):1130–55.

40. Izquierdo-Garcia D, Catana C. MR Imaging-Guided Attenuation Correction of PET Data in PET/MR Imaging. Pet Clin 2016;11(2):129–49.

41. Allen TJ, Henze Bancroft LC, Kumar M, et al. Gadolinium-based contrast agent attenuation does not impact PET quantification in simultaneous dynamic contrast enhanced breast PET/MR. Med Phys 2022;49(8):5206–15.

42. Martinez-Moller A, Souvatzoglou M, Delso G, et al. Tissue classification as a potential approach for attenuation correction in whole-body PET/MRI: evaluation with PET/CT data. J Nucl Med 2009;50(4):520–6.

43. Beyer T, Lassen ML, Boellaard R, et al. Investigating the state-of-the-art in whole-body MR-based attenuation correction: an intra-individual, inter-system, inventory study on three clinical PET/MR systems. Magma 2016;29(1):75–87.

44. Arabi H, Rager O, Alem A, et al. Clinical assessment of MR-guided 3-class and 4-class attenuation correction in PET/MR. Mol Imaging Biol 2015;17(2):264–76.

45. Andersen FL, Ladefoged CN, Beyer T, et al. Combined PET/MR imaging in neurology: MR-based attenuation correction implies a strong spatial bias when ignoring bone. Neuroimage 2014;84:206–16.

46. Khalife M, Fernandez B, Jaubert O, et al. Subject-specific bone attenuation correction for brain PET/MR: can ZTE-MRI substitute CT scan accurately? Phys Med Biol 2017;62(19):7814–32.

47. Cabello J, Lukas M, Forster S, et al. MR-based attenuation correction using UTE pulse sequences in dementia patients. J Nucl Med 2015;56(3):423–9.

48. Delso G, Fernandez B, Wiesinger F, et al. Repeatability of ZTE bone maps of the head. IEEE Trans Radiat Plasma Med Sci 2017;2(3):244–9.

49. Arabi H, Zaidi H. Comparison of atlas-based techniques for whole-body bone segmentation. Med Image Anal 2017;36:98–112.

50. Bogdanovic B, Gafita A, Schachoff S, et al. Almost 10 years of PET/MR attenuation correction: the effect on lesion quantification with PSMA: clinical evaluation on 200 prostate cancer patients. Eur J Nucl Med Mol Imaging 2021;48(2):543–53.

51. Arabi H, Zaidi H. MRI-guided attenuation correction in torso PET/MRI: Assessment of segmentation-, atlas-, and deep learning-based approaches in the presence of outliers. Magn Reson Med 2022;87(2):686–701.

52. Mehranian A, Zaidi H, Reader AJ. MR-guided joint reconstruction of activity and attenuation in brain PET-MR. Neuroimage 2017;162:276–88.

53. Fuin N, Pedemonte S, Catalano OA, et al. PET/MRI in the Presence of Metal Implants: Completion of the Attenuation Map from PET Emission Data. J Nucl Med 2017;58(5):840–5.

54. Nuyts J, Bal G, Kehren F, et al. Completion of a truncated attenuation image from the attenuated PET emission data. IEEE Trans Med Imaging 2013;32(2):237–46.

55. Arabi H, Zaidi H. Applications of artificial intelligence and deep learning in molecular imaging and radiotherapy. Eur J Hybrid Imaging 2020;4(1):1–23.

56. Zaidi H, El Naqa I. Quantitative molecular Positron Emission Tomography imaging using advanced deep learning techniques. Annu Rev Biomed Eng 2021;23:249–76.

57. Chen X, Liu C. Deep-learning-based methods of attenuation correction for SPECT and PET. J Nucl Cardiol 2022. https://doi.org/10.1007/s12350-022-03007-3.

58. Arabi H, Bortolin K, Ginovart N, et al. Deep learning-guided joint attenuation and scatter correction in multitracer neuroimaging studies. Hum Brain Mapp 2020;41(13):3667–79.

59. Arabi H, Zaidi H. Deep learning-guided estimation of attenuation correction factors from time-of-flight PET emission data. Med Image Anal 2020;64:101718.

60. Hwang D, Kim KY, Kang SK, et al. Improving the Accuracy of Simultaneously Reconstructed Activity and Attenuation Maps Using Deep Learning. J Nucl Med 2018;59(10):1624–9.

61. Dong X, Wang T, Lei Y, et al. Synthetic CT generation from non-attenuation corrected PET images for whole-body PET imaging. Phys Med Biol 2019;64(21):215016.

62. Eldib M, Bini J, Faul DD, et al. Attenuation Correction for Magnetic Resonance Coils in Combined PET/MR Imaging: A Review. Pet Clin 2016;11(2):151–60.

63. Frohwein LJ, Heß M, Schlicher D, et al. PET attenuation correction for flexible MRI surface coils in hybrid PET/MRI using a 3D depth camera. Phys Med Biol 2018;63(2):025033.

64. Aizaz M, Moonen RPM, van der Pol JAJ, et al. PET/MRI of atherosclerosis. Cardiovasc Diagn Ther 2020;10(4):1120–39.

65. Oehmigen M, Lindemann ME, Lanz T, et al. Integrated PET/MR breast cancer imaging: Attenuation correction and implementation of a 16-channel RF coil. Med Phys 2016;43(8):4808.

66. Lee YH, Song KH, Yang J, et al. Fabrication and evaluation of bilateral Helmholtz radiofrequency coil for thermo-stable breast image with reduced artifacts. J Appl Clin Med Phys 2022;23(1):e13483.

67. Lindemann ME, Gratz M, Blumhagen JO, et al. MR-based truncation correction using an advanced HUGE method to improve attenuation correction in PET/MR imaging of obese patients. Med Phys 2022;49(2):865–77.

68. Arabi H, Zaidi H. Truncation compensation and metallic dental implant artefact reduction in PET/MRI attenuation correction using deep learning-based object completion. Phys Med Biol 2020;65(19):195002.

69. Liu F, Jang H, Kijowski R, et al. Deep Learning MR Imaging-based Attenuation Correction for PET/MR Imaging. Radiology 2018;286(2):676–84.

70. Catana C. Attenuation correction for human PET/MRI studies. Phys Med Biol 2020;65(23):23tr02.

71. Schramm G, Ladefoged CN. Metal artifact correction strategies in MRI-based attenuation correction in PET/MRI. BJR Open 2019;1(1):20190033.

72. Kudura K, Oblasser T, Ferraro DA, et al. Metal artifact reduction in (68)Ga-PSMA-11 PET/MRI for prostate cancer patients with hip joint replacement using multiacquisition variable-resonance image combination. Eur J Hybrid Imaging 2020;4(1):6.

73. Rezaei A, Schramm G, Willekens SMA, et al. A Quantitative Evaluation of Joint Activity and Attenuation Reconstruction in TOF PET/MR Brain Imaging [published online ahead of print 2019/04/14]. J Nucl Med 2019;60(11):1649–55.

74. Guo R, Xue S, Hu J, et al. Using domain knowledge for robust and generalizable deep learning-based CT-free PET attenuation and scatter correction [published online ahead of print 2022/10/07]. Nat Commun 2022;13(1):5882.

75. Chen Z, Sforazzini F, Baran J, et al. MR-PET head motion correction based on co-registration of multi-contrast MR images. Hum Brain Mapp 2021;42(13):4081–91.

76. Lassen ML, Rasul S, Beitzke D, et al. Assessment of attenuation correction for myocardial PET imaging using combined PET/MRI. J Nucl Cardiol 2019;26(4):1107–18.

77. Brown R, Kolbitsch C, Delplancke C, et al. Motion estimation and correction for simultaneous PET/MR using SIRF and CIL. Philos Trans A Math Phys Eng Sci 2021;379(2204):20200208.

78. Munoz C, Kunze KP, Neji R, et al. Motion-corrected whole-heart PET-MR for the simultaneous visualisation of coronary artery integrity and myocardial viability: an initial clinical validation. Eur J Nucl Med Mol Imaging 2018;45(11):1975–86.

79. Einspänner E, Jochimsen TH, Harries J, et al. Evaluating different methods of MR-based motion correction in simultaneous PET/MR using a head phantom moved by a robotic system. EJNMMI Phys 2022;9(1):15.

80. Benz DC, Buechel RR. The winding road towards respiratory motion correction: is this just another dead-end or do we finally get breathing under control? [published online ahead of print 2019/03/08]. J Nucl Cardiol 2020;27(6):2231–3.

81. Chen KT, Salcedo S, Chonde DB, et al. MR-assisted PET motion correction in simultaneous PET/MRI studies of dementia subjects. J Magn Reson Imaging 2018;48(5):1288–96.

82. Shiyam Sundar LK, Iommi D, Muzik O, et al. Conditional Generative Adversarial Networks Aided Motion Correction of Dynamic (18)F-FDG PET Brain Studies. J Nucl Med 2021;62(6):871–9.

83. Polycarpou I, Soultanidis G, Tsoumpas C. Synergistic motion compensation strategies for positron emission tomography when acquired simultaneously with magnetic resonance imaging. Philos Trans A Math Phys Eng Sci 2021;379(2204):20200207.

84. Ippoliti M, Lukas M, Brenner W, et al. Respiratory motion correction for enhanced quantification of hepatic lesions in simultaneous PET and DCE-MR imaging. Phys Med Biol 2021;66(9).

85. Mehranian A, Belzunce MA, Niccolini F, et al. PET image reconstruction using multi-parametric anato-functional priors. Phys Med Biol 2017;62(15):5975–6007.

86. Bland J, Mehranian A, Belzunce MA, et al. MR-Guided Kernel EM Reconstruction for Reduced Dose PET Imaging. IEEE Trans Radiat Plasma Med Sci 2018;2(3):235–43.

87. Belzunce MA, Mehranian A, Reader AJ. Enhancement of Partial Volume Correction in MR-Guided PET Image Reconstruction by Using MRI Voxel Sizes. IEEE Trans Radiat Plasma Med Sci 2019;3(3):315–26.

88. Nguyen VG, Lee SJ. Incorporating anatomical side information into PET reconstruction using nonlocal regularization. IEEE Trans Image Process 2013;22(10):3961–73.

89. Sanaat A, Shooli H, Böhringer AS, et al. A cycle-consistent adversarial network for brain PET partial volume correction without prior anatomical information. Eur J Nucl Med Mol Imaging 2023. https://doi.org/10.1007/s00259-023-06152-0 [published online ahead of print 20230220].

90. Matsubara K, Ibaraki M, Kinoshita T. for the Alzheimer's Disease Neuroimaging I. DeepPVC: prediction of a partial volume-corrected map for brain positron emission tomography studies via a deep convolutional neural network. EJNMMI Phys 2022;9(1):50.

91. Alavi A, Werner TJ, Hoilund-Carlsen PF, et al. Correction for partial volume effect Is a must, not a luxury, to fully exploit the potential of quantitative PET imaging in clinical oncology. Mol Imaging Biol 2018;20(1):1–3.

Update on Positron Emission Tomography/ Magnetic Resonance Imaging
Cancer and Inflammation Imaging in the Clinic

Paniz Sabeghi, MD[a,1], Sanaz Katal, MD, MPH[b,1], Michelle Chen, BA[a], Farzaneh Taravat, MD[a], Thomas J. Werner, MS[c], Babak Saboury, MD, MPH[c,d], Ali Gholamrezanezhad, MD[a], Abass Alavi, MD[c,*]

KEYWORDS

• PET/MRI • PET/CT • Cancer • Inflammation • Metastasis • Recurrence • Staging

KEY POINTS

- PET/MRI has high accuracy and specificity in the detection, classification, staging, and treatment response evaluation of malignant lesions.
- Despite the high cost, PET/MRI provides high spatial resolution and high tissue contrast images along with significantly reduced overall radiation exposure when compared to PET/CT.
- Contrary to sequential PET/MRI or PET/CT systems, hybrid PET/MRI simultaneously acquires PET and MRI data, overcoming motion artifacts and enabling dynamic motion correction based on "time-dependent" attenuation information from MRI.
- Using PET/MRI prevents potential future secondary malignancies due to the absence of ionizing radiation, making it a highly desirable imaging modality for pediatric patients, pregnant women, and patients requiring repeated imaging.

INTRODUCTION

Multimodal molecular imaging has revolutionized both clinical practice and biomedical research. PET/CT performed using the positron emission tomography (PET) radiotracer 18F-fluorodeoxyglucose (^{18}F-FDG) has become a pivotal modality for imaging a variety of pathologies and is particularly useful in the detection and evaluation of cancers. Hybrid whole-body PET/CT yields complementary sets of structural data and metabolic or functional information in one harmonious setting and allows for successful utilization in clinical settings with results superior to both PET and CT individually.

However, despite its many benefits as an imaging modality, ^{18}F-FDG PET/CT has several limitations, most notably being the ionizing radiation and lower soft tissue resolution associated with CT. In this setting, where high spatial resolution, soft-tissue contrast, or radiation exposure are

[a] Department of Radiology, Keck School of Medicine of University of Southern California, Health Science Campus, 1500 San Pablo Street, Los Angeles, CA 90033, USA; [b] Medical Imaging Department of St. Vincent's Hospital, Melbourne, Victoria, Australia; [c] Department of Radiology, Hospital of the University of Pennsylvania, 3400 Spruce Street, Philadelphia, PA 19104, USA; [d] Department of Radiology and Imaging Sciences, Clinical Center, National Institutes of Health, 9000 Rockville Pike, Bethesda, MD 20892, USA
[1] These authors contributed equally to work and should be considered as co-first authors. The Authors have nothing to disclose.
* Corresponding author. Department of Radiology, Hospital of the University of Pennsylvania, 3400 Spruce Street, Philadelphia, PA 19104.
E-mail address: abass.alavi@pennmedicine.upenn.edu

Magn Reson Imaging Clin N Am 31 (2023) 517–538
https://doi.org/10.1016/j.mric.2023.07.001
1064-9689/23/© 2023 Elsevier Inc. All rights reserved.

issues, the novel PET/MRI may be indicated to attain optimal clinical management. PET/MRI aims to capitalize on the unique features of MRI, including excellent soft tissue contrast and functional MR capabilities such as diffusion-weighted imaging (DWI), DCE, (functional)magnetic resonance imaging (fMRI), and MR spectroscopy. In addition, the routine use of respiratory gating in PET/MRI protocols provides high temporal spatial registration and superior image fusion when compared to PET/CT.[1] A distinct advantage of recent hybrid simultaneous PET/MRI systems over PET/CT or sequential PET/MRI systems is the truly simultaneous manner of obtaining PET and MRI data. The spatial and temporal matching allows for dynamic motion correction during PET data acquisition,[2] with the "time-dependent" attenuation data from MRI allowing for attenuation correction for different motion states rather than for a static map.[3] Additionally, the lack of ionizing radiation in PET/MRI makes this imaging modality particularly appealing in pediatric practice, imaging of pregnant women, and in care of patients who need to be repeatedly imaged.

Integrated PET/MRI was first introduced to clinical use in 2008, decades after it was first proposed in 1980 to 1990s.[4] Its development was far slower than that of PET/CT due to technical difficulties related to electromagnetic interference and the resultant artifacts and signal-to-noise (SNR) reduction.[5] This was overcome with the utilization of avalanche photodiode solid-state PET detectors in modern MR-compatible PET scanners. Subsequent advances in silicon photomultipliers and image reconstruction with more rapid and robust MRI sequences brought promise for future application in the field of personalized medicine. Integrated whole-body PET/MRI systems for clinical purposes are now commercially available.

Equipment and operational costs and logistics also account for slower adoption of PET/MRI. Since 2008, only about 115 systems have been installed worldwide, mostly in academic institutions.[6] Currently, there are only approximately 30 PET/MRI scanners across the United States, compared with over 1600 PET/CT systems,[7] although this number is slowly increasing with more widespread adoption of the imaging technique.

PET/MRI is currently at the frontier in molecular imaging and rapidly making its way into clinical practice. While the added value of PET/MRI is established in many neurology, cardiology and oncology cases, it has yet to become widely validated in clinical practice. Here, we aim to review the current state of hybrid PET/MR imaging in a variety of different pathologies where it has shown promise, and to outline its potential for future application.[1–6]

ONCOLOGY

PET/MRI modality allows for simultaneous regional and whole-body imaging, which allows for lower-radiation exposure use than PET/CT in a wide spectrum of cancers. In addition, PET/MRI can accurately differentiate benign lesions from malignant ones.[7] PET/MRI results are comparable to PET/CT regarding fast lesion detection, classification, and staging cancer, but require significantly less overall radiation exposure. According to a prospective study with mixed oncologic patients, choosing PET/MRI over PET/CT despite the higher cost allows for more effective treatment strategies based on brain and liver metastases not detected by PET/CT.[8]

Whilst the role of PET/MRI is already established in the imaging of brain and certain pelvic cancers, recent studies support using ^{18}F-FDG PET/MRI in other forms of cancer as well, such as nasopharyngeal cancer, high-risk breast cancers, prostate cancer recurrence, liver metastases in colorectal malignancies, and local cervical tumor invasion.[9] Multi-parametric PET/MRI may also benefit the location of bone metastases and determination of intra-prostatic neoplasm localization.[10]

GYNECOLOGY

Endometrial carcinoma: Biopsy is considered the gold standard for endometrial carcinoma staging, but alternative modalities of staging have become more attractive due to patient discomfort from invasive procedures, lack of accuracy in staging deep myometrial invasion, and high rates of nearby organ involvement. PET/CT, which has high sensitivity and specificity and high positive predictive value in the determination of metastases, is commonly utilized for endometrial carcinoma staging prior to surgery. However, pitfalls such as relatively low soft-tissue resolution and lack of capability to detect primary endometrial tumor are increasing demand for a more accurate imaging modality. ^{18}F-FDG PET/MRI can be applied in staging gynecologic malignancies due to its high resolution and ability to obtain functional information about metabolic processes (Fig. 1).[11] It possesses comparable accuracy for endometrial carcinoma stage II and III and pelvic nodal metastasis detection by FIGO classification, but has outstanding diagnostic performance in stage I staging when compared to PET/CT. In addition, it performs more accurate detection of cervical invasion detection. Among the many quantitative PET/MRI parameters, the strongest correlation between clinicopathological features was reported for standardized uptake value (SUV)max/apparent

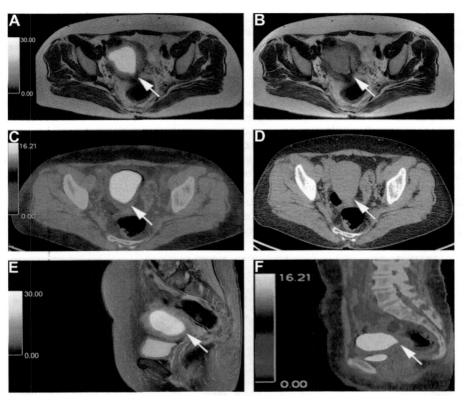

Fig. 1. FIGO stage II pathologically confirmed moderately differentiated adenocarcinoma in a 57-year-old female patient. (*A*) Axial PET/MR images. (*B*) Axial MR T2-weighted images. (*C*) Axial PET/CT images. (*D*) Axial CT images. (*E*) Sagittal PET/MR images. (*F*) Sagittal PET/CT images. PET/MRI and MRI show the endometrial carcinoma invading the cervical stroma. PET/CT also shows the endometrial carcinoma invading the cervical stroma, while CT is difficult to determine the extension of the tumor. The PET/MRI and PET/CT staging were consistent with the pathologic stage, namely FIGO stage II. The white arrow indicates endometrial carcinoma. FIGO, International Federation of Gynecology and Obstetrics; PET, positron emission tomography; MRI, magnetic resonance imaging; CT, computed tomography. (Reproduced from Yu Y et al.,[11] an open access article under the CC BY license).

diffusion coefficient (ADC)min.[11,12] ^{18}F-FDG PET/MRI without gadolinium-based contrast agents provides considerably higher diagnostic value for predicting myometrial invasion and T staging than ^{18}F-FDG PET/CT, contrast-enhanced computed tomography (ceCT), and /contrast-enhanced magnetic resonance imagingceMRI, which makes it a possible alternative technique for staging and diagnosis in patients allergic to contrast agent or with severe renal dysfunction.[13] While both PET/CT and PET/MRI have 100% accuracy for primary tumor diagnosis, PET/MRI has higher sensitivity and specificity in detecting adjacent lymph nodes and distant metastases, with far shorter scanning time needed.[14]

Ovarian cancer: Ovarian cancer, one of the highest mortality gynecologic malignancies, is classified into epithelial, germ cell, sex-cord stromal, and other types of tumors. Due to its non-exclusive serum biomarkers and nonspecific symptoms at early stages, patients are often diagnosed first-time at an advanced stage, with poor prognosis and a less than 5-year survival rate. It is also easy to miss ovarian cancer or produce a false-negative by ultrasound due to small size of the tumor, lack of invasion beyond the ovary, and lack of early-stage morphologic ovarian changes. ^{18}F-FDG PET/CT offers structural and functional information about tumor cells even at the molecular stage, and therefore, allow for early detection of these lesions.[15] ^{18}F-FDG PET/MRI provides even higher sensitivity and specificity for the characterization of ovarian tumors than ^{18}F-FDG CT, as well as other modalities. Overall, ^{18}F-FDG PET/MRI is a feasible alternative for ceMRI to discover and diagnose endometrial cancer and ovarian malignancies, as well as vaginal neoplasms.[13]

Cervical cancer: ^{18}F-FDG PET/MRI has superior diagnostic accuracy with improved functional imaging compared to other diagnostic tools in the evaluation of cervical cancer. In comparison with MRI and CT independently, this new modality offers equal diagnostic value in local extent evaluation but preferable sensitivity and specificity in nodal metastasis detection.[16,17]

HEAD AND NECK

PET/MRI is a clinically accepted modality in the evaluation of head and neck cancers, with higher accuracy in diagnosing malignant lesions compared to both MRI alone and PET/CT (Fig. 2). [18–20] Hybrid PET/MRI also demonstrates higher sensitivity in predicting histopathological characteristics of head and neck squamous cell carcinoma (HNSCC). It can also accurately assess Ki-67 and tumor cellularity and expression of HIF-1α in HNSCC, thus obtaining additional information about tumor

biological features such as metabolic activity, cellularity, and vascularity which provide additional parameters for the prediction of invasion and growth of the cancer.[21–23] Lastly, hybrid PET/MRI is excellent for the detection and T-classification of HNSCC recurrence after chemoradiotherapy, which aids salvage surgery planning after radiotherapy.[24]

BREAST CANCER

^{18}F-FDG PET/MRI is extremely valuable for whole-body staging and response monitoring in breast cancer.[25] PET/MRI had superior accuracy and better detection rate in nodal metastasis localization from axillary level I to III, internal mammary, and supraclavicular lymph nodes.[26,27]

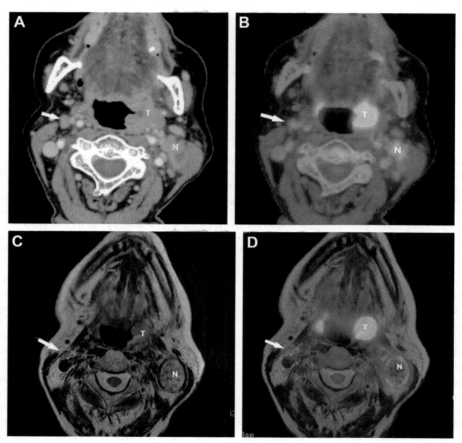

Fig. 2. A patient with an SCC in the left tonsil and ipsilateral metastasis. The right-sided node (*arrow*) was judged as metastatic on PET/CT (false positive) but not on PET/MRI (true negative). US-FNAC of the node revealed no malignant cells, and the node was at considered reactive at the MDC. Arrow = contralateral reactive node. (*A*) CT scan reveals slightly enlarged, rounded right-sided node (*arrow*). (*B*) An FDG-PET/CT hybrid image shows the node (*arrow*) has an elevated FDG-tracer uptake (SUVmax 5.4). (*C*) On T2W MRI, the node (*arrow*) has a normal fusiform appearance. (*D*) FDG PET/MRI hybrid image demonstrates mild FDG-tracer uptake (SUVmax 4.5) in the node (*arrow*). CT, computed tomography; MDC, multidisciplinary conference; MRI, magnetic resonance imaging; N, metastatic ipsilateral node; PET, positron emission tomography; SCC, squamous cell carcinoma; T, tumor; T2W, T2-weighted; US-FNAC, ultrasound-guided fine-needle aspiration cytology. (Reproduced from Flygare L et al.,[18] an open access article under the CC BY license).

Diffusion-weighted contrast-enhanced whole-body PET/MR is also more sensitive for distant metastases to the liver and bone; it also allows for the capture of brain metastases, for less than half of the radiation dose required for PET/CT.[28]

In addition, PET/MRI holds promise for novel analytical methods, such as machine learning methods such as convolutional neural networks, to accurately predict response to neoadjuvant chemotherapy in advanced breast cancer.[29-31] Lastly, recent studies proposed that multiparametric PET/MRI allows for high-quality radiomics analysis to predict breast cancer subtype, hormone receptor status, proliferation rate, and disease spread, which are beneficial to risk-stratify patients and to guide further surgical management.[32]

PROSTATE CANCER

^{68}Ga-PSMA-11 PET/CT and ^{68}Ga-PSMA PET/MRI show equivalent performance in biochemical recurrence prediction in prostate cancer. A systematic review on PET/MRI efficacy for prostate cancer, however, claims the application of PET/MRI in primary neoplasm diagnosis, tumor invasion prediction, and monitoring is superior to use of PET/CT in facilitating biopsy targeting and targeted therapies and earlier identification of recurrent malignancy.[33,34] Hybrid ^{68}Ga-PSMA-11 PET/MRI provides excellent diagnostic value in recurrent prostate cancer, lymph node, and detection of distant metastases, and has superior performance in local recurrence and prostate-specific membrane antigen (PSMA)-positive lesions even at low serum prostate-specific antigen (PSA) levels.[35-37] PSMA PET/MRI is also a promising modality to reduce unnecessary biopsies and allow for accurate image-guided biopsies when needed, in addition to the prevention of missed clinically significant prostate cancer due to higher accuracy detection features (Fig. 3).[38-40]

GASTROINTESTINAL

Gastric cancer: fibroblast activation protein inhibitor (FAPi) as a quinoline-based PET tracer with CT/MRI exhibited diagnostic sensitivity, with low physiologic uptake and higher uptake and expression in different cancer types. ^{68}Ga-FAPI-PET CT/MRI thus provides more sensitive images of lymph node metastasis due to higher affinity for ^{68}Ga-FAPI-PET in fibroblast reticular cells. [68 Ga] Ga-FAPI-04 PET has a higher detection rate of primary gastric cancer, peritoneal metastasis and nodal metastasis than does ^{18}F-FDG PET MRI/CT, which has low affinity in primary gastric cancer. Qin and colleagues recently compared the performance

of ^{68}Ga-DOTA-FAPI-04 PET/MRI with that of ^{18}F-FDG PET/CT for the diagnosis of primary tumor and metastatic lesions in 20 patients with gastric carcinomas and found that ^{68}Ga-FAPI PET/MR outperformed ^{18}F-FDG PET/CT in visualizing primary and most of the metastatic lesions of gastric cancer. Hence, FAPI PET/MR may be a promising tool in the evaluation of gastric cancer, although additional study is needed.[41-43]

Liver: ^{18}F-FDG PET/MRI can assist with primary hepatic neoplasm grading, intrahepatic lesion type differentiation, and microvascular invasion prediction before surgical intervention (Fig. 4).[44-46] Additionally, ^{18}F-FDG PET/MRI can more accurately differentiate hepatic metastases read by MRI as indeterminate lesions (Fig. 5).[47,48]

Whole-body (WB)-PET/MRI modality greatly enhances the sensitivity and diagnostic accuracy for metastatic staging in hepatocellular carcinoma and is considered a "one-stop-shop." It can help with managing patients who have locally advanced B-cell lymphoma by detecting metastases and reducing uncertainty in the diagnosis and treatment strategy.[49,50] Delayed liver PET/MR scans also offer more valuable diagnostic information than PET/CT in lesion identification.[51] ^{18}F-FDG PET is 89% sensitive and 100% specific in recurrent cholangiocarcinoma and gallbladder cancer. In one case report,[68]Ga-FAPI-04-PET/CT was able to capture high tumor uptake in cholangiocarcinoma, with lower background uptake by liver, brain, and other abdominal organ tissue. Increased ^{18}F-FDG PET uptake was also suggestive of malignancy in intraductal papillary mucinous neoplasms, while negligible ^{18}F-FDG PET uptake could be interpreted as a likely benign tumor.[52] Similarly, to earlier comparisons of malignancy diagnostics, PET/MRI shows excellent performance in hepatic and extrahepatic lesions as well. A combination of PET/MRI and CT is superior in determining the overall resectability of biliary tract cancers as well as in the surveillance of postoperative local recurrence than use of CT alone.[50,53,54]

Rectal cancer: ^{18}F-FDG uptake assessment in PET/MRI can accurately distinguish between rectal adenocarcinoma with and without mucinous components. Unlike hybrid PET/MRI, PET/CT utilization alone or with separate MRI is insufficient for the differentiation of glycolytic metabolism within mucinous and nonmucinous components, leading to misdiagnosis of primary rectal adenocarcinoma in regional and distant metastatic lesions.[55] Hybrid PET/CT and PET/MRI in conjunction with clinical findings is thus preferable for rectal cancer staging and restaging.[56]

Pancreatic cancer: ^{18}F-FDG PET/CT and PET/MRI, both routine imaging tests in the work-up of

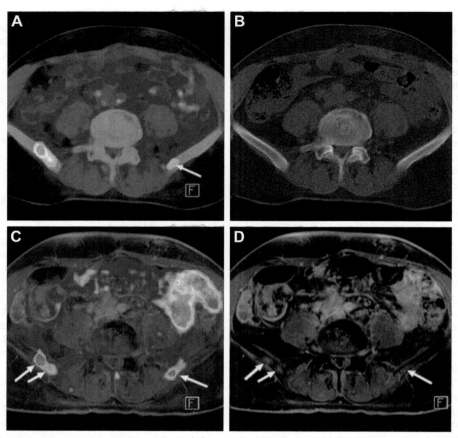

Fig. 3. ^{68}Ga-PSMA PET/CT (*A*, *B*) and PET/MRI (*C*, *D*) images in a patient with prostate cancer. This is an example of the potential of MRI to clarify even moderate PSMA tracer accumulations visible on PET/CT. Tracer accumulation is visible on the PET/CT image (a yellow *arrow*) without correlation on the CT image (*B*), but pathologic signals are visible on the PET/MR image (*C white arrows*) with correlation on the MR image (*D white arrows*) indicating bone metastases. a PET/CT fusion image, b CT image without contrast medium, c PET/MRI fusion image, d MR image (T1 with contrast medium and fat saturation). (Reprinted with permission from Afshar-Oromieh A et al.[38].)

pancreatic malignancy, significantly improve the management of pancreatic ductal adenocarcinoma in patients. Both demonstrate high specificity in the evaluation of lymph node metastasis and high specificity and sensitivity in distal metastases assessment; however, ^{18}F-FDG PET/MRI is valuable for its capacity for the early estimation of chemotherapy response in pancreatic ductal adenocarcinoma.[57–59]

Esophageal cancer: Tumor invasion depth is a critical factor in determining the treatment of esophageal cancer. Conventional modalities are limited in evaluating this aspect. ^{18}F-FDG PET/MRI has a higher accuracy rate (86.7%) than CT (77.8%) or endoscopic ultrasound (83.3%) in T staging. Additionally, ^{18}F-FDG PET/MRI is superior in lymph node staging compared to other modalities, with an area under the curve (AUC) of 0.883 and a sensitivity of 78.3%. As a result, ^{18}F-FDG PET/MRI may be used to supplement or as a standalone alternative to other techniques for T and N staging.[60]

Neuroendocrine tumors: Both ^{68}Ga-DOTA-TOC PET/CT and PET/MRI have high specificity and sensitivity in diagnosis of neuroendocrine tumors, but Ga-DOTA-TOC PET/MRI allows for improved spatial resolution, simultaneous image access, noise reduction, increased smaller lesion sensitivity, and artifact avoidance.[61]

Lung cancer

Accurate preoperative imaging-based staging is crucial to successful surgical resection in lung cancer. ^{18}F-FDG PET/CT and ^{18}F-FDG PET/MRI are equally sufficient for T and N staging in patients with non-small cell lung cancer (NSCLC). However, NSCLC mainly metastasizes to the brain, liver, and bones, which are better assessed using PET/MRI. Therefore, PET/MRI

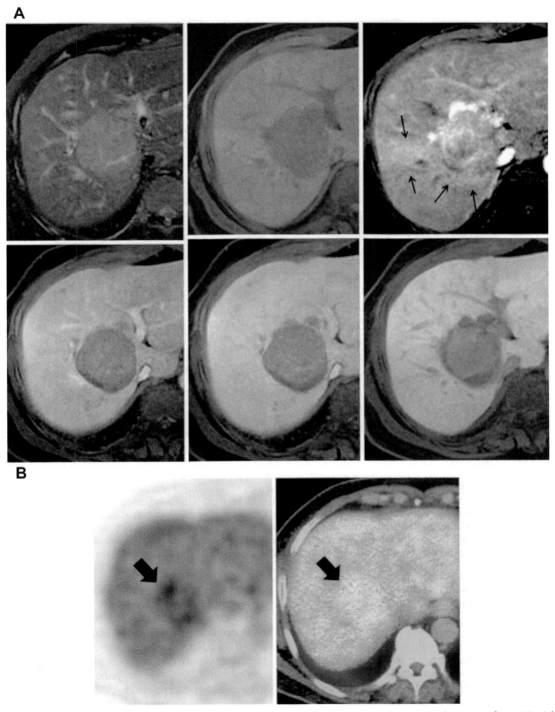

Fig. 4. A 64-year-old male with chronic C viral hepatitis and who underwent liver transplantation for HCC with microvascular invasion. (A) Axial respiratory-triggered, T2-weighted, fast-spin-echo (FSE) images, gadoxetic acid-enhanced fat-suppressed T1-weighted 3D gradient-recalled echo MR images obtained at the pre-contrast-phase, arterial-phase, portal-phase, delayed-phase, and hepatobiliary-phase images are arranged in order. 5.9-cm sized HCC in the Rt. lobe of the liver shows peritumoral enhancement (*arrow*) on arterial-phase imaging. (B) PET and fusion scans of the same patient with MVI-positive HCC. The SUVmax, TSUVmax/LSUVmax, and TSUVmax/LSUV-mean were 4.97, 1.13, and 1.22, respectively. (Reprinted with permission from Ann YS et al.[44].)

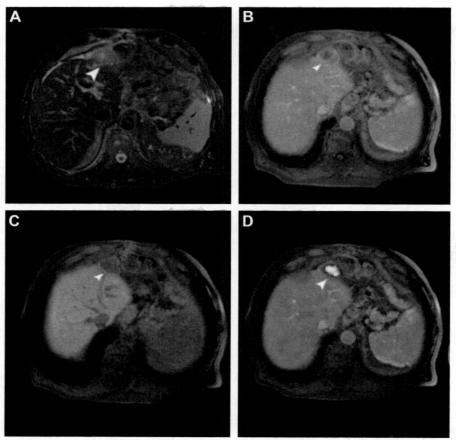

Fig. 5. An 82-y-old gastric cancer patient after left hemihepatectomy. (*A*) On T2-weighted fast spin-echo MRI, subcapsular lesion (*arrowhead*) is hyperintense. (*B*) Lesion shows slight rim-like contrast uptake during portal venous phase. (*C*) Lesion shows no contrast medium uptake during hepatobiliary phase after the injection of gadolinium ethoxybenzyl diethylenetriamine pentaacetic acid (Gd-EOB-DTPA). Based on MRI findings, lesion was graded as probably malignant (grade 4). (*D*) When information from PET was added to MRI, 18F-FDG uptake indicated that lesion was definitely malignant (grade 5). Histopathology confirmed diagnosis of hepatic metastasis from gastric carcinoma. (This research was originally published in JNM. Donati OF, Hany TF, Reiner CS, et al. Value of retrospective fusion of PET and MR images in detection of hepatic metastases: comparison with 18F-FDG PET/CT and Gd-EOB-DTPA-enhanced MRI. Journal of nuclear medicine : official publication, Society of Nuclear Medicine 2010;51:692-699. © SNMMI.)

may serve as a valuable alternative to PET/CT in the thoracic staging of NSCLC (**Fig. 6**).[62–66]

Bone marrow

Multiple Myeloma: Imaging is crucial in the diagnosis and follow-up of multiple myeloma due to its characteristic bone involvement. Hybrid PET/MRI, the most sensitive all-in-one test used in multiple myeloma diagnosis, provides combined information on metabolic activity and morphology, bone marrow cellularity, fat content, and vascularization. Furthermore, PET/MRI is the optimal modality for staging, treatment response evaluation, lesion complication detection, and prognosis prediction.[67,68]

Osseous metastases: 18F-NaF/18F-FDG PET/MRI is more sensitive in detecting skeletal lesions in prostate and breast cancer than 99mTc-methyl-diphosphonate whole-body bone scintigraphy, with the added value of extra-skeletal disease identification, which can improve treatment management (**Fig. 7**). [69–71] In patients with current diagnoses of prostate cancer,68Ga-PSMA PET provides higher sensitivity detection of bone marrow metastases when comparing PSMA and WB-MRI. In addition, PET/MRI offers superior specificity and positive predictive value (PPV) in joint evaluation, while WB-MRI shows superior specificity and PPV in whole-body evaluation. Thus, the combination of PSMA-PET and WB-MRI seems beneficial for prostate cancer management.[72]

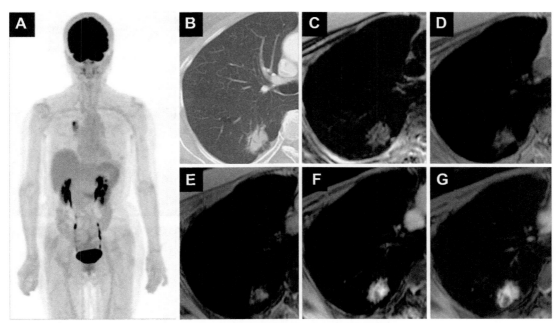

Fig. 6. CT and PET/MRI images of a 69-year-old woman. (*A*) PET/MRI maximum intensity projection image shows an accumulation on the right hilar side of the lung. (*b*) Axial thin-slice CT using lung windows image shows a pulmonary nodule in the lower lobe of the right lung. The same nodule is relatively clearly depicted on the following axial MRI images; (*C*) T2-weighted image, (*D*) in-phase T1-weighted image, (*E*) opposed-phase T1-weighted image, and f post-contrast water (fat-sat) T1-weighted image. (*G*) PET/MRI fusion images show high glucose uptake consistent with the nodule. The final diagnosis of this nodule was adenocarcinoma. (Reprinted with permission from Kajiyama A et al.[62].)

Chemical shift imaging on MRI and ^{18}F-FDG PET both allow for convenient differentiation of intertrabecular metastasis from hematopoietic bone marrow hyperplasia and are comparable in sensitivity, although the ^{18}F-FDG PET has superior specificity.[73,74]

Sarcoma

^{18}F-FDG PET/MRI, demonstrates excellent diagnosis and accurate prediction of histopathological response of tumors when used to evaluate treatment response in patients with soft-tissue sarcoma and showed that isolated limb perfusion was more effective as a neoadjuvant than MR-adapted Choi criteria and RECIST. Therefore, hybrid PET/MRI is a beneficial tool for pre-therapeutic and preoperative evaluation in addition to the monitoring of treatment strategies.[75] Additionally, evaluation of early metabolic changes, exact neoplasm location and accurate differentiation between tumor, necrosis, and hematoma by PET/MRI allows for early staging and prevents probable overtreatment, such as unnecessary limb amputation. PET/MRI is unique in its ability to allow for these due to accurate delineation of edema and

inflammation of tumor margins when compared to ceMRI alone. Concomitant morphologic and metabolic data derived from PET/MRI also helps better orient tumor biopsy procedures than PET/CT.[76]

Hybrid PET/MRI offers reliable recurrence tracking results in soft-tissue and bone sarcomas, specifically in primary patients with Ewing sarcoma, through the assessment of metabolic activity and local staging of tumors in addition to the identification of metabolic spread.[77,78]

Lymphoma

^{18}F-FDG PET/MR demonstrates excellent agreement with PET/CT regarding staging and response assessment in Hodgkin lymphoma, high-grade B-cell lymphoma, and diffuse large B-cell lymphoma. However, ^{18}F-FDG PET/MR shows lower overall specificity and sensitivity for evaluating extranodal regions. Discrepancies exist in the most challenging sites for staging, such as hilar, mediastinal, and infra-clavicular lymph nodes, which can be explained by poor quality of DWI sequences and poor arm positioning.

Treatment response assessment of both nodal and extranodal regions has 100% sensitivity and

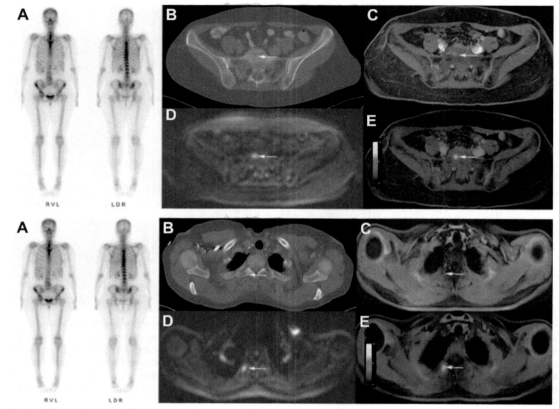

Fig. 7. Fifty-eight-year-old woman with breast cancer and histologically proven bone metastases in the os sacrum and the second right rib. Clear evidence of metastatic infestation in fused [18F]FDG PET/MRI (*E*) and in DWI-sequences (*D*). In T1 fs Vibe the lesions are hard to detect (*C*). No signs of malignancy were seen in CT and bone scintigraphy (*A, B*). (Reproduced from Bruckmann NM et al.,[69] an open access article under the CC BY license.)

99.9% specificity by ^{18}F-FDG PET/MRI. Despite the highly reliable SUV_{max} and SUV_{peak} of ^{18}F-FDG uptake in both modalities, median SUV_{max} is slightly superior in PET/MRI.[79]

A combination of ^{18}F-FDG PET/MRI with DWI in evaluating response of relapsed/refractory large B-cell lymphoma to chimeric antigen receptor (CAR) T-cell therapy is a promising alternative for PET/CT; it strongly predicts overall and progression-free survival by providing reliable parameters of bone marrow ^{18}F-FDG uptake, total tumor burden, and tumor mean ADC_{mean} which has a higher sensitivity for post-therapy prognosis prediction than ^{18}F-FDG alone.[80]

INFLAMMATION
Cardiovascular

Ability to detect inflammation is one of the critical goals of medical imaging advancements. PET/MRI is potentially more useful in detecting inflammation than other modalities. This is particularly useful in evaluating cardiopulmonary inflammatory

diseases, which include a broad spectrum of diseases defined by their multisystem expression.[81,82] PET/MRI can provide a more improved multimodal analysis of vascular lumen, aortic wall inflammation, and vascular activity in severe and non-severe Large Vessel Vasculitis than other modalities can, especially in challenging cases.[83]

Atherosclerosis: Conventional imaging methods such as ultrasound and CT are of limited value in the detection of early stages of atherosclerosis, as they can only detect structural changes in later or end-stage disease. Molecular imaging with PET allows for the identification of the metabolically active plaques at early, molecular, and active phases. Prior studies have shown that arterial ^{18}F-FDG uptake can predict cardiovascular risk and identify individuals likely to benefit from early intervention. However, several factors compromise the ^{18}F-FDG imaging of plaques and detection of inflammation, such as low specificity and significant physiologic myocardial uptake. Therefore, much effort has been taken to apply other PET tracers with high plaque affinity and minimal uptake in the adjacent structures to refine imaging. Alternative radiotracers for ^{18}F-FDG in diagnosing atherosclerosis disease by PET include as 18F-sodium fluoride (NaF), known for its arterial wall micro and macro-calcification affinity. NaF-PET is superior to ^{18}F-FDG PET for detecting and characterizing this arterial disease and may become the future technique of choice for the early detection of atherosclerosis. However, while the molecular imaging of coronary artery atherosclerosis is very promising, PET/CT has its own limitations, such as disruption by cardiac and respiratory motion during image acquisition. Thus, hybrid PET/MRI shows promise in providing additional capability for atherosclerotic imaging, through the utilization of the excellent soft tissue contrast of MRI. Using various tracers, such as ^{18}F-FDG, NaF, or [68]GaPentixafor (for the imaging of atherosclerosis through CXCR4 targeting), with PET/MRI has immense potential for the characterization of molecular changes, and discovery of intraplaque hemorrhage and neoangiogenesis, and can therefore better predict the progression of early-stage atherosclerotic plaques. Future studies are still needed before more widespread use given quantitative uncertainty in parameters measured by this tool.[84-93]

Sarcoidosis: Active cardiac sarcoidosis has a high mortality rate due to left ventricle (LV) dysfunction, arrhythmia, and conduction abnormalities created by granuloma formation and inflammation. PET/MRI is among the most helpful modalities for the measurement of LV wall thickness and detection of injuries in the myocardium. Research results demonstrate that hybrid 18F-FDG PET/MRI provides complementary diagnostic data with high specificity, including the detection of active inflammation, determination of the pattern of injury, and thus the prediction of the prognosis of sarcoidosis. Simultaneous hybrid 18F-FDG PET/MRI imaging provides an optimal noninvasive imaging tool to improve both the detection of cardiac sarcoidosis and its activity level in a single scan (Fig. 8).[94-98]

Amyloidosis: Cardiac amyloidosis, which can occasionally cause heart failure, is often asymptomatic in early stages. Several hybrid PET/MRI studies using radiotracers targeting amyloid such as ^{18}F-florbetaben, or ^{18}F-NaF, and FAPI produced more accurate results than PET/CT did when diagnosing and evaluating cardiac amyloidosis.[99,100]

Myocarditis: Recent studies show that ^{18}F-FDG PET/MRI is comparable to and can work in conjunction with cardiac MR imaging findings (Fig. 9).[101] ^{18}F-FDG PET/MRI can detect focal myocardial inflammation induced by the COVID-19 mRNA vaccine injected 5 days prior with good visualization.[102,103] Another study investigated the potential application of a combination of ^{18}F-FDG

and Gd-DTPA constant infusion to measure extracellular volume (ECV) and inflammation post-MI from 3 days to 40 days after the incident in canines, which found a remarkable ECV increase in remote tissue, likely due to ongoing inflammation early weeks post-MI; this modality could be utilized in patients as well.[104]

SPECIFIC APPLICATIONS
Pregnancy positron emission tomography

^{18}F-FDG PET/MRI performed on a large group of pregnant women demonstrated minimal radiation absorption by the fetus, with the highest estimate being 3.2 mGy during early pregnancy and an average of 1.1 ± 0.5 mGy throughout the rest of pregnancy. Despite the radiation dose, however low, benefits of the test for both the fetus and mother were thought to be greater than any probable risks. Additionally, the radiation dose calculation was based on assumed radiation needed, thus possibly influencing final results. The actual radiation dose was lower than expected in 8 of 11 fetuses due to possible ethnicity and fetal visibility differences.[105]

Pediatrics

Hybrid PET/MRI has shown significant clinical value in the diagnosis, staging, restaging, personalized treatment, and response monitoring of pediatric malignancies (Fig. 10).[106] Using hybrid PET/MRI decreases the need for repetitive anesthesia and overall scanning time when compared with the application of two separate techniques, and decreases exposure to ionizing radiation, which plays a vital role in preventing potential future secondary malignancies.[106-109]

Kurch and colleagues proposed that ^{18}F-FDG PET/MRI may serve as a valuable method for staging of pediatric non-Hodgkin lymphoma, especially in the evaluation of the skeleton, Waldeyer's ring, pleura, and lymph nodes.[110] Additional studies have proposed the potential of ^{18}F-FDG PET/MRI in other pediatric tumors. 18F-FDG PET/MRI has been shown to be valuable for imaging pediatric bone tumors, with the ability to assess the primary tumor and whole-body metastases in a single session. Limitations include time-consuming image acquisition, need for additional chest CT for lung assessment, and false-positive results from unrelated disease processes, such as osteomyelitis. New advancements such as usage of [11C]-(R)-PK11195 tracer to image activated macrophages, ^{18}F-FTC-146 to detect inflammatory markers in chronic pain, and ^{18}F-metafluorobenzylguanidine and ^{18}F-DOPA as off-label radiotracers to evaluate neuroendocrine malignancies have made ^{18}F-FDG PET/MRI more effective in

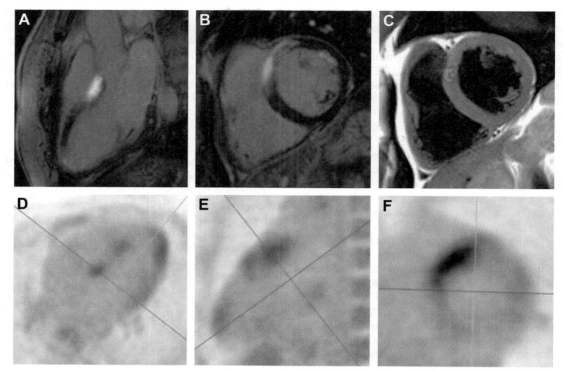

Fig. 8. Cardiac sarcoidosis. Combined PET/MRI in a male patient with active cardiac sarcoidosis presenting with onset of ventricular tachycardia several months ago as well as right bundle branch block but preserved left ventricular function (left ventricular ejection fraction in MRI 67%). The patient was prepared with a 24 h low-carb, high-fat diet combined with 50 I/E unfractionated heparin loading 15 min prior to tracer injection. PET overlay in three-chamber view (A), and basal short-axis view (B) of late gadolinium enhancement MRI depicts focal granulomatous hyper-enhancement in the anterior and antero-septal wall as well as in the lateral wall and apex. T1-weighted native MRI in corresponding basal short-axis view reveals structural myocardial changes in the antero-lateral wall (C). PET overlay indicates active corresponding inflammation in antero-lateral wall and apex (A, B, D, E, F) but rather inactive scar in anterior and lateral wall (B). (Reproduced from Krumm P et al.,[94] an open access article under the CC BY license.)

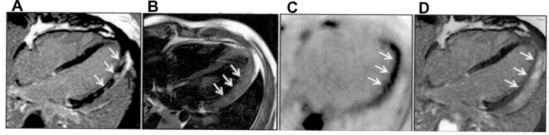

Fig. 9. (A), Intramyocardial nodules (*white arrows*) as well as diffuse subepicardial late gadolinium enhancement (blue *arrow*) can be detected with MRI in the lateral wall 10 minutes after the injection of gadolinium chelate using an inversion-recovery sequence. (B), T2-weighted acquisitions on MRI show a weak intramyocardial as well as diffuse subepicardial signal representing areas of edema (*white arrows*). (C), An intense 18F-fluoro-deoxyglucose (FDG) uptake (*white arrows*) can be detected in the lateral wall with PET. (D), Fused images of cardiac MRI and PET images confirm the colocalization of FDG uptake with regions showing late gadolinium enhancement (*white arrows*). (Reprinted with permission from von Olshausen G et al.[101].)

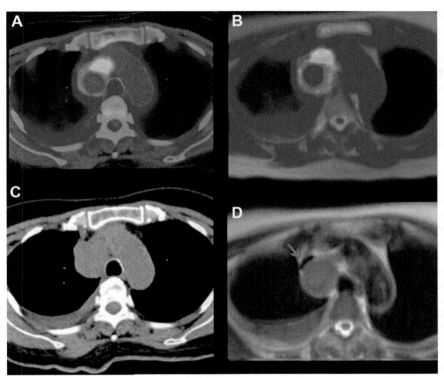

Fig. 10. Pediatric patient with Rhabdomyosarcoma. (A) ^{18}F-FDG PET/CT chest scan, (B) PET/MRI, (C) non-contrast CT, (D) MRI. Figure demonstrates centrally necrotic right upper paratracheal nodal deposit and compressed superior vena cava not discernible on the CT scan but well delineated on the MR images (red arrow). (Reprinted with permission from Sepehrizadeh T et al.[106].)

diagnosing and monitoring pediatric disease.[111] ^{18}F-FDG PET/MRI was 97% aligned with DWI-MRI results in 60-day post-chemotherapy scans showed increased correlation over time; however, imaging in patients with sarcoma shows higher correlation than in those with lymphoma. Tumor metabolic changes also preceded proton-diffusion changes in some patients, indicating the ability of ^{18}F-FDG PET/MRI to provide earlier assessment of treatment effectiveness.[112]

Nuclear medicine techniques, hybrid PET/MRI, and radiopharmaceutical utilization in pediatric diagnosis are generally comparable to those in adults with few significant differences. Combined PET/MRI usage in pediatric and neonatal disease management is still relatively new but expanding. Pediatric PET/MRI imaging has a wide range of clinical uses in cardiovascular, central nervous system, infectious, and chronic inflammatory disease, and can also be applied to cancer and renal disorders.[106]

Musculoskeletal

Arthritis/spondylitis: Anti-TNF antibody treatment causes a significant decrease in osteoblastic activity within 3 to 6 months, leading to symptomatic improvement as well as regression of radiographic changes in patients with active disease. In this setting, ^{18}F-NaF PET/MRI may be useful for monitoring the effect of tumor necrosis factor (TNF) on osteoblastic activity in disease-specific lesions.[113–116]

Bone Stress and Loading: There are limited imaging modalities in analysis of osteoarthritis and altered joint function., ^{18}F-NaF PET/MRI is among the few, and is well-known for its ability to evaluate the effect of bone stress like in exercise's effect on osteoarthritic knees, which leads to acute large bone physiology changes.[117,118]

Degeneration/OA: Osteoarthritis is a common degenerative disorder without a definitive treatment that manifests as articular cartilage degeneration with associated hypertrophic bone alteration, subchondral sclerosis, synovial abnormalities, joint space narrowing, and bone turnover.[119] Bone-cartilage interaction and synovial abnormalities have been implicated as the common driving factors behind OA progression,[120,121] and are easily detectable using advanced methods of MRI in most cases of OA knees via molecular evaluation of whole joint pathology. PET/MRI method in vivo can evaluate functional details of synovitis via DCE; additional assessment of ^{18}F-NaF uptake offers information regarding peripheral bone metabolism (Fig. 11).[122] This method can localize actively mineralizing regions through ion exchange with exposed hydroxyapatite.[119] Studies focused on evaluating the bone-synovium interface and changes in bone metabolism using PET/MRI have shown positive correlation between detected cartilage biochemical change and bone remodeling.[123,124]

Osteoporosis: The most prevalent metabolic bone disorder is osteoporosis. This systemic skeletal disorder weakens bones and raises fracture risk, due to the deterioration of the bone microarchitecture and osteoblast, osteoclast, and osteocyte dysregulation, leading to reduction in bone mineral density and trabecular connectivity. Using PET with ^{18}F-NaF as a radiotracer allows for the evaluation of treatment response in osteoporotic patients and the assessment of fracture risk and bone morphology in patients. ^{18}F-NaF PET/CT scan is the most feasible and straightforward modality used to sensitively assess bone turnover assessment in the skeleton, bone metabolism, and response to therapy. Dynamic ^{18}F-NaF PET/CT might also offer valuable research data such as the 3D view reconstruction of bone turnover in addition to the evaluation of osteoblast activity, bone perfusion estimation, and precise extra cellular fluid (ECF) volume assessment.[125]

Osteomyelitis: periprosthetic joint infection (PJI) due to dislocation or loosening is the third most frequent hip or knee post-arthroplasty complication. Early diagnosis and prompt action are vital in reducing morbidity by distinguishing between aseptic loosening and bacterial infection, which affects surgical management. Conventional radiologic modalities to detect typical late signs of PJI cannot detect the metabolic changes that precede morphologic changes. Metabolic changes can be evaluated by scintigraphic methods such as anti-granulocyte scintigraphy and ^{18}F-FDG PET/MRI. Between these two methods, ^{18}F-FDG PET/MRI provides significantly higher early detection of morphologic changes in the infectious bone or soft tissue with few false-negative results. This advantage makes simultaneous ^{18}F-FDG PET/MRI the most efficient diagnostic modality for spinal infections as well.[126,127]

18F-FDG PET/MRI shows comparable results and additional soft tissue data when compared to 18F-FDG PET/CT, which can be helpful in surgical planning in the treatment of chronic osteomyelitis.[128] Researchers have proposed that ^{18}F-FDG PET/MRI is thus an excellent alternative to ^{18}F-FDG PET/CT in the diagnosis of osteomyelitis.[129]

A combination of C-reactive protein and ^{18}F-FDG PET can help detect residual pyogenic vertebral osteomyelitis after initial therapy with increased diagnostic accuracy through analysis of the pattern of ^{18}F-FDGuptake.[130]

Fracture: PET/MRI is an effective tool for diagnosing pelvic insufficiency fracture (PIF) as a late sequela of cervical cancer radiotherapy. As PIF is often accompanied by restricted mobility and intractable pain, particularly in the sacrum, early diagnosis and treatment can improve cancer survivors' quality of life. In addition, PET/MRI is the best modality for radiation reduction, which is essential for avoiding excessive radiation in patients who need repetitive imaging for the detection and monitoring of recurrent disease.[131]

Pain: complex regional pain syndrome (CRPS) causes extreme pain sensation in the extremities. It is classified into two types: CRPS type I, with an unknown cause of nerve injury, and CRPS type II, correlated with a clear history of nerve damage. Because of the uncertain history of nerve damage in type I, it is challenging to individualize the source of pain and provide precise, suitable treatment. Despite use of MRI in examining pathologic changes within the musculoskeletal and nervous system, more accurate imaging is needed to derive a better understanding of the disease mechanism and localized changes in CRPS. Thus, using ^{18}F-FDG PET imaging, with its notable strength in detecting inflammation with minimal ionizing radiation, allows for the detection of metabolic and physiologic abnormalities in a broad spectrum of CRPS origin sources such as neurovascular bundles, muscle abnormalities, and skin inflammatory status, which may also assist with the specific staging of the disease.[132]

Gastrointestinal

IBD: PET-MR enterography is a unique, noninvasive diagnostic approach with higher accuracy and specificity than MR morphological criteria (MRmorph) and DWI in evaluating active inflammation in Crohn's disease and ulcerative colitis, and it does not require prior bowel preparation.[133,134] Prior studies on the diagnostic performance of hybrid ^{18}F-FDG PET/MRI in ulcerative colitis (UC) and Crohn's disease suggest that it is excellent at assessing disease activity, differentiating mixed or inflammatory responses from fibrotic strictures, and providing more accurate diagnostic assessment.[135–137]

Acute intestinal graft versus host disease (GvHD): allogenic stem cell transplantation (alloSCT) is the gold standard of curative treatment for numerous hematological diseases. One of the frequent complications of alloSCT is GvHD, which causes non-specific clinical symptoms and has a

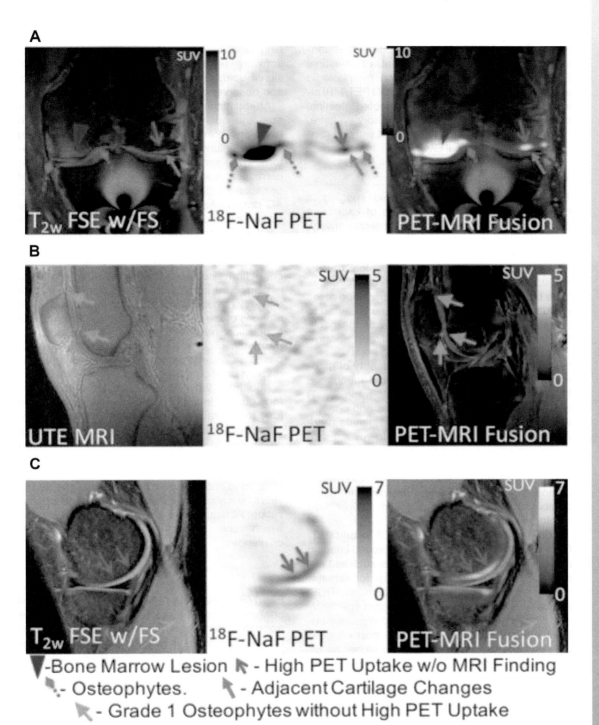

Fig. 11. (*A–C*) In patients with osteoarthritis, 18F-NaF PET-MRI demonstrates reactive bone marrow as well as other degenerative changes including osteophyte formation and associated osteoblastic activity. FS: fat saturation; FSE: fast spin echo; UTE: ultrashort echo time. (Modified with permission from Kogan F et al.[122].)

high mortality rate. Recent studies have found that hybrid ^{18}F-FDG PET/MRI is an accurate and non-invasive tool for the assessment of intestinal GvHD, with higher sensitivity than morphologic and metabolic imaging alone. ^{18}F-FDG PET/MRI allows for analysis of the number of affected intestinal segments and metabolic/inflammatory volume, both of which can then be correlated with the clinical severity of intestinal GvHD.[138]

Parathyroid adenoma

The main objective of parathyroid imaging is determining the accurate location of excessive parathyroid hormone secretion preoperatively, to better inform definitive surgical strategy. Several new imaging modalities allow for better analysis of parathyroid adenomas before or during surgical planning, and combined techniques have been the most successful. Ultrasound relies exclusively on structural features and is limited to the superficial acoustic evaluation of the neck. Single-photon emission computerized tomography (SPECT) with various radiotracers assesses cellular physiology, such as the quantity of mitochondria present in parathyroid adenomas. Four-dimensional computed tomography (CT) and MRI improve structural features and characteristics, distinguishing parathyroid glands more precisely from nearby structures. However, these modalities often expose the parathyroid gland to a higher dose of radiation. Therefore, the acquisition of complete functional and structural information gained in a single examination using combined molecular imaging with CT or MRI would be preferred.

Compared to SPECT or SPECT/CT, hybrid PET/CT is widely available and offers improved imaging and quantification. Novel PET tracers, such as 11C-choline and ^{18}F-Fluorocholine, allow for simultaneous dynamic contrast enhancement (DCE) anatomic imaging and PET acquisition in a perfectly coregistered manner, and thus hold immense potential for revolutionarily safe and cost-effective parathyroid imaging. PET/MRI with higher sensitivity is particularly suitable for parathyroid imaging, especially in pediatric populations and more challenging cases, such as patients with secondary hyperparathyroidism. However, as choline also traces general neoplastic activity and does not specifically target the parathyroid glands, there is need for the future development of a more specific parathyroid tissue biomarker.[139,140]

Pitfalls

PET/MRI is a sophisticated imaging method, but it possesses some limitations and challenges. These

include high costs, limited availability, long scanning time, lack of protocol standardization, and software limitations. Other challenges include signal voids, metal artifacts, motion correction, and observer dependency.

Attenuation correction (AC), essential for accurate and quantitative data, has been limited in bone and brain imaging, including in converting bremsstrahlung radiation to mono-energetic photons, non-simultaneity, and beam hardening correction, specifically in the presence of dental or metallic artifacts, pathologies, and air cavities. AC drawbacks in oncology include field-of-view constraint and gradient-field. The most critical pitfall in thoracic and neurologic imaging is bone and non-target tissue radiation absorption.

The ability of PET/MRI to process motion correction also faces challenges. This challenge is significant particularly with patients who have difficulty remaining still during the scan and when motions of the abdomen and thorax during image acquisition have a significant artifact, such as mismatch of a patient's diaphragm during MR-based attenuation correction with normal diaphragm position during longer PET application.

Additional limitations include patient discomfort during imaging, limited patient selection (due to contraindications such as medical conditions, body size, claustrophobia, or cooperation), challenges in the photo-detection process, and the effect of PET radioactive material on MRI. Nevertheless, there have been tremendous technical and scientific advancements in recent years, such as improved correction and optimization, AI usage, and interdisciplinary teamwork, which have helped minimize these potential challenges.[141,142]

SUMMARY

PET/MRI is evolving rapidly. The initial technical challenges have been overcome, and the future appears promising. This newly integrated solution holds unique advantages over existing imaging modalities, including decreased usage of radiation, improved accuracy due to perfectly coregistered data, and precise analytical techniques such as those used in motion correction. Growing evidence suggests that PET/MRI is extremely valuable in a variety of clinical fields such as neurology, cardiology, oncology, and pediatric imaging, and may in fact be preferred over PET/CT in many clinical situations. However, additional technological barriers must be addressed before more widespread usage and adoption for definitive use as a diagnostic mainstay.

CLINICS CARE POINTS

- 18F-FDG PET/MRI is a valuable method for staging pediatric non-Hodgkin lymphoma, particularly for evaluating the skeleton, Waldeyer's ring, pleura, and lymph nodes.
- PET/MRI enables early intervention and risk prediction in atherosclerosis, diagnosing and prognosticating of cardiac sarcoidosis, and assessment of myocarditis and post-myocardial infarction inflammation.
- 18F-FDG PET/MRI is an alternative to contrast-enhanced MRI for discovering and diagnosing endometrial cancer, ovarian malignancies, and vaginal neoplasms.
- Choosing PET/MRI over PET/CT enables more effective treatment strategies through the detection of brain and liver metastases missed by PET/CT.
- 18F-FDG PET/MRI is a potential alternative for staging and diagnosis in patients allergic to iodinated contrast or with severe renal dysfunction.

AUTHOR CONTRIBUTIONS

P. Sabeghi and S. Katal drafted the survey for the present study. M. Chen managed the survey edits. A. Gholamrezanezhad and A. Alavi proposed the idea, survey design and draft review. A. Gholamrezanezhad facilitated network outreach. P. Sabeghi and S. Katal drafted the article. Prior to submission all authors provided edits.

REFERENCES

1. Broski SM, Goenka AH, Kemp BJ, et al. Clinical PET/MRI: 2018 Update. AJR American journal of roentgenology 2018;211:295–313.
2. Yang ZL, Zhang LJ. PET/MRI of central nervous system: current status and future perspective. Eur Radiol 2016;26:3534–41.
3. Ouyang J, Li Q, El Fakhri G. Magnetic resonance-based motion correction for positron emission tomography imaging. Semin Nucl Med 2013;43:60–7.
4. Mannheim JG, Schmid AM, Schwenck J, et al. PET/MRI Hybrid Systems. Semin Nucl Med 2018;48:332–47.
5. Sollini M, Berchiolli R, Kirienko M, et al. PET/MRI in Infection and Inflammation. Semin Nucl Med 2018;48:225–41.
6. Ehman EC, Johnson GB, Villanueva-Meyer JE, et al. PET/MRI: Where might it replace PET/CT? J Magn Reson Imag : JMRI 2017;46:1247–62.
7. Galgano SJ, Calderone CE, Xie C, et al. Applications of PET/MRI in abdominopelvic oncology41. Radiographics : a review publication of the Radiological Society of North America, Inc; 2021. p. 1750–65.
8. Mayerhoefer ME, Prosch H, Beer L, et al. PET/MRI versus PET/CT in oncology: a prospective single-center study of 330 examinations focusing on implications for patient management and cost considerations. Eur J Nucl Med Mol Imag 2020;47:51–60.
9. Morsing A, Hildebrandt MG, Vilstrup MH, et al. Hybrid PET/MRI in major cancers: a scoping review. Eur J Nucl Med Mol Imag 2019;46:2138–51.
10. Spick C, Herrmann K, Czernin J. 18F-FDG PET/CT and PET/MRI Perform Equally Well in Cancer: Evidence from Studies on More Than 2,300 Patients. Journal of nuclear medicine : official publication, Society of Nuclear Medicine 2016;57:420–30.
11. Yu Y, Zhang L, Sultana B, et al. Diagnostic value of integrated (18)F-FDG PET/MRI for staging of endometrial carcinoma: comparison with PET/CT. BMC Cancer 2022;22:947.
12. Bezzi C, Zambella E, Ghezzo S, et al. 18 F-FDG PET/MRI in endometrial cancer: systematic review and meta-analysis. Clin Trans Imag 2021;1–14.
13. Tsuyoshi H, Tsujikawa T, Yamada S, et al. Diagnostic value of (18)F-FDG PET/MRI for staging in patients with endometrial cancer. Cancer Imag 2020;20:75.
14. Bian LH, Wang M, Gong J, et al. Comparison of integrated PET/MRI with PET/CT in evaluation of endometrial cancer: a retrospective analysis of 81 cases. PeerJ 2019;7:e7081.
15. Hu X, Li D, Liang Z, et al. Indirect comparison of the diagnostic performance of (18)F-FDG PET/CT and MRI in differentiating benign and malignant ovarian or adnexal tumors: a systematic review and meta-analysis. BMC Cancer 2021;21:1080.
16. Tsuyoshi H, Tsujikawa T, Yamada S, et al. Diagnostic Value of (18)F-FDG PET/MRI for Revised 2018 FIGO Staging in Patients with Cervical Cancer. Diagnostics 2021;11.
17. Ahangari S, Hansen NL, Olin AB, et al. Toward PET/MRI as one-stop shop for radiotherapy planning in cervical cancer patients. Acta oncologica (Stockholm, Sweden) 2021;60:1045–53.
18. Flygare L, Erdogan ST, Söderkvist K. PET/MR versus PET/CT for locoregional staging of oropharyngeal squamous cell cancer. Acta radiologica (Stockholm, Sweden : 1987) 2022. 2841851221140668.
19. Huellner MW. PET/MR in Head and Neck Cancer - An Update. Semin Nucl Med 2021;51:26–38.
20. Park J, Pak K, Yun TJ, et al. Diagnostic Accuracy and Confidence of [18F] FDG PET/MRI in comparison with PET or MRI alone in Head and Neck Cancer. Sci Rep 2020;10:9490.

21. Surov A, Meyer HJ, Höhn AK, et al. Combined Metabolo-Volumetric Parameters of (18)F-FDG-PET and MRI Can Predict Tumor Cellularity, Ki67 Level and Expression of HIF 1alpha in Head and Neck Squamous Cell Carcinoma: A Pilot Study. Translational oncology 2019;12:8–14.

22. Samolyk-Kogaczewska N, Sierko E, Dziemianczyk-Pakiela D, et al. Usefulness of Hybrid PET/MRI in Clinical Evaluation of Head and Neck Cancer Patients. Cancers 2020;12.

23. Cheng Y, Bai L, Shang J, et al. Preliminary clinical results for PET/MR compared with PET/CT in patients with nasopharyngeal carcinoma. Oncol Rep 2020;43:177–87.

24. Becker M, Varoquaux AD, Combescure C, et al. Local recurrence of squamous cell carcinoma of the head and neck after radio(chemo)therapy: Diagnostic performance of FDG-PET/MRI with diffusion-weighted sequences. Eur Radiol 2018;28:651–63.

25. Bruckmann NM, Morawitz J, Fendler WP, et al. A Role of PET/MR in Breast Cancer? Semin Nucl Med 2022;52:611–8.

26. Morawitz J, Bruckmann NM, Dietzel F, et al. Comparison of nodal staging between CT, MRI, and [(18)F]-FDG PET/MRI in patients with newly diagnosed breast cancer. Eur J Nucl Med Mol Imag 2022;49:992–1001.

27. Lu XR, Qu MM, Zhai YN, et al. Diagnostic role of 18F-FDG PET/MRI in the TNM staging of breast cancer: a systematic review and meta-analysis. Ann Palliat Med 2021;10:4328–37.

28. Melsaether AN, Raad RA, Pujara AC, et al. Comparison of Whole-Body (18)F FDG PET/MR Imaging and Whole-Body (18)F FDG PET/CT in Terms of Lesion Detection and Radiation Dose in Patients with Breast Cancer. Radiology 2016;281:193–202.

29. Choi JH, Kim HA, Kim W, et al. Early prediction of neoadjuvant chemotherapy response for advanced breast cancer using PET/MRI image deep learning. Sci Rep 2020;10:21149.

30. Han S, Choi JY. Impact of 18F-FDG PET, PET/CT, and PET/MRI on Staging and Management as an Initial Staging Modality in Breast Cancer: A Systematic Review and Meta-analysis. Clin Nucl Med 2021;46:271–82.

31. Bruckmann NM, Sawicki LM, Kirchner J, et al. Prospective evaluation of whole-body MRI and (18)F-FDG PET/MRI in N and M staging of primary breast cancer patients. Eur J Nucl Med Mol Imag 2020;47:2816–25.

32. Carmona-Bozo JC, Manavaki R, Woitek R, et al. Hypoxia and perfusion in breast cancer: simultaneous assessment using PET/MR imaging. Eur Radiol 2021;31:333–44.

33. Huo H, Shen S, He D, et al. Head-to-head comparison of (68)Ga-PSMA-11 PET/CT and (68)Ga-PSMA-11 PET/MRI in the detection of biochemical recurrence of prostate cancer: summary of head-to-head comparison studies, Prostate Cancer Prostatic Dis 2022;26(1):16–24.

34. Evangelista L, Zattoni F, Cassarino G, et al. PET/MRI in prostate cancer: a systematic review and meta-analysis. Eur J Nucl Med Mol Imag 2021;48:859–73.

35. Kranzbühler B, Müller J, Becker AS, et al. Detection Rate and Localization of Prostate Cancer Recurrence Using (68)Ga-PSMA-11 PET/MRI in Patients with Low PSA Values ≤ 0.5 ng/mL. J Nuc Med 2020;61:194–201.

36. Guberina N, Hetkamp P, Ruebben H, et al. Whole-Body Integrated [(68)Ga]PSMA-11-PET/MR Imaging in Patients with Recurrent Prostate Cancer: Comparison with Whole-Body PET/CT as the Standard of Reference. Mol Imag Biol 2020;22:788–96.

37. Jentjens S, Mai C, Ahmadi Bidakhvidi N, et al. Prospective comparison of simultaneous [(68)Ga]Ga-PSMA-11 PET/MR versus PET/CT in patients with biochemically recurrent prostate cancer. Eur Radiol 2022;32:901–11.

38. Afshar-Oromieh A, Haberkorn U, Schlemmer HP, et al. Comparison of PET/CT and PET/MRI hybrid systems using a 68Ga-labelled PSMA ligand for the diagnosis of recurrent prostate cancer: initial experience. Eur J Nucl Med Mol Imag 2014;41:887–97.

39. Ferraro DA, Becker AS, Kranzbühler B, et al. Diagnostic performance of (68)Ga-PSMA-11 PET/MRI-guided biopsy in patients with suspected prostate cancer: a prospective single-center study. Eur J Nucl Med Mol Imag 2021;48:3315–24.

40. Chen M, Zhang Q, Zhang C, et al. Combination of (68)Ga-PSMA PET/CT and Multiparametric MRI Improves the Detection of Clinically Significant Prostate Cancer: A Lesion-by-Lesion Analysis. Journal of nuclear medicine : official publication, Society of Nuclear Medicine 2019;60:944–9.

41. Qin C, Shao F, Gai Y, et al. 68Ga-DOTA-FAPI-04 PET/MR in the Evaluation of Gastric Carcinomas: Comparison with (18)F-FDG PET/CT. Journal of nuclear medicine : official publication, Society of Nuclear Medicine 2022;63:81–8.

42. Liu Y, Zheng D, Liu JJ, et al. Comparing PET/MRI with PET/CT for Pretreatment Staging of Gastric Cancer. Gastroenterology research and practice 2019;2019:9564627.

43. Wang Y, Luo W, Li Y. [(68)Ga]Ga-FAPI-04 PET MRI/CT in the evaluation of gastric carcinomas compared with [(18)F]-FDG PET MRI/CT: a meta-analysis. European journal of medical research 2023;28:34.

44. Ahn SY, Lee JM, Joo I, et al. Prediction of microvascular invasion of hepatocellular carcinoma using gadoxetic acid-enhanced MR and (18)F-FDG PET/CT. Abdom Imaging 2015;40:843–51.

45. Çelebi F, Yaghouti K, Cindil E, et al. The Role of 18F-FDG PET/MRI in the Assessment of Primary Intrahepatic Neoplasms. Acad Radiol 2021;28:189–98.

46. Çelebi F, Görmez A, Ilgun AS, et al. The value of 18F-FDG PET/MRI in prediction of microvascular invasion in hepatocellular carcinoma. European journal of radiology 2022;149:110196.

47. Donati OF, Hany TF, Reiner CS, et al. Value of retrospective fusion of PET and MR images in detection of hepatic metastases: comparison with 18F-FDG PET/CT and Gd-EOB-DTPA-enhanced MRI. Journal of nuclear medicine : official publication, Society of Nuclear Medicine 2010;51:692–9.

48. Akkus Gunduz P, Ozkan E, Kuru Oz D, et al. Clinical value of fluorine-18-fluorodeoxyglucose PET/MRI for liver metastasis in colorectal cancer: a prospective study. Nucl Med Commun 2023;44:150–60.

49. Vermersch M, Mulé S, Chalaye J, et al. Impact of the (18)F-FDG-PET/MRI on Metastatic Staging in Patients with Hepatocellular Carcinoma: Initial Results from 104 Patients. J Clin Med 2021;10.

50. Hong SB, Choi SH, Kim KW, et al. Diagnostic performance of [(18)F]FDG-PET/MRI for liver metastasis in patients with primary malignancy: a systematic review and meta-analysis. Eur Radiol 2019;29:3553–63.

51. Zhou N, Meng X, Zhang Y, et al. Diagnostic Value of Delayed PET/MR in Liver Metastasis in Comparison With PET/CT. Frontiers in oncology 2021;11:717687.

52. Siripongsatian D, Promteangtrong C, Kunawudhi A, et al. 68)Ga-FAPI-46 PET/MR Detects Recurrent Cholangiocarcinoma and Intraductal Papillary Mucinous Neoplasm in a Patient Showing Increasing CEA with Negative (18)F-FDG PET/CT and Conventional CT. Nuclear medicine and molecular imaging 2021;55:257–60.

53. Yoo J, Lee JM, Yoon JH, et al. Additional Value of Integrated (18)F-FDG PET/MRI for Evaluating Biliary Tract Cancer: Comparison with Contrast-Enhanced CT. Korean J Radiol 2021;22:714–24.

54. Cohen D, Kesler M, Muchnik Kurash M, et al. A lesson in humility: the added values of PET-MRI over PET-CT in detecting malignant hepatic lesions. Eur J Nucl Med Mol Imag 2023;50(5):1423–33.

55. Queiroz MA, Naves A, Dreyer PR, et al. PET/MRI Characterization of Mucinous Versus Nonmucinous Components of Rectal Adenocarcinoma: A Comparison of Tumor Metabolism and Cellularity. AJR American journal of roentgenology 2021;216:376–83.

56. Rutegård MK, Båtsman M, Axelsson J, et al. PET/MRI and PET/CT hybrid imaging of rectal cancer - description and initial observations from the RECTOPET (REctal Cancer trial on PET/MRI/CT) study. Cancer Imag 2019;19:52.

57. Lee JW, O JH, Choi M, et al. Impact of F-18 Fluorodeoxyglucose PET/CT and PET/MRI on Initial Staging and Changes in Management of Pancreatic Ductal Adenocarcinoma: A Systemic Review and Meta-Analysis. Diagnostics 2020;10.

58. Furtado FS, Ferrone CR, Lee SI, et al. Impact of PET/MRI in the Treatment of Pancreatic Adenocarcinoma: a Retrospective Cohort Study. Mol Imag Biol 2021;23:456–66.

59. Harder FN, Jungmann F, Kaissis GA, et al. [(18)F] FDG PET/MRI enables early chemotherapy response prediction in pancreatic ductal adenocarcinoma. EJNMMI Res 2021;11:70.

60. Wang F, Guo R, Zhang Y, et al. Value of (18)F-FDG PET/MRI in the Preoperative Assessment of Resectable Esophageal Squamous Cell Carcinoma: A Comparison With (18)F-FDG PET/CT, MRI, and Contrast-Enhanced CT. Frontiers in oncology 2022;12:844702.

61. Prado-Wohlwend S, Ballesta-Moratalla M, Torres-Espallardo I, et al. Same-day comparative protocol PET/CT-PET/MRI [(68) Ga]Ga-DOTA-TOC in paragangliomas and pheochromocytomas: an approach to personalized medicine. Cancer Imag : the official publication of the International Cancer Imaging Society 2023;23:4.

62. Kajiyama A, Ito K, Watanabe H, et al. Consistency and prognostic value of preoperative staging and postoperative pathological staging using (18)F-FDG PET/MRI in patients with non-small cell lung cancer. Ann Nucl Med 2022;36:1059–72.

63. Zhang A, Meng X, Yao Y, et al. Predictive Value of 18 F-FDG PET/MRI for Pleural Invasion in Solid and Subsolid Lung Adenocarcinomas Smaller Than 3 cm. J Magn Reson Imaging 2023;57(5):1367–75.

64. Wang ML, Zhang H, Yu HJ, et al. An initial study on the comparison of diagnostic performance of (18) F-FDG PET/MR and (18)F-FDG PET/CT for thoracic staging of non-small cell lung cancer: Focus on pleural invasion. Rev Española Med Nucl Imagen Mol 2023;42:16–23.

65. Kirchner J, Sawicki LM, Nensa F, et al. Prospective comparison of (18)F-FDG PET/MRI and (18)F-FDG PET/CT for thoracic staging of non-small cell lung cancer. Eur J Nucl Med Mol Imag 2019;46:437–45.

66. Biondetti P, Vangel MG, Lahoud RM, et al. PET/MRI assessment of lung nodules in primary abdominal malignancies: sensitivity and outcome analysis. Eur J Nucl Med Mol Imag 2021;48:1976–86.

67. Mulé S, Reizine E, Blanc-Durand P, et al. Whole-Body Functional MRI and PET/MRI in Multiple Myeloma. Cancers 2020;12.

68. Lecouvet FE, Boyadzhiev D, Collette L, et al. MRI versus (18)F-FDG-PET/CT for detecting bone marrow involvement in multiple myeloma: diagnostic performance and clinical relevance. Eur Radiol 2020;30:1927–37.

69. Bruckmann NM, Kirchner J, Umutlu L, et al. Prospective comparison of the diagnostic accuracy

of 18F-FDG PET/MRI, MRI, CT, and bone scintigraphy for the detection of bone metastases in the initial staging of primary breast cancer patients. Eur Radiol 2021;31:8714–24.

70. Sonni I, Minamimoto R, Baratto L, et al. Simultaneous PET/MRI in the Evaluation of Breast and Prostate Cancer Using Combined Na[(18)F] F and [(18)F]FDG: a Focus on Skeletal Lesions. Mol Imag Biol 2020;22:397–406.

71. Husseini JS, Amorim BJ, Torrado-Carvajal A, et al. An international expert opinion statement on the utility of PET/MR for imaging of skeletal metastases. Eur J Nucl Med Mol Imag 2021;48:1522–37.

72. Asa S, Ozgur E, Uslu-Besli L, et al. Hybrid Ga-68 prostate-specific membrane antigen PET/MRI in the detection of skeletal metastasis in patients with newly diagnosed prostate cancer: Contribution of each part to the diagnostic performance. Nucl Med Commun 2023;44:65–73.

73. Oki N, Ikebe Y, Koike H, et al. FDG-PET vs. chemical shift MR imaging in differentiating intertrabecular metastasis from hematopoietic bone marrow hyperplasia. Jpn J Radiol 2021;39:1077–85.

74. Behzadi AH, Raza SI, Carrino JA, et al. Applications of PET/CT and PET/MR Imaging in Primary Bone Malignancies. Pet Clin 2018;13:623–34.

75. Grueneisen J, Schaarschmidt B, Demircioglu A, et al. (18)F-FDG PET/MRI for Therapy Response Assessment of Isolated Limb Perfusion in Patients with Soft-Tissue Sarcomas. Journal of nuclear medicine : official publication, Society of Nuclear Medicine 2019;60:1537–42.

76. Cassarino G, Evangelista L, Giraudo C, et al. 18F-FDG PET/MRI in adult sarcomas. Clinical and Translational Imaging 2020;8:405–12.

77. Chodyla M, Barbato F, Dirksen U, et al. Utility of Integrated PET/MRI for the Primary Diagnostic Work-Up of Patients with Ewing Sarcoma: Preliminary Results. Diagnostics 2022;12.

78. Erfanian Y, Grueneisen J, Kirchner J, et al. Integrated 18F-FDG PET/MRI compared to MRI alone for identification of local recurrences of soft tissue sarcomas: a comparison trial. Eur J Nucl Med Mol Imag 2017;44:1823–31.

79. Husby T, Johansen H, Bogsrud T, et al. A comparison of FDG PET/MR and PET/CT for staging, response assessment, and prognostic imaging biomarkers in lymphoma. Ann Hematol 2022; 101:1077–88.

80. Sjöholm T, Korenyushkin A, Gammelgård G, et al. Whole body FDG PET/MR for progression free and overall survival prediction in patients with relapsed/refractory large B-cell lymphomas undergoing CAR T-cell therapy. Cancer Imag 2022; 22:76.

81. Nikpanah M, Katal S, Christensen TQ, et al. Potential Applications of PET Scans, CT Scans, and MR Imaging in Inflammatory Diseases: Part II: Cardiopulmonary and Vascular Inflammation. Pet Clin 2020;15:559–76.

82. Saboury B, Morris MA, Borja AJ, et al. The Future of PET-MRI Beyond "PET Plus MRI": Initial Failure of Utilization Potential and Pathways to Success. Adv Clin Radiol 2020;2:165–90.

83. Paravastu SS, Theng EH, Morris MA, et al. Artificial Intelligence in Vascular-PET:: Translational and Clinical Applications. Pet Clin 2022;17:95–113.

84. Fernández-Friera L, Fuster V, López-Melgar B, et al. Vascular Inflammation in Subclinical Atherosclerosis Detected by Hybrid PET/MRI. J Am Coll Cardiol 2019;73:1371–82.

85. Li X, Heber D, Leike T, et al. [68Ga]Pentixafor-PET/ MRI for the detection of Chemokine receptor 4 expression in atherosclerotic plaques. Eur J Nucl Med Mol Imag 2018;45:558–66.

86. Li X, Yu W, Wollenweber T, et al. [(68)Ga]Pentixafor PET/MR imaging of chemokine receptor 4 expression in the human carotid artery. Eur J Nucl Med Mol Imag 2019;46:1616–25.

87. Senders ML, Hernot S, Carlucci G, et al. Nanobody-Facilitated Multiparametric PET/MRI Phenotyping of Atherosclerosis. JACC Cardiovascular imaging 2019;12:2015–26.

88. Sahota A, Naidu S, Jacobi A, et al. Atherosclerosis inflammation and burden in young adult smokers and vapers measured by PET/MR. Atherosclerosis 2021;325:110–6.

89. Lu X, Calabretta R, Wadsak W, et al. Imaging Inflammation in Atherosclerosis with CXCR4-Directed [(68)Ga]PentixaFor PET/MRI-Compared with [(18)F]FDG PET/MRI. Life 2022;12.

90. Kazimierczyk R, Szumowski P, Nekolla SG, et al. Prognostic role of PET/MRI hybrid imaging in patients with pulmonary arterial hypertension. Heart (British Cardiac Society) 2021;107:54–60.

91. Wurster TH, Landmesser U, Abdelwahed YS, et al. Simultaneous [18F]fluoride and gadobutrol enhanced coronary positron emission tomography/magnetic resonance imaging for in vivo plaque characterization. European heart journal Cardiovascular Imaging 2022;23:1391–8.

92. Andrews JPM, MacNaught G, Moss AJ, et al. Cardiovascular (18)F-fluoride positron emission tomography-magnetic resonance imaging: A comparison study. J Nucl Cardiol : official publication of the American Society of Nuclear Cardiology 2021; 28:1–12.

93. Saboury B, Edenbrandt L, Piri R, et al. Alavi-Carlsen Calcification Score (ACCS): A Simple Measure of Global Cardiac Atherosclerosis Burden. Diagnostics 2021;11.

94. Krumm P, Mangold S, Gatidis S, et al. Clinical use of cardiac PET/MRI: current state-of-the-art and potential future applications. Jpn J Radiol 2018;36:313–23.

95. Wisenberg G, Thiessen JD, Pavlovsky W, et al. Same day comparison of PET/CT and PET/MR in patients with cardiac sarcoidosis. J Nucl Cardiol : official publication of the American Society of Nuclear Cardiology 2020;27:2118–29.
96. Dweck MR, Abgral R, Trivieri MG, et al. Hybrid Magnetic Resonance Imaging and Positron Emission Tomography With Fluorodeoxyglucose to Diagnose Active Cardiac Sarcoidosis. JACC Cardiovascular imaging 2018;11:94–107.
97. Greulich S, Gatidis S, Gräni C, et al. Hybrid Cardiac Magnetic Resonance/Fluorodeoxyglucose Positron Emission Tomography to Differentiate Active From Chronic Cardiac Sarcoidosis. JACC Cardiovascular imaging 2022;15:445–56.
98. Cheung E, Ahmad S, Aitken M, et al. Combined simultaneous FDG-PET/MRI with T1 and T2 mapping as an imaging biomarker for the diagnosis and prognosis of suspected cardiac sarcoidosis. European journal of hybrid imaging 2021;5:24.
99. Kircher M, Ihne S, Brumberg J, et al. Detection of cardiac amyloidosis with (18)F-Florbetaben-PET/CT in comparison to echocardiography, cardiac MRI and DPD-scintigraphy. Eur J Nucl Med Mol Imag 2019;46:1407–16.
100. Abulizi M, Sifaoui I, Wuliya-Gariepy M, et al. F-sodium fluoride PET/MRI myocardial imaging in patients with suspected cardiac amyloidosis. J Nucl Cardiol : official publication of the American Society of Nuclear Cardiology 2021;28:1586–95, 18.
101. von Olshausen G, Hyafil F, Langwieser N, et al. Detection of acute inflammatory myocarditis in Epstein Barr virus infection using hybrid 18F-fluoro-deoxyglucose-positron emission tomography/magnetic resonance imaging. Circulation 2014;130:925–6.
102. Nensa F, Kloth J, Tezgah E, et al. Feasibility of FDG-PET in myocarditis: Comparison to CMR using integrated PET/MRI. J Nucl Cardiol : official publication of the American Society of Nuclear Cardiology 2018;25:785–94.
103. Lee CH, Kong EJ. FDG PET/MRI of Acute Myocarditis After mRNA COVID-19 Vaccination. Clin Nucl Med 2022;47:e421–2.
104. Wilk B, Smailovic H, Wisenberg G, et al. Tracking the progress of inflammation with PET/MRI in a canine model of myocardial infarction. J Nucl Cardiol : official publication of the American Society of Nuclear Cardiology 2022;29:1315–25.
105. Zanotti-Fregonara P, Ishiguro T, Yoshihara K, et al. (18)F-FDG Fetal Dosimetry Calculated with PET/MRI. Journal of nuclear medicine : official publication, Society of Nuclear Medicine 2022;63:1592–7.
106. Sepehrizadeh T, Jong I, DeVeer M, et al. PET/MRI in paediatric disease. European journal of radiology 2021;144:109987.
107. Baratto L, Hawk KE, States L, et al. PET/MRI Improves Management of Children with Cancer. Journal of nuclear medicine : official publication, Society of Nuclear Medicine 2021;62:1334–40.
108. Qi J, Thakrar PD, Browning MB, et al. Clinical utilization of whole-body PET/MRI in childhood sarcoma. Pediatr Radiol 2021;51:471–9.
109. States LJ, Reid JR. Whole-Body PET/MRI Applications in Pediatric Oncology. AJR American journal of roentgenology 2020;215:713–25.
110. Kurch L, Kluge R, Sabri O, et al. Whole-body [(18)F]-FDG-PET/MRI for staging of pediatric non-Hodgkin lymphoma: first results from a single-center evaluation. EJNMMI Res 2021;11:62.
111. Padwal J, Baratto L, C A, et al. PET/MR of pediatric bone tumors: what the radiologist needs to know. Skeletal Radiol 2023;52:315–28.
112. Theruvath AJ, Siedek F, Muehe AM, et al. Therapy Response Assessment of Pediatric Tumors with Whole-Body Diffusion-weighted MRI and FDG PET/MRI. Radiology 2020;296:143–51.
113. Katal S, Gholamrezanezhad A, Nikpanah M, et al. Potential Applications of PET/CT/MR Imaging in Inflammatory Diseases: Part I: Musculoskeletal and Gastrointestinal Systems. Pet Clin 2020;15:547–58.
114. Hancin EC, Borja AJ, Nikpanah M, et al. PET/MR Imaging in Musculoskeletal Precision Imaging - Third wave after X-Ray and MR. Pet Clin 2020;15:521–34.
115. Sawicki LM, Lütje S, Baraliakos X, et al. Dual-phase hybrid (18) F-Fluoride Positron emission tomography/MRI in ankylosing spondylitis: Investigating the link between MRI bone changes, regional hyperaemia and increased osteoblastic activity. Journal of medical imaging and radiation oncology 2018;62:313–9.
116. Bruckmann NM, Rischpler C, Tsiami S, et al. Effects of Anti-Tumor Necrosis Factor Therapy on Osteoblastic Activity at Sites of Inflammatory and Structural Lesions in Radiographic Axial Spondyloarthritis: A Prospective Proof-of-Concept Study Using Positron Emission Tomography/Magnetic Resonance Imaging of the Sacroiliac Joints and Spine. Arthritis Rheumatol 2022;74:1497–505.
117. Haddock B, Fan AP, Uhlrich SD, et al. Assessment of acute bone loading in humans using [(18)F]NaF PET/MRI. Eur J Nucl Med Mol Imag 2019;46:2452–63.
118. Watkins LE, Haddock B, MacKay JW, et al. [(18)F] Sodium fluoride PET-MRI detects increased metabolic bone response to whole-joint loading stress in osteoarthritic knees. Osteoarthritis Cartilage 2022;30:1515–25.
119. Spirig JM, Hüllner M, Cornaz F, et al. [18F]-sodium fluoride PET/MR for painful lumbar facet joint degeneration - a randomized controlled clinical

trial. Spine J : official journal of the North American Spine Society 2022;22:769–75.

120. MacKay JW, Watkins L, Gold G, et al. [(18)F]NaF PET-MRI provides direct in-vivo evidence of the association between bone metabolic activity and adjacent synovitis in knee osteoarthritis: a cross-sectional study. Osteoarthritis Cartilage 2021;29:1155–62.

121. Jena A, Taneja S, Rana P, et al. Emerging role of integrated PET-MRI in osteoarthritis. Skeletal Radiol 2021;50:2349–63.

122. Kogan F, Fan AP, McWalter EJ, et al. PET/MRI of metabolic activity in osteoarthritis: A feasibility study. J Magn Reson Imag : JMRI 2017;45:1736–45.

123. Tibrewala R, Pedoia V, Bucknor M, et al. Principal Component Analysis of Simultaneous PET-MRI Reveals Patterns of Bone-Cartilage Interactions in Osteoarthritis. J Magn Reson Imag : JMRI 2020;52:1462–74.

124. Tibrewala R, Bahroos E, Mehrabian H, et al. [18F]-Sodium Fluoride PET/MR Imaging for Bone–Cartilage Interactions in Hip Osteoarthritis. A Feasibility Study 2019;37:2671–80.

125. Sheppard AJ, Paravastu SS, Wojnowski NM, et al. Emerging Role of (18)F-NaF PET/Computed Tomographic Imaging in Osteoporosis: A Potential Upgrade to the Osteoporosis Toolbox. Pet Clin 2023;18:1–20.

126. Henkelmann J, Henkelmann R, Denecke T, et al. Simultaneous (18)F-FDG-PET/MRI for the detection of periprosthetic joint infections after knee or hip arthroplasty: a prospective feasibility study. Int Orthop 2022;46:1921–8.

127. Gholamrezanezhad A, Basques K, Batouli A, et al. Clinical Nononcologic Applications of PET/CT and PET/MRI in Musculoskeletal, Orthopedic, and Rheumatologic Imaging. AJR American journal of roentgenology 2018;210:W245–63.

128. Hulsen DJW, Geurts J, Arts JJ, et al. Hybrid FDG-PET/MR imaging of chronic osteomyelitis: a prospective case series. European journal of hybrid imaging 2019;3:7.

129. Hulsen DJW, Mitea C, Arts JJ, et al. Diagnostic value of hybrid FDG-PET/MR imaging of chronic osteomyelitis. European journal of hybrid imaging 2022;6:15.

130. Jeon I, Kong E, Kim SW, et al. Assessment of Therapeutic Response in Pyogenic Vertebral Osteomyelitis Using (18)F-FDG-PET/MRI. Diagnostics 2020;10.

131. Azumi M, Matsumoto M, Suzuki K, et al. PET/MRI is useful for early detection of pelvic insufficiency fractures after radiotherapy for cervical cancer. Oncol Lett 2021;22:776.

132. Yoon D, Xu Y, Cipriano PW, et al. Neurovascular, Muscle, and Skin Changes on [18F]FDG PET/MRI in Complex Regional Pain Syndrome of the Foot: A Prospective Clinical Study. Pain Med 2022;23:339–46.

133. Li Y, Schaarschmidt B, Umutlu L, et al. (18)F-FDG PET-MR enterography in predicting histological active disease using the Nancy index in ulcerative colitis: a randomized controlled trial. Eur J Nucl Med Mol Imag 2020;47:768–77.

134. Li Y, Langhorst J, Koch AK, et al. Assessment of Ileocolonic Inflammation in Crohn's Disease: Which Surrogate Marker Is Better-MaRIA, Clermont, or PET/MR Index? Initial Results of a Feasibility Trial. Journal of nuclear medicine : official publication, Society of Nuclear Medicine 2019;60:851–7.

135. Langhorst J, Umutlu L, Schaarschmidt BM, et al. Diagnostic Performance of Simultaneous [(18)F]-FDG PET/MR for Assessing Endoscopically Active Inflammation in Patients with Ulcerative Colitis: A Prospective Study. J Clin Med 2020;9.

136. Tenhami M, Virtanen J, Kauhanen S, et al. The value of combined positron emission tomography/magnetic resonance imaging to diagnose inflammatory bowel disease: a prospective study. Acta radiologica (Stockholm, Sweden: 1987) 2021;62:851–7.

137. Shih IL, Wei SC, Yen RF, et al. PET/MRI for evaluating subclinical inflammation of ulcerative colitis. J Magn Reson Imag : JMRI 2018;47:737–45.

138. Roll W, Schindler P, Masthoff M, et al. 18)F-FDG-PET-MRI for the assessment of acute intestinal graft-versus-host-disease (GvHD). BMC Cancer 2021;21:1015.

139. Morris MA, Saboury B, Ahlman M, et al. Parathyroid Imaging: Past, Present, and Future. Front Endocrinol 2021;12:760419.

140. Gholamrezanejhad A, Mirpour S, Mariani G. Future of nuclear medicine: SPECT versus PET. Journal of nuclear medicine : official publication, Society of Nuclear Medicine 2009;50:16N–8N.

141. Afaq A, Faul D, Chebrolu VV, et al. Pitfalls on PET/MRI. Semin Nucl Med 2021;51:529–39.

142. Bogdanovic B, Solari EL, Villagran Asiares A, et al. PET/MR Technology: Advancement and Challenges. Semin Nucl Med 2022;52:340–55.

PET/MR Imaging in Head and Neck Cancer

Minerva Becker, MD[a],*, Claudio de Vito, MD[b], Nicolas Dulguerov, MD[c], Habib Zaidi, PhD[d,e,f,g]

KEYWORDS

• Head and neck cancer • Staging • PET/MR imaging • MR imaging • Diffusion-weighted imaging

KEY POINTS

• In patients with head and neck (HN) tumors, FDG PET/MR imaging shows a similar performance as PET/CT in terms of image quality, fusion quality, lesion conspicuity, anatomic location, and number of detected lesions.
• Studies investigating the T and N staging accuracy of PET/MR imaging compared with PET/CT in HN squamous cell carcinoma (HNSCC) have yielded conflicting results, nevertheless with a trend toward improved assessment of locoregional spread with PET/MR imaging. As most studies were based on small patient samples, larger studies are necessary to firmly establish the role of PET/MR imaging in this clinical setting.
• FDG PET/diffusion-weighted imaging (DWI) MR imaging with precisely defined diagnostic criteria including T2 signal and DWI characteristics yields excellent results for the detection of residual/recurrent HNSCC after radiotherapy with an excellent agreement between imaging-based and pathologic T stage.
• FDG PET/MR imaging has an excellent and similar diagnostic performance as FDG PET/CT for detecting distant metastases and distant second primary cancers in HNSCC patients; distant malignant lesions occur more often in the posttreatment surveillance group than in patients imaged for primary tumor staging.

INTRODUCTION

The rationale behind the integration of PET and MR imaging lies in the complementary strengths of each modality. PET provides metabolic information using radiotracers, whereas MR imaging offers detailed anatomic imaging with excellent soft tissue contrast, as well as functional information based on diffusion-weighted imaging (DWI), dynamic contrast-enhanced (DCE) perfusion imaging and magnetic resonance spectroscopy. By combining these modalities, PET/MR imaging can offer a comprehensive and synergistic qualitative and quantitative approach to better characterize tumors.

When hybrid PET/MR imaging technology was introduced in academic centers over a decade ago, the radiologic and nuclear medicine community had high expectations for oncologic head and neck (HN) imaging in terms of tumor characterization, localization and staging, detection of lymph nodes, distant metastases and recurrent disease,

[a] Diagnostic Department, Division of Radiology, Unit of Head and Neck and Maxillofacial Radiology, Geneva University Hospitals, University of Geneva, Rue Gabrielle-Perret-Gentil 4, Geneva 14 1211, Switzerland; [b] Diagnostic Department, Division of Clinical Pathology, Geneva University Hospitals, Rue Gabrielle-Perret-Gentil 4, Geneva 14 1211, Switzerland; [c] Department of Clinical Neurosciences, Clinic of Otorhinolaryngology, Head and Neck Surgery, Unit of Cervicofacial Surgery, Geneva University Hospitals, Rue Gabrielle-Perret-Gentil 4, Geneva 14 1211, Switzerland; [d] Diagnostic Department, Division of Nuclear Medicine and Molecular Imaging, Geneva University Hospitals, University of Geneva, Rue Gabrielle-Perret-Gentil 4, Geneva 14 1211, Switzerland; [e] Geneva University Neurocenter, University of Geneva, Geneva, Switzerland; [f] Department of Nuclear Medicine and Molecular Imaging, University of Groningen, University Medical Center Groningen, Groningen, Netherlands; [g] Department of Nuclear Medicine, University of Southern Denmark, Odense, Denmark
* Corresponding author.
E-mail address: Minerva.Becker@hcuge.ch

Magn Reson Imaging Clin N Am 31 (2023) 539–564
https://doi.org/10.1016/j.mric.2023.08.001
1064-9689/23/© 2023 Elsevier Inc. All rights reserved.

and tumor segmentation for radiotherapy planning.[1,2] Furthermore, imaging biomarkers extracted from PET/MR imaging, such as the apparent diffusion coefficient (ADC), maximum and mean standardized uptake values (SUV_{max}, SUV_{mean}), total lesion glycolysis (TLG), and vascular permeability constants (eg, volume transfer constant, K_{trans}), were shown to correlate with tumor grade and stage,[3,4] and in combination with clinical risk factors—they can predict the survival of HNSCC patients thus outperforming the traditional tumor node metastasis (TNM) system.[5]

Even if hybrid PET/MR imaging equipment is today not as widely available as stand-alone MR imaging and PET/CT technology, the research on combined PET and MR imaging information including DWI or perfusion imaging has led to an increasing understanding of HN cancer biology and to an improved diagnosis in challenging areas, for example, posttreatment evaluation.[6,7] Furthermore, combined PET and MR imaging information— whether derived from hybrid PET/MR imaging systems or from standalone MR imaging and PET/CT technology—is complementary and pitfalls of image interpretation can thus be avoided.[6–8] MR imaging can help to avoid FDG PET/CT pitfalls related to high physiologic FDG uptake of normal structures (eg, muscles, salivary glands) and it can also detect lesions with low FDG uptake (hypometabolic tumors, necrotic lymph nodes, or tumors located in vicinity of areas with high FDG metabolism), which can be missed on PET/CT[8] (Fig. 1). Vice versa, PET/ CT can facilitate the detection of metastatic neck nodes and it can reveal neck carcinoma of unknown primary (NCUP), a more challenging task at MR imaging[9,10] (Fig. 2).

The primary aim of this review is to critically summarize the current literature on PET/MR imaging in HN cancer and to offer the interested reader a comprehensive appraisal of what has been achieved during the past decade while at the same time providing an outlook on future directions in the implementation and clinical use of multiparametric PET/MR imaging. The focus of this article is on HN squamous cell carcinoma (HNSCC).

HEAD AND NECK SQUAMOUS CELL CARCINOMA: IMAGING INDICATIONS AND PET/MR IMAGING PROTOCOLS

Squamous cell carcinoma (SCC) is the most common malignant tumor originating in the HN. It is the sixth most common tumor worldwide and its incidence is increasing with an anticipated rise by 30% by 2030.[11] Despite ongoing advances in radiotherapy, surgery, chemotherapy and immunotherapy, 5-year survival rates remain under

50%.[12] HNSCC arises either from the mucosal lining of the upper aerodigestive tract or from the skin. Tobacco and alcohol consumption are typically associated with SCC of the oral cavity, larynx, and hypopharynx.[11,13] In contrast, infection with the human papilloma virus (HPV)—mainly HPV-16—is typically associated with SCC of the oropharynx, whereas infection with the Epstein– Barr virus (EBV) is an important etiologic factor in SCC of the nasopharynx.[11] Finally, exposure to ultraviolet light plays an important role in the etiology of SCC of the skin and lip.

Staging of primary HNSCC of the upper aerodigestive tract includes clinical examination, panendoscopy, and cross-sectional imaging. Contrast-enhanced CT and MR imaging are the most commonly used cross-sectional imaging modalities to assess locoregional disease, and CT is also used to detect distant metastases or second primary tumors. Whether contrast-enhanced PET/ CT should be used routinely for the initial HNSCC staging is still a matter of debate. However, in most institutions, PET/CT is recommended for the initial staging of locally advanced HNSCC (because of an increased risk of distant metastases) and in NCUP. Furthermore, PET/CT is also recommended for radiotherapy planning (see below).

For the follow-up of HNSCC patients, although PET/CT is routinely used in the posttreatment setting in different institutions, many institutions prefer MR imaging or CT for the locoregional assessment and an additional CT for the evaluation of the chest, whereas other institutions prefer to combine MR imaging and PET/CT or—if available—they perform PET/MR imaging. Irrespective of the imaging modality used, a baseline posttreatment surveillance study is carried out at 12 weeks after treatment, after which surveillance is done depending on local preferences given the paucity of literature demonstrating a clear benefit from surveillance imaging beyond the baseline posttreatment examination in asymptomatic patients.[14] However, in patients with a history of smoking, lung screening with chest CT is usually carried out during the first 2 to 5 years after treatment.

In clinical practice, most patients with HNSCC imaged with PET/MR imaging are selected by needing a dedicated HN MR imaging examination as well as whole body staging with PET.[15]

Imaging protocols for MR imaging and PET/MR imaging vary significantly from one institution to another. Nevertheless, a dedicated MR imaging examination of the HN region should include T1W, T2W, contrast-enhanced T1W sequences and a DWI acquisition. Some authors use fat-saturated T2W and fat-saturated post-contrast T1W images, whereas others do not recommend

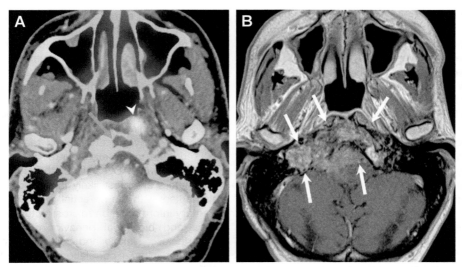

Fig. 1. (A) Axial PET/CT image shows asymmetric uptake behind the nasopharynx (*arrowhead*) and expected high uptake in the explored hindbrain. A lytic lesion in the clivus with well-defined sclerotic borders and without FDG uptake is also detected (*arrow*). The remaining of the total body PET/CT was normal. FDG uptake in the left longus colli muscle (*arrowhead*) was interpreted as physiologic. (B) Corresponding axial contrast-enhanced T1-weighted MR image obtained in the same patient illustrates an infiltrative, poorly delineated tumor invading the clivus, the right jugular fossa, the right petrous apex, and the brainstem (*arrows*), not revealed by PET/CT. Subsequent biopsy of the clivus, intracranially and of the nasopharynx showed a primary adenocarcinoma of the skull base. The increased FDG uptake in the left nasopharynx seen in A corresponds to tumor invasion of the longus colli muscle. Owing to intratumoral areas with variable FDG avidity and tumor vicinity to the highly metabolic brain parenchyma, this lesion is less well depicted by PET/CT than MR imaging. (*Reproduced from* Purohit et al.[8])

fat saturation.[13,16] An additional DCE perfusion imaging sequence is not recommended in clinical routine mainly because of a lack of consensus regarding relevant quantitative parameters.

PET/MR imaging examinations take longer than PET/CT examinations. Therefore, due to costs constraints and limited patient cooperation, different PET/MR imaging protocols for patients with HN cancer have been proposed; these protocols reflect institutional preferences for sequences and imaging planes.[17–19] Nevertheless, most investigators have proposed the sole acquisition of

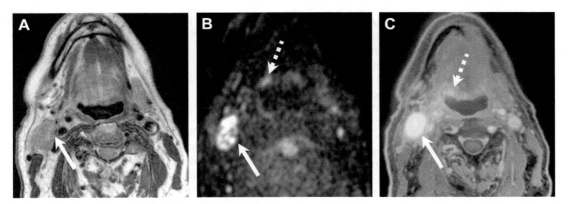

Fig. 2. Unknown primary cancer detected on PET/MR imaging. (A) T2W image shows a large level II lymph node metastasis (*arrow*) in a 63-year-old man. Ultrasonography-guided fine needle aspiration cytology revealed p16 positive squamous cell carcinoma (SCC). (B) Corresponding b1000 image from DWI. (C) FDG PET fused with the fat-saturated T1W contrast-enhanced image obtained at the same level. The metastatic lymph node (*arrows*) is equally well seen in (A, B) and (C). The small base of the tongue tumor is detected on DWI and PET (*dashed arrows*). Note, however, improved lesion conspicuity on PET due to increased FDG uptake. Endoscopic biopsy-confirmed HPV-positive SCC.

anatomic MR imaging sequences,[17,20–23] which can be used for PET attenuation correction and orientation (typically a Dixon-type T1W sequence ± intravenous (IV) contrast and a T2W sequence ± fat saturation in the HN and a Dixon-type T1W sequence or a periodically rotating overlapping parallel lines with enhanced reconstruction (PROPELLER) type sequence for the lung and abdomen), whereas only a minority of investigators has proposed a full diagnostic HN MR imaging protocol including DWI ± DCE perfusion imaging followed by anatomic MR imaging sequences for the chest, abdomen, and pelvis.[6,18,24] Using the MR imaging part of PET/MR imaging mainly for anatomic imaging makes sense given the superior soft tissue discrimination of MR imaging in comparison to CT, especially in the HN. However, if MR imaging is only employed for anatomic orientation, the full potential of PET/MR imaging is not used.[25]

DETECTION OF FOCAL LESIONS AND QUANTIFICATION ON PET/MR IMAGING

Most early publications on PET/MR imaging in HN cancer have focused on lesion detection and quantification in comparison to PET/CT.[19,26–29] Based on these publications, the following conclusions can be drawn.

- In patients with HN tumors, PET/MR imaging shows a similar performance to PET/CT in terms of image quality, fusion quality, lesion conspicuity or anatomic location, number of detected lesions, and number of patients with and without malignant lesions.
- There is an excellent correlation for SUV measurements on both modalities, nevertheless SUVs measured in malignant lesions, benign lesions, and organs on PET/MR imaging are underestimated compared with PET/CT.
- Differences in SUVs can be partly attributed to what kind of MR imaging-based attenuation correction map was used and partly to tracer kinetics, as PET/MR imaging and PET/CT were performed sequentially after administration of a single [18F] Fluorodeoxyglucose dose.
- Intra- and interobserver agreement for ADC and SUV measurements is very good.

CORRELATION BETWEEN PET/MR IMAGING-DERIVED BIOMARKERS

HNSCC typically have an increased FDG uptake, which reflects their increased glucose metabolism and they display restricted diffusivity at DWI, which corresponds to increased cellularity, lower ADC values depicting higher tumor cellularity. ADC values show a significant correlation with tumor differentiation, a higher grade tumor showing more restriction than a lower grade tumor.[30,31]

Several investigators have evaluated the correlation between quantitative FDG PET parameters and ADC values to find out whether there is a correlation between metabolic tumor activity (SUV_{max}, SUV_{mean}, TLG) and tumor cellularity (ADC values). Based on studies including 35 to 71 HNSCC patients, most investigators found that quantitative FDG uptake parameters were not significantly correlated with ADC values; therefore, the two parameters are most likely independent imaging biomarkers with the potential to provide complementary information on microstructural characteristics and biological behavior of HNSCC.[30–36] Nevertheless, Nakajo and colleagues reported a significant inverse correlation between SUV and ADC values in a series of 26 HNSCC patients.[37] Likewise, Han and colleagues reported a significant inverse correlation between ADC_{min} and TLG in 34 patients. However, the reported correlations were moderate to low with correlation coefficients varying between −0.56 and −0.35, respectively.[37,38] Moreover, several investigators have reported significant correlations between perfusion parameters (K_{trans}, K_{ep}, V_e) and PET parameters on the one hand, and between perfusion parameters and DWI parameters on the other hand.[3,31,38]

In conclusion, the relationships between DWI, FDG PET and DCE perfusion parameters rather suggest complex interactions and the reported data cannot be considered as evident with the exception of a most likely absent correlation between metabolism and cellularity in HNSCC. Nevertheless, if we expect to apply deep learning (DL) models for precise tumor segmentation and evaluation of prognostic factors further studies on larger patient cohorts are mandatory.

STAGING OF PRIMARY HEAD AND NECK SQUAMOUS CELL CARCINOMA
Local Tumor Evaluation (T Staging)

In primary HNSCC, tumor size, thickness and depth of invasion are directly correlated with tumor aggressiveness.[12] Correctly evaluating deep tumor spread and T stage in HNSCC has direct implications for treatment planning and prognosis.

Both primary and recurrent HNSCC have characteristic PET/DWI MR imaging features, which include an intermediate signal intensity on T1W, T2W, or fat-saturated T2W sequences, moderate enhancement after intravenous (IV) administration of contrast material, restricted diffusivity with ADC values less than 1.2 to 1.3 × 10^{-3} mm^2/s, and increased FDG uptake with SUV_{max} values usually greater than 3 (**Fig. 3**).

To validate PET/MR imaging findings, correlation with cross-sectional whole-organ histologic slices is the ideal approach (**Fig. 4**). However, this is quite difficult to achieve in a busy clinical setting and because many patients do not undergo surgery. Most studies evaluating the diagnostic performance of FDG PET/MR imaging for local tumor staging of primary HNSCC are based on small sample sizes.[39–41] Moreover, not all authors precisely specify the standard of reference, and functional MR imaging sequences were not used. Also, some studies compared PET/MR imaging with PET/CT results, whereas other studies lacked comparative data with PET/CT.

Among these studies, Schaarschmidt and colleagues found no significant difference in T and N staging among PET/MR imaging, PET/CT, and MR imaging alone in 12 patients with primary HNSCC, histopathology of the resected tumors serving as the standard of reference.[39] In a study including 20 patients with hypopharyngeal SCC (with histopathology of the surgical specimen in 11 patients), Huang and colleagues found that the T staging accuracy of PET/MR imaging, PET/CT, and MR imaging alone was similar, that is, 82%, 64%, and 73%, respectively.[40] Sekine and colleagues compared the diagnostic accuracy of PET/MR imaging and PET/CT for the initial staging of 27 patients with newly diagnosed HNSCC and reported a comparable TNM staging accuracy with both modalities, although there was a trend toward higher sensitivity and specificity with PET/MR imaging.[41] In contrast, Samolyk-Kogaczewska and colleagues reported a superior T staging accuracy with PET/MR imaging in comparison to CT in 21 patients with HNSCC.[42] In a retrospective study including 36 patients with oropharyngeal SCC, Flygare and colleagues found no significant differences in T staging or in measurement of maximum tumor diameter between PET/DWIMR imaging and

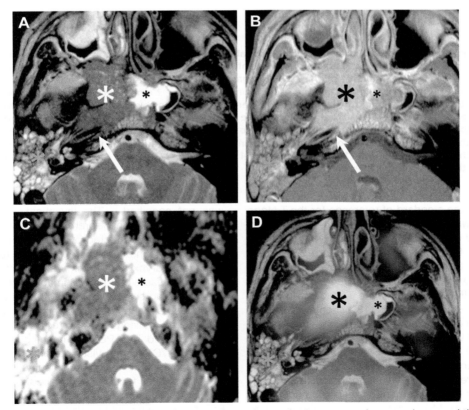

Fig. 3. Characteristic PET/DWIMR imaging features of an advanced primary nasopharyngeal cancer. (*A*) T2W image. (*B*) Contrast-enhanced T1W image. (*C*) ADC map from DWI. (*D*) Fused PET and T2W image. Infiltrating tumor (*large asterisks*) with an intermediate signal intensity on T2W images, enhancement after IV administration of contrast-material and restricted diffusion (ADC = 0.86×10^{-3} mm²/s). High FDG uptake (SUV_{max} = 11). Skull base invasion reaching the right carotid canal (*arrows*). Blue asterisks indicate fluid retention in the right mastoid air cells. Small asterisks indicate fluid retention in the sphenoid sinus.

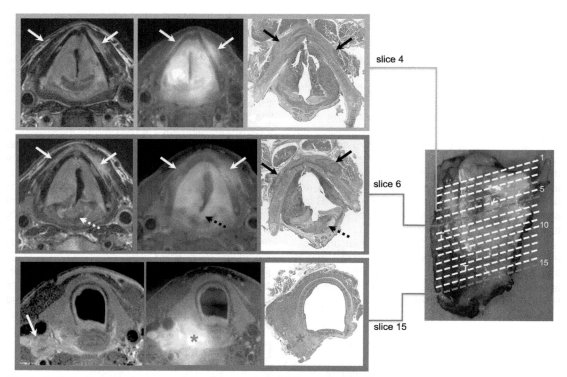

Fig. 4. Radiologic -pathologic correlation protocol enabling precise slice by slice correlation between MR imaging, PET, and whole-organ serial histology. Contrast-enhanced T1W images: left column. Fused PET and contrast-enhanced Dixon sequence: middle column. Whole-organ serial histology: right column. After surgical resection, whole-organ slices are obtained parallel to the imaging plane every 3 mm. Selected slices are shown. Slice 4: supraglottic larynx. Slice 6: glottic larynx. Slice 15: cervical trachea. In this figure with a bilateral transglottic SCC of the larynx, there is invasion of the anterior (*blue asterisks*) and posterior commissure (*dashed arrows*), paraglottic space bilaterally and there is tumor spread into the strap muscles (arrows in slice 4 and 6). The tumor has invaded the tracheoesophageal groove (red asterisks on slice 15). Metastatic lymph with extranodal spread is also seen on the contrast-enhanced T1W image at the level of the trachea (*arrow on slice 15*). Note variation in SUV values with locally higher values on slice 4 and 15.

PET/CT; the standard of reference for the T stage was, however, not specified.[43] In the study of Flygare and colleagues, the interobserver agreement between two readers was higher for PET/DWIMR imaging than for PET/CT. However, there was only a weak agreement between PET/CT and PET/DWIMR imaging for the T stage.[43] In a prospective study including 113 patients with nasopharyngeal carcinoma, Chan and colleagues reported that PET/MR imaging was more accurate than MR imaging and PET/CT for the staging of nasopharyngeal cancer, however, the investigators did not report any *P* values for pairwise comparisons; for the assessment of deep submucosal tumor spread, MR imaging served as the standard of reference.[44] Kuhn and colleagues found slight advantages of PET/MR imaging over PET/CT for the local assessment of HNSCC, especially for invasion of adjacent structures and PNS; however, the standard of reference for deep tumor spread

was not specified.[45] The investigators also reported that tumors in the oral cavity and oropharynx were more often affected by artifacts on PET/CT (because of dental hardware), whereas tumors in the hypopharynx and larynx were affected more often by artifacts on PET/MR imaging (because of breathing and swallowing) (Fig. 5). In a cohort of 35 patients with nasopharyngeal carcinoma, Cheng and colleagues reported that T2W and non-enhanced T1W PET/MR imaging were superior to PET/CT for the visualization of primary lesions due to higher lesion conspicuity.[36]

Other studies focused on the local assessment of HNSCC and on whether MR imaging and/or PET parameters could predict local tumor resectability. Among these studies, Meerwein and colleagues evaluated tumor fixation to the prevertebral space in 59 patients with advanced SCC of the hypopharynx.[46] Neoplastic invasion of the prevertebral space renders a tumor unresectable;

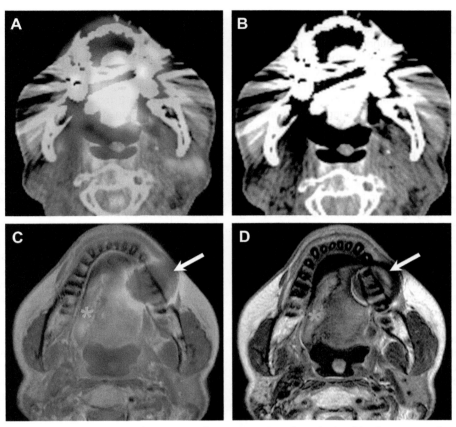

Fig. 5. (A, B) FDG PET/CT images. (C, D) Corresponding PET/MR imaging obtained in the same patient after surgery and radiotherapy for SCC of the oral cavity. Owing to dental hardware, the oral cavity can be hardly evaluated on PET/CT; however, on PET/MR imaging, no recurrent disease can be identified. Note the relatively limited artifact due to metal implant on the left (arrows). Normal flap used to reconstruct the floor of the mouth on the right (asterisks).

prevertebral space invasion can be diagnosed by exploratory cervicotomy or by palpation during panendoscopy. Both the MR imaging feature "complete obliteration of the retropharyngeal fat" and the combination of PET-based parameters "focal FDG uptake of prevertebral muscles and increased SUV_{max} of the primary tumor" independently predicted fixation to the prevertebral space with an accuracy of 98%.[46] In a series of 58 patients with primary and recurrent HNSCC, Sekine and colleagues evaluated further factors affecting local tumor resectability (eg, invasion of the mediastinum, mandible and laryngeal cartilages, or perineural spread [PNS]) and found that both contrast-enhanced PET/CT and PET/MR imaging with a fully diagnostic regional MR imaging protocol (but without DWI or perfusion imaging) performed equally well, although there was a slight but nonsignificant trend toward more accurate results with PET/MR imaging.[47] The standard of reference in this study consisted in clinical

findings, intraoperative results and/or histopathology, which was, however, available only in 51% of cases.

PNS along the cranial nerves has a major impact on prognosis, risk stratification, staging, and treatment planning in a variety of HN tumors; however, it is often underdiagnosed clinically. HNSCC and adenoid cystic carcinoma have the highest incidence of PNS, followed by desmoplastic melanoma, mucoepidermoid carcinoma, and lymphoma.[48,49] Contrast-enhanced MR imaging is considered the most appropriate imaging modality to detect PNS and invasion of the skull base.[50] Primary MR imaging findings in PNS include thickening, nodularity, nerve enhancement, and fat pad obliteration, and secondary MR imaging findings are denervation of muscles as well as changes of the superficial muscular aponeurotic system.[50] PNS can also be detected on FDG PET—if tumors are FDG avid or in the presence of extensive PNS—and correlation with anatomic imaging improves the assessment of PNS presence and extent and skull base invasion.[49,51] Although some investigators highly recommend FDG PET/CT to assess PNS, others suggest using PET/MR imaging or PET/CT only as problem-solving tools in posttreatment surveillance as MR imaging has a high diagnostic performance in the assessment of PNS.[50,52] As suggested by several investigators and based on our own experience, PNS lesions can be missed on PET/CT scans and combining PET with MR imaging improves the detection of PNS (Fig. 6).[44,47,51] Nevertheless, there are currently no studies comparing the diagnostic performance of PET/MR imaging with PET/CT or MR imaging alone specifically addressing PNS, and further research is necessary to establish more conclusive comparisons.

Lymph Node Evaluation (N Staging)

The presence of lymph node metastases in HNSCC is one of the most important parameters affecting prognosis, one single positive node already decreasing survival by 50%.[53] Other factors affecting survival include the number of metastatic nodes, their location in the neck (upper vs lower neck), and the presence of extranodal extension (ie, cancer extending beyond the nodal capsule). Therefore, early detection and accurate

staging of lymph node metastases are crucial for determining appropriate treatment strategies to improve patient outcome.

To diagnose metastatic lymph nodes in HNSCC, the following PET/DWI/MR imaging criteria are applied (Figs. 7 and 8): morphologic MR imaging criteria (size > 10 mm, rounded shape, irregular margins, inhomogeneous enhancement, central nodal necrosis); restricted diffusivity (ADC values in metastatic nodes are lower than in reactive nodes; however, no uniform cutoff value is available in the literature); and increased glucose metabolism (focal FDG uptake of metastatic nodes, but no uniform cutoff value, occasionally absent FDG uptake in entirely necrotic nodes).

Most studies evaluating the diagnostic performance of FDG PET/MR imaging for the N staging of HNSCC are either based on relatively small sample sizes or there is no histopathologic correlation to confirm the N stage. Among the few studies with neck dissection specimen as standard of reference, a comparable N staging accuracy with PET/MR imaging and PET/CT was reported by Sekine and colleagues in 14 HNSCC patients, by Schaarschmidt and colleagues in 25 HNSCC patients, and by Huang and colleagues in 11 patients with hypopharyngeal SCC, respectively.[39,40,41] Huang and colleagues also reported that PET/MR imaging, PET/CT, and MR imaging alone had a

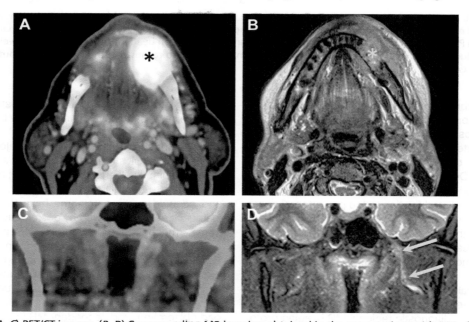

Fig. 6. (A, C) PET/CT images. (B, D) Corresponding MR imaging obtained in the same patient with SCC of the oral cavity (asterisks) invading the horizontal branch of the mandible. SUV$_{max}$, 18. The coronal PET/CT image (C) does not show any PNS along the mandibular nerve (V3). However, the corresponding coronal Short-TI Inversion Recovery (STIR) image (D) clearly shows thickening of V3 (arrows) extending up to the foramen ovale and corresponding to PNS. After IV administration of contrast material, enhancement of the thickened V3 was seen (not shown). Six months after surgery and radiochemotherapy, PNS progressed intracranially.

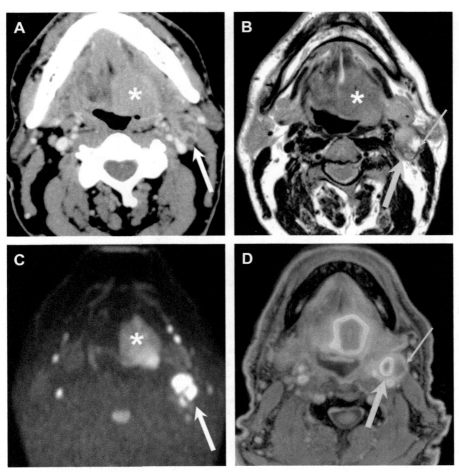

Fig. 7. Characteristic aspect of metastatic lymph nodes on CT and PET/MR imaging. (*A*) Contrast-enhanced CT image obtained in a 58-year-old patient with an HPV positive base of the tongue SCC (*asterisk*). Note an ipsilateral enlarged level II metastatic node (*arrow*) with peripheral rim enhancement and necrotic portions. Corresponding PET/MR imaging obtained at the same level (*B*). T2W image (*C*) b 1000 image from DWI. (*D*) Fused PET and contrast-enhanced Dixon image. The tumor (*asterisks in B and C*) invades the extrinsic tongue muscles and has an intermediate signal intensity on T2, restricted diffusion and increased FDG uptake (SUV$_{max}$ = 15). The solid portions of the level II metastatic node (*thick yellow arrows*) show increased FDG uptake (SUVmax = 14), whereas the necrotic portions (*thin arrows*) show no relevant uptake.

similar sensitivity, specificity, and accuracy in the per-patient analysis (*n* = 11), per-nodal level analysis (*n* = 54), and per-node analysis (*n* = 464), respectively.[40] Inter-reader agreement for PET/MR imaging, PET/CT, and MR imaging was perfect with Cohen kappa values greater than 0.9.[40] Likewise, Platzek and colleagues found no significant differences between PET/MR imaging, PET alone, and MR imaging alone in terms of sensitivity, specificity, and accuracy in their analysis of 391 dissected lymph node levels in 38 patients with HNSCC.[54] In contrast, based on a series of 44 HNSCC patients with clinically N0 necks and neck dissections, Cebeci and colleagues found that PET/MR imaging had a superior sensitivity and

negative predictive value (NPV) in comparison to MR imaging alone (sensitivity = 83% vs 50%; NPV = 97% vs 92%, *P* < .05).[55] Likewise, based on the analysis of 865 lymph nodes obtained from neck dissections in 26 patients, Crimi and colleagues found that compared with contrast-enhanced MR imaging alone or PET alone, PET/MR imaging had a superior diagnostic performance.[56] Furthermore, PET/MR imaging with a SUV$_{max}$ cutoff of 5.7 combined with size and/or morphologic MR imaging criteria reached high values for accuracy (98.2%), NPV (98.2%), and positive predictive value (PPV) (95.2%).[56]

Among the studies using the N stage set at the multidisciplinary tumor board (MDTB) as standard

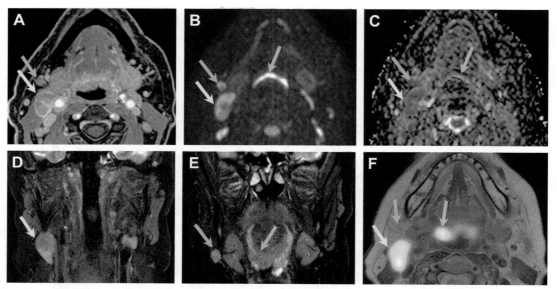

Fig. 8. PET/DWIMR imaging features of metastatic lymph nodes seen in a patient with NCUP. (A) Contrast-enhanced Dixon sequence. (B) b 1000 image from DWI. (C) ADC map from DWI. (D, E) Coronal STIR images. (F). Fused PET and T2W image. The patient presented with a level II palpable node (*yellow arrows*) which has the characteristic features of a metastatic lymph node (increased size, restricted diffusion with ADC = 0.85 × 10–3 mm^2/s, inhomogeneous enhancement and increased FDG uptake, SUV$_{max}$ = 16). The smaller level Ib node on the right (*green arrows*) is suspicious on MR imaging (rounded shape, irregular contour, low ADC, and inhomogeneous enhancement) but shows no FDG uptake due to its small size. On (F), a lesion is seen in the right base of the tongue (*blue arrows*), which was retrospectively also identified on the coronal STIR (E). Owing to geometric distortion on DWI, the base of the tongue lesion is not seen. Biopsy-revealed HPV-negative SCC in the base of the tongue. Ultra-sonography-guided fine needle aspiration cytology (US FNAC) of level II and level Ib nodes was positive for SCC.

of reference, Flygare and colleagues found that PET/MR imaging was more accurate than PET/CT in 40 patients with oropharyngeal SCC.[43] In the series of Chan and colleagues (113 patients with nasopharyngeal cancer), the standard of reference consisted of the N stage set at the MDTB after having performed ultrasonography-guided fine needle aspiration cytology (US FNAC) or biopsy in cases with discordant imaging findings.[44] The investigators found that the sensitivity of PET/MR imaging (99.5%) was higher than that of PET/CT (91%) or MR imaging alone (94%); PET/MR imaging was particularly useful for distinguishing retropharyngeal nodal metastases from nasopharyngeal tumors.[44]

The above-mentioned studies are based on PET and morphologic MR imaging criteria, and data on the combined PET/DWIMR imaging assessment of lymph nodes in HNSCC are still lacking. In several publications, DWIMR imaging has been shown to have a high diagnostic accuracy for detecting lymph node metastases, including subcentimeter metastatic lymph nodes.[57–60] In a systematic review, Driessen and colleagues reported that the accuracy of DWIMR imaging was 85% to 91% and the NPV was higher than 91% for

the assessment of metastatic lymph nodes.[61] Belfiore and colleagues concluded that ADC values can be reliably used to assess metastatic lymph nodes in the neck and that the sensitivity, specificity, and area under the curve (AUC) of a narrower region of interest (ROI) for recognizing metastases were greater compared with the ADC value of the whole node.[62] Several studies on PET, DWI, and MR imaging characteristics of HNSCC lymph nodes have assessed differences between normal and metastatic neck nodes without reporting the diagnostic performance of the respective modalities for N staging.[63,64] From a clinical point of view, it would be very useful to know whether combining morphologic MR imaging criteria with DWI and PET criteria could improve the N staging accuracy in HNSCC.

Detection of Distant Metastases (M staging) and Second Primary Cancers

Distant tumor spread includes hematogenous spread to distant organs and lymphatic spread to distant lymph nodes. Up to 28% of patients with primary and recurrent HNSCC have metastases or second primary cancers at the time of diagnosis.[24,65,66] These second primary cancers originate within the HN region or in distant sites (eg, lung, esophagus, or colon). Most of the HNSCC metastases are found in the lungs or mediastinum, whereas bone and liver metastases are uncommon. In a prospective study evaluating distant metastases and second primary cancers in 82 HNSCC patients undergoing PET/MR imaging and PET/CT, Katirtzidou and colleagues reported that patients imaged for follow-up/suspected HNSCC recurrence had a higher incidence of distant malignant lesions compared with patients with primary tumors or NCUP; the standard of reference was histology and follow-up greater than 2 years or until death.[24]

In the past, HNSCC patients with distant metastases were treated only palliatively and screening for distant metastases aimed to avoid aggressive locoregional treatment. However, in recent years, as oligometastases are treated by metastasectomy or stereotactic radiotherapy, the therapeutic paradigm in HNSCC patients has changed.[67] In addition, there is a growing body of evidence supporting the implementation of whole-body MR imaging or FDG PET/MR imaging for the detection of distant metastases.[67–69]

In a prospective study enrolling 198 patients with primary oropharyngeal and hypopharyngeal SCC, Yeh and colleagues found a similar PET/MR imaging and PET/CT sensitivity for the detection of second primary cancers and metastases to neck nodes and distant sites (73.5% vs 69.9%, $P = .08$) and there were no significant differences in terms of diagnostic capability between MR imaging and PET/CT (AUC = 0.905 vs 0.917, $P = .469$) and between PET/MR imaging and PET/CT (AUC = 0.930 vs 0.917, $P = .062$), respectively; the standard of reference was biopsy and follow-up greater than 1 year or until death.[66]

In contrast to the study of Yeh and colleagues, Katirtzidou and colleagues specifically focused on malignant lesions outside the HN area. In a prospective study including 103 examinations in 82 HNSCC patients with 183 distant lesions, the investigators reported that PET/MR imaging had a similar and high diagnostic performance as PET/CT for the detection of distant malignant lesions (metastases and second primary cancers), regardless of the type of analysis conducted (AUC per patient = 0.947 vs 0.975; AUC per examination = 0.965 vs 0.968; AUC per lesion = 0.957 vs 0.944, $P > .05$) (Figs. 9–11). Depending on the analysis type (per patient, per examination, per lesion), the sensitivity, specificity, and accuracy varied between 94%–96%, 85%–90%, and 89%–91% for PET/MR imaging and 90%–96%, 86%–93%, and 88%–93% for PET/CT,

respectively; all pairwise comparisons yielded P values > 0.05.[24] Furthermore, the findings in this study suggested that due to the high occurrence of distant metastases and second primary cancers during follow-up, imaging with FDG PET/CT or FDG PET/MR imaging outside the HN area should be considered more frequently. As FDG PET/MR imaging has shown excellent results in detecting local recurrence after radio(chemo)therapy,[13] the investigators suggested that whole-body PET/MR imaging could reliably complement locoregional PET/MR imaging assessment.[24]

Based on a meta-analysis including 14 studies (1042 patients), Zhang and colleagues reported a higher sensitivity of FDG PET/MR imaging compared with PET/CT (0.87 vs 0.81), a higher AUC value (0.98 vs 0.95), and similar specificity (0.97 vs 0.97) for detecting distant metastases.[70] This meta-analysis included, however, different cancer types, for example, breast and lung cancer, which are known to be more commonly associated with bone metastases than HNSCC.[71] The investigators also noted that FDG PET/MR imaging and PET/CT had different diagnostic performances in different tumors types, for example, the accuracy of PET/MR imaging was higher in patients with breast cancer, whereas the accuracy of PET/CT was higher in patients with lung cancer.[70]

As most HNSCC patients develop distant malignant lesions in the lungs (and rarely in the bones), it is important to be aware of the diagnostic PET/MR imaging performance for lung nodules. Several investigators have suggested that PET/MR imaging can reliably detect and characterize FDG-avid pulmonary lesions.[68,69,72] In a study involving patients with different types of primary cancers, Chandarana and colleagues showed that PET/MR imaging had a high sensitivity for the detection of FDG-avid nodules (96%) and nodules greater than 0.5 cm in diameter (89%), with a low sensitivity for small non-FDG-avid nodules.[68] Likewise, Lee and colleagues reported a high detection rate for FDG-avid pulmonary nodules (sensitivity = 98%) with PET/MR imaging in a series of 51 patients with different cancer types, whereas the sensitivity for non-FDG-avid small nodules was only 35%.[69] The FDG-avidity of tumors is influenced by their histology, which impacts the diagnostic performance of FDG PET. Therefore, it is essential for studies to consider this aspect. As metastases and distant second primary cancers in HNSCC patients are mostly FDG-avid, the detection rate in HNSCC is high and similar with PET/MR imaging and PET/CT. Furthermore, the study of Katirtzidou and colleagues found that FDG-negative lung nodules ≤8 mm in HNSCC patients were predominantly benign.[24] It is worthwhile mentioning that

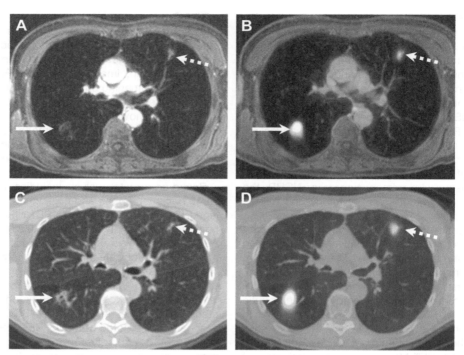

Fig. 9. Lung metastases correctly diagnosed on PET/MR imaging (*A, B*) and PET/CT (*C, D*) in a 60-year old woman with nodal recurrence after radiochemotherapy for oropharyngeal HPV-negative SCC. The right upper lobe metastasis (*arrows*) shows a combination of high focal FDG uptake (SUVmax on PET/MR imaging = 7.7 and SUV-max on PET/CT = 9.3) and an excavated aspect on the contrast-enhanced fat-saturated MR image and on the corresponding CT image. The left upper lobe metastasis (*dashed arrows*) displays minor focal FDG uptake (SUVmax on PET/MR imaging = 1.7 and SUVmax on PET/CT = 2.1) and clustered nodules on the corresponding morphologic MR imaging/CT images. Both lesions were rated with a score of 5 (highly suspicious) on PET/MR imaging and PET/CT. (*Reproduced from* Katirtzidou et al.[24])

false positive evaluations due to high FDG uptake can also occur (especially in the mediastinum) and depending on the clinical situation, biopsy is mandatory (**Fig. 12**).

In conclusion, the current literature suggests that both PET/MR imaging and PET/CT have a high and comparable diagnostic performance for the detection of distant metastases and distant second primary cancers in HNSCC patients.

NECK CARCINOMA OF UNKNOWN PRIMARY

Historically, 1%–9% of HNSCC were considered as NCUP.[73] However, during the past decades, the incidence of NCUP has increased due to the increasing incidence of HPV-positive oropharyngeal SCC, which often presents clinically as NCUP. The 8th edition of the TNM staging manual classifies HPV-positive NCUP as HPV-positive oropharyngeal SCC.[74]

The guidelines for the workup of NCUP include US FNAC or US-guided biopsy of the enlarged neck node (with p16 immunohistochemistry and direct HPV testing), PET/CT, MR imaging,

endoscopic biopsy under general anesthesia, tonsillectomy, and more recently narrow band imaging and tongue base mucosectomy.[73,75] Narrow band imaging uses blue and green light with different wavelengths to optimize visualization of mucosal microvascular changes as seen in dysplasia and malignancy.

In most studies, the reported rates of NCUP identification with FDG PET/CT remain below 55%.[73,76–78] In contrast, only one study including 30 NCUP patients reported a sensitivity of 94%.[10] Most investigators agree that FDG PET/CT has a relatively high number of false positives (up to 40%) due to the physiologic uptake of oropharyngeal lymphoid tissue.[10,73,78] Nevertheless, FDG PET/CT enables the detection of additional metastatic lymph nodes and distant metastases.[78] Recently, Noji and colleagues reported that the sensitivity and specificity of qualitative and quantitative analysis with DWIMR imaging and FDG PET/CT were similar; however, adding DWIMR imaging did not improve the accuracy of FDG PET/CT.[10] An important limitation of most published studies is the fact that most series

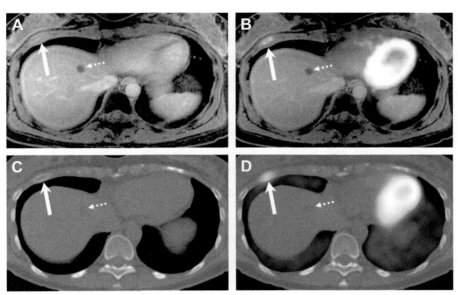

Fig. 10. Rib metastasis detected on both PET/MRI (*A, B*) and PET/CT (*C, D*) in a 42-year old female without loco-regional recurrence after radiochemotherapy for an SCC of the paranasal sinuses. The rib lesion (arrows on all images) shows a combination of high focal FDG uptake (SUVmax on PET/MR imaging = 6.3 and SUVmax on PET/CT = 4.7) and an expansile aspect on MR imaging/CT. Note lesion enhancement on the contrast enhanced fat saturated MR image. The lesion was rated with a score of 5 (highly suspicious) on PET/MR imaging and with a score of 4 (moderately suspicious) on PET/CT. Dashed arrows point at a liver cyst. (*Reproduced from Katirtzidou et al.[24]*)

included only a small number of patients. In the only study published so fat directly comparing the diagnostic performance of FDG PET/CT with PET/MR imaging (without DWI), Ruhlmann and colleagues found a similar diagnostic ability for the detection of primary cancer and metastases in 20 patients with NCUP.[78]

Based on the current literature, no evidence-based conclusion can be drawn about the role of PET/MR imaging ± DWI in the workup of NCUP and further studies are warranted.

TUMOR SEGMENTATION

Curative treatment options for patients with HNSCC include surgery and radio(chemo)therapy. Regardless of the chosen treatment, precise and accurate delineation of tumor margins and, therefore, tumor volume are fundamental for effectively managing patients with HNSCC. In surgical procedures, a delicate trade-off must be achieved between a limited tumor resection with the risk of positive or close margins (associated with poorer prognosis) and a wide resection (leading to unsatisfactory functional and cosmetic outcomes).

In terms of tumor volume, radiation oncologists distinguish between gross tumor volume (GTV, which is the delineated radiologically measurable tumor), clinical target volume (CTV, which adds a

margin to the GTV to cover areas of potential microscopic disease), and planning target volume (PTV, defined as the CTV surrounded by adequate margins to account for organ and patient motion or variation in patient position). Although the adoption of intensity-modulated radiation therapy protocols has reduced irradiation volumes on the one hand (thus avoiding irradiation of organs at risk), it has also increased the importance of precise GTV delineation on the other hand.[79-81] Precise delineation of GTVs has not only a direct impact on patient outcome but it can also jeopardize the robustness of quantitative metrics, including radiomics features.[82]

Although contrast-enhanced CT is a standard imaging technique for radiation therapy planning in HNSCC, it falls short in precisely delineating GTVs of primary tumors and lymph node metastases. Incorporating PET data into radiation therapy planning offers several advantages over using CT alone.[79] By using FDG PET, the risk of inaccurately targeting radiation delivery to the intended volumes is reduced.[83,84] In addition, the use of other radiotracers, such as 18F-fluoromisonidazole, a biomarker for hypoxia, can identify tissues that require intensified treatment approaches.[85] Beyond PET biomarkers, functional MR imaging biomarkers provide the ability to characterize cellularity, vascularity, and permeability of tumors,

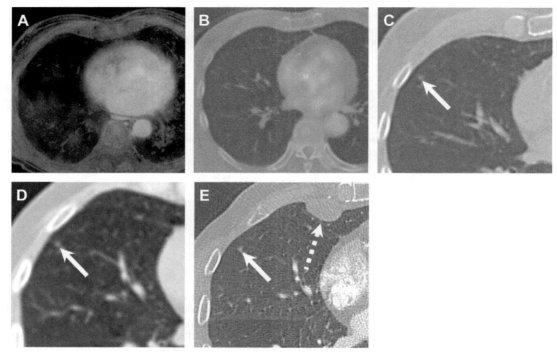

Fig. 11. False-negative PET/MR imaging (*A*) and PET/CT (*B*) in an 89-year-old man with primary SCC of the oral cavity. Both PET/MR imaging and PET/CT were rated as negative for distant metastases or second primary cancers (diagnostic score = 1). PET/MR imaging (*A*) shows no lesion. PET/CT (*B*) and detail of the corresponding CT component of the PET/CT (*C*) show a non-FDG avid 5 mm solid lung nodule (*arrow* in *C*), which was considered as benign according to diagnostic criteria (no FDG uptake and ≤8 mm in size). The lesion was rated with a score of 1 on PET/MR imaging and PET/CT. Follow-up CT obtained 2 months later (*D*) showed no change in size and shape of the 5 mm nodule (*arrow*). CT obtained 7 months later (*E*) revealed no change in the 5 mm nodule (*arrow*), however, a pleural metastasis (*dashed arrow*) that was confirmed histologically. As the pleural metastasis occurred within the 2-year follow-up, both PET/CT and PET/MR imaging were considered as false negative. In this study, criteria for progression were an increase in lesion size during follow-up or the appearance of new lesions within 2 years. A greater than 2-year follow-up period was chosen as distant metastases/second primary cancers may be subclinical at initial imaging, and depending on tumor kinetics and patient immune status, they may show only minimal changes over time. (*Reproduced from* Katirtzidou et al.[24])

thus leading to a more accurate representation of the biological tumor volume.[30,86]

Against this background, the focus of attention has recently shifted toward multimodality PET/MR imaging or PET/CT/MR imaging-guided estimation of GTV.[79,87] Nevertheless, published data on this topic are very scarce. Moreover, most studies are based on small series without histopathologic correlation and GTVs defined on planning CT or on morphologic MR images were used as standard of reference (ground truth). In a prospective study including 11 patients with HNSCC, Wang and colleagues compared primary and nodal GTVs delineated on CT (ground truth) with the corresponding GTVs delineated on PET/MR imaging; the investigators found that PET/MR imaging- and CT-derived GTVs were similar. However, the Dice similarity coefficient (DSC), a metric evaluating the spatial overlap between two

measured volumes, was only 0.63 to 0.69 (DSC range = 0–1, with 1 indicating perfect match), and the modified Hausdorff distance (ie, the orthogonal distance difference between CT and PET/MR imaging segmentation) was 1.6 to 2.3 mm.[88] Samolyk-Kogaczewska and colleagues evaluated the usefulness and accuracy of PET/MR imaging GTV delineation by radiation oncologists in 10 patients with SCC of the tongue.[89] The GTVs for primary tumors and lymph nodes defined on CT (ground truth) were compared with the GTVs delineated on PET/MR imaging. The investigators found that in 7/10 patients, the volumes were smaller on PET/MR imaging than on CT. The investigators also analyzed which SUV_{max} threshold best matched the ground truth, and they reported best results for 30% SUV_{max} for tumors and 30%–40% SUV_{max} for lymph nodes, respectively.[89] Bird and colleagues found significant

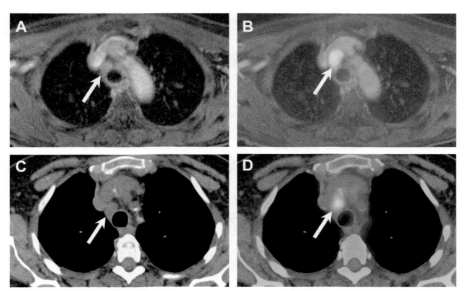

Fig. 12. False-positive PET/MR imaging (*A,B*) and PET/CT (*C,D*) in a 63-year old woman imaged for follow-up of an SCC of the larynx (T3N1) treated with radiochemotherapy. Both PET/MR imaging and PET/CT were rated as positive for distant mediastinal lymph node metastases. An enlarged mediastinal lymph node (*arrows*) shows a combination of high focal FDG uptake (SUVmax on PET/MR imaging = 7.5 and SUVmax on PET/CT = 6.7) and slightly heterogeneous contrast enhancement on the contrast-enhanced fat-saturated MR image. On the corresponding CT image, due to the absence of contrast enhancement, only lymph node enlargement was present (13 × 15 × 17 mm). The lymph node was rated with a score of 5 (highly suspicious) on PET/MR imaging and a score of 4 (moderately suspicious) on PET/CT. However, mediastinoscopy with biopsy-revealed sarcoidosis. (*Reproduced from* Katirtzidou et al.[24])

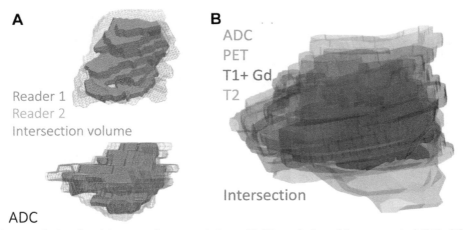

Fig. 13. The complexity of multiparametric segmentation with 3D rendering of the segmented GTVs. (*A*) Segmentation of an oropharyngeal SCC based on the ADC map. Two different readers (a radiation oncologist and a specialized head and neck radiologist) segmented the tumor. The intersection volume is indicated in blue. (*B*) Segmentation of the same oropharyngeal SCC by one reader based on a multiparametric PET/MR imaging acquisition (ADC, PET, contrast-enhanced T1 and T2 images). The intersection volume is rendered in dark red. Note that there is neither a perfect overlap between the GTVs contoured on the different modalities nor between the two readers.

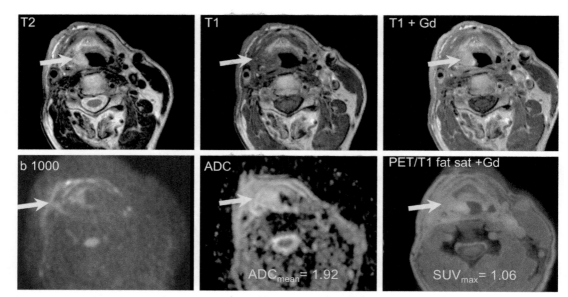

Fig. 14. Posttreatment inflammatory edema in a patient with radiochemotherapy and neck dissection for an SCC of the oral cavity. Note a poorly delineated area with high signal intensity on T2, major contrast enhancement, no restriction of diffusion and no relevant FDG uptake (*yellow arrows*).

differences in mean GTVs between CT, MR imaging, PET, and combinations thereof in 11 patients with locally advanced oropharyngeal SCC with no single imaging technique encompassing all potential GTV regions.[90] The investigators also found that the use of MR imaging reduced interobserver variability.

In the only study published so far using histopathology of the resected specimen as ground truth and GTV contoured on a modern PET/MR imaging hybrid system, Terzidis and colleagues compared the pathologic GTVs obtained from 13 surgical HNSCC specimens (GTV$_{patho}$) with the corresponding CTVs delineated on PET/MR imaging in

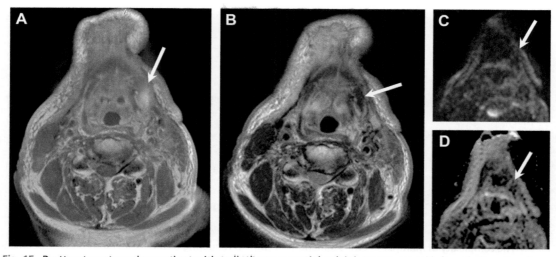

Fig. 15. Posttreatment scar in a patient with radiotherapy, partial pelviglossectomy and left neck dissection for an SCC of the oral cavity. Images obtained from a PET/DWIMR imaging examination. (*A*) Fused PET with contrast-enhanced T1W image (*arrow*). (*B*) Corresponding T2W image. (*C*) b 1000 image. (*D*) ADC map. Note an area of focal uptake on the fused PET and contrast-enhanced T1W image. SUV$_{max}$ = 9. The T2W image shows an area with very low signal intensity (*arrow*) corresponding to mature scar tissue. On DWI, a T2 black-out effect (*arrows*) is seen resulting in a low ADC value (ADC = 0.93 × 10–3 mm^2/s).

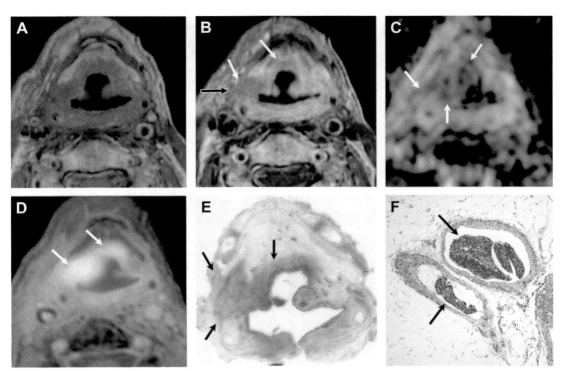

Fig. 16. True positive evaluation with combined PET/DWIMR imaging (positive concordant findings on MR imaging, DWI, and PET). A 69-year-old man with pain 4 years after radiochemotherapy for SCC of the hypopharynx. Unenhanced T1 (*A*): poorly defined hypointensity in both aryepiglottic folds, pre-epiglottic space, and retropharyngeal space. Contrast-enhanced T1 (*B*): infiltrative, moderately enhancing lesion (*white arrows*) in the right paraglottic and pre-epiglottic space with invasion into the soft tissues of the neck (*black arrow*) suggesting recurrence. Note strongly enhancing retropharyngeal space and left aryepiglottic fold due to inflammatory edema. (*C*) ADC map: restricted diffusion on the right (*arrows*, ADCmean = 0.997×10^{-3} mm^2/s) consistent with recurrence. High signal in the left paraglottic space and retropharyngeal space (ADCmean = 1.815×10^{-3} mm^2/s) due to inflammatory edema. (*D*) PET/MR imaging (PET fused with gadolinium-enhanced Dixon) consistent with recurrence (*arrows*, SUVmean = 4.417; SUVmax = 5.518). (*E*) Corresponding whole-organ axial histologic section (hematoxylin-eosin, HE) confirms recurrence on the right (*arrows*) and inflammatory edema on the left and in the retropharyngeal space. (*F*) Section from right specimen periphery (HE, original magnification 100 ×) depicts venous tumor thrombi (*arrows*). T stage on PET/DWIMR imaging was T4a. Pathologic stage was pT4a. (*Reproduced from* Becker et al 2018.[6])

combination with clinical information (GTV$_{oncologic}$).[80] The mean tumor volume defined by PET/MR imaging and clinical information (GTV$_{oncologic}$) was larger than the tumor volume defined at histopathology. The mean mismatch between the GTV$_{patho}$ and the GTV$_{oncologic}$ (ie, the percentage of GTV$_{patho}$ not encompassed in the GTV$_{oncologic}$) was 27.9% and in 12/13 patients GTV$_{patho}$ was not fully encompassed in the GTV$_{oncologic}$. Nevertheless, an isotropic 5 mm expansion to GTV$_{oncologic}$ was sufficient to cover the GTV$_{patho}$.[80] The investigators concluded that despite modern PET/MR imaging technology, a mismatch between imaging and GTV$_{patho}$ was observed in all patients.[80] They also pointed out that reducing margins by even 1 mm may increase the proportion of tumor outside the radiotherapy

target volume, which could explain recurrences at the periphery of GTVs delineated for radiotherapy treatment planning.[80]

In routine clinical work, GTVs and CTVs are contoured manually by radiation oncologists. However, this time-consuming task suffers from subjectivity, interobserver variability, and other factors affecting human expertise. For example, recent publications have shown that the review of oncologist-delineated radiotherapy target volumes by specialized HN radiologists changes 52%–55% of volumes delineated on CT or MR imaging.[91,92] Moreover, Adjogatse and colleagues reported that MR imaging-based peer review by specialized HN radiologists altered 76% of GTVs and 41.5% of gross nodal volumes with 55% of GTV and 67% of gross nodal volume alterations classified as

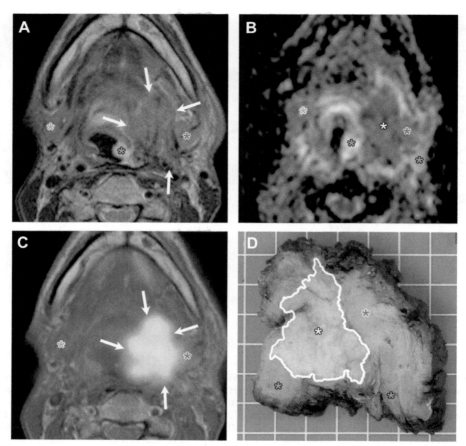

Fig. 17. True positive evaluation with combined PET/DWIMR imaging (positive concordant findings on MR imaging, DWI, and PET). A 48-year-old man with reflex otalgia 1 year after radiochemotherapy for SCC of the base of the tongue. Endoscopy: edema and intact mucosa. T2 (*A*) infiltrative tumor recurrence with intermediate signal (*arrows*) in the left tongue base, extrinsic tongue muscles, vallecula, and parapharyngeal space. Suspected invasion of the left submandibular gland (*pink asterisk*). Submucosal edema with very high T2 signal (*green asterisk*). Normal right submandibular gland (*blue asterisk*). ADC map (*B*) restricted diffusion suggesting recurrence (*white asterisk*, ADCmean = 1.127 $\times$ 10^{-3} mm^2/s). High ADC signal surrounding the tumor (*green asterisks*, ADC-mean = 1.789–1.965 $\times$ 10^{-3} mm^2/s) due to edema. Left and right submandibular glands (*pink and blue asterisks*). (*C*) PET/MR imaging (PET fused with T1) suggests recurrence (increased FDG uptake, *arrows*, SUVmean = 7.688; SUVmax = 12.11). Left and right submandibular glands (*pink and blue asterisks*). (*D*) Whole-organ axial section from surgical specimen (same orientation) confirms recurrence (*white asterisk*) invading the above-described structures. Submandibular gland (*pink asterisk*). Tumor margins contoured by pathologist (*white line*). Green asterisks: *inflammatory edema*. T-stage on PET/DWIMR imaging was T4a. Pathologic stage was pT4a. (*Reproduced from* Becker et al 2018.[6])

"major." Undercontouring of soft tissue involvement and unidentified lymph nodes were main reasons for change.[81] Therefore, some institutions have already introduced a formal MR imaging-based radiology review of oncologist-delineated target volumes into the radiotherapy workflow for patients with HNSCC.[81]

As we can see from these different studies, manual tumor segmentation has inherent drawbacks related not only to factors affecting human expertise but also because of lacking availability of specialized manpower for peer review of contoured GTVs. Therefore, advanced computational approaches such as DL models hold promise to standardize and fully automatize tumor segmentation and to improve consistency and accuracy in target definition for radiotherapy.[93] As the development of DL models requires very large data sets, which usually cannot be obtained in a single center and as data acquired in a single center may be too homogeneous, therefore impeding generalizability, current DL approaches for HNSCC segmentation are based on centralized or on federated frameworks, which incorporate data from many different

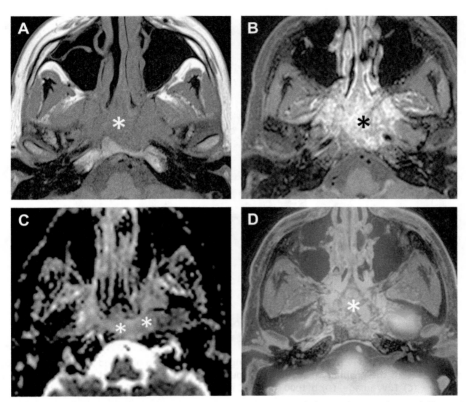

Fig. 18. PET/MR imaging obtained 6 months after proton therapy and chemotherapy for undifferentiated sino-nasal carcinoma. Recurrence in the nasopharynx was suspected clinically. (A) Axial T1W image shows a large hy-pointense nasopharyngeal mass (asterisk). (B) Corresponding fat-saturated gadolinium-enhanced T1W shows that the nasopharyngeal mass (asterisk) invades the clivus and central skull base, suggesting recurrence versus radiation-induced inflammation. (C) ADC map reveals restricted diffusivity (ADC$_{mean}$, 0.98 × 10–3 mm^2/s) suggest-ing recurrence (asterisks). (D) Corresponding fused PET and gadolinium-enhanced fat-saturated T1 reveal absent FDG uptake (asterisk) suggesting inflammation. Surgical biopsy and follow-up greater than 3 years revealed in-flammatory tissue. (Images B, C, and D reproduced from Becker et al 2014.[1])

centers.[82,94–96] In the centralized framework, the centers send their data to a central server with sig-nificant computational power, whereas in the federated framework, the users train DL models locally and then send the data to a central server; the central server then aggregates the local up-dates into a global network. The decentralized federated framework has the advantage of addressing privacy concerns as well as ethical and legal issues.[97] Based on PET images only, Shiri and colleagues have shown that the performance of DL approaches for the segmentation of HNSCC is nearly identical for the centralized and federated approach, both approaches having a DSC of 0.84 and a negligible percent relative error for SUV$_{max}$ compared with manual specialist tumor segmenta-tion. In addition, PET/CT information fusion has been shown to outperform segmentation tasks based on PET only and CT only images, conven-tional image level, and DL fusions achieving

competitive results.[96] Future challenges for DL-based segmentation of HNSCC include segmenta-tion tasks based on multimodality PET/DWI/MR imaging information (Fig. 13).

EVALUATION OF TREATMENT RESPONSE AND DETECTION OF RECURRENT DISEASE

Recurrence in HNSCC is relatively common and depends on patient age, tumor subsite and stage, histologic differentiation, and treatment type. Most recurrences occur at the site of the primary tumor within 2 to 3 years after treatment. Irrespective of tumor type, early detection of recurrent disease is crucial. However, endoscopic and clinical follow-up may miss recurrent disease, especially after radiotherapy due to radiation-induced changes (edema, fibrosis, soft tissue, cartilage, or bone necrosis).

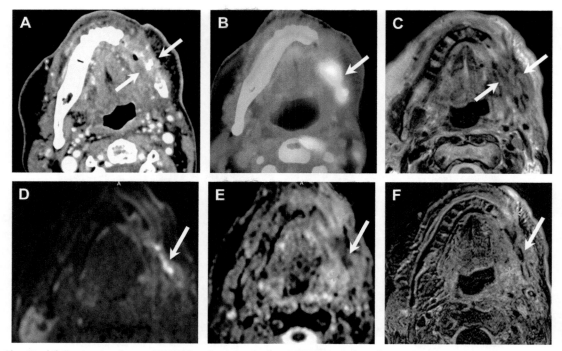

Fig. 19. (*A*) Contrast-enhanced PET/CT and corresponding DWIMR imaging obtained in a 70-year-old patient with radiotherapy for SCC of the oropharynx 3 years previously. (*A*) Contrast-enhanced CT. (*B*) Fused PET and unenhanced CT image. (*C*) T2W image. (*D*) b 1000. (*E*) ADC map. (*F*) Subtraction image (T1W image was subtracted from the contrast-enhanced T1W image). On CT, an enhancing lesion (*arrows*) surrounding the fragmented horizontal branch of mandible is seen on the left. Strong FDG uptake (SUV$_{max}$, 16). On PET/CT, it is difficult to distinguish between osteoradionecrosis and recurrent SCC or a combination of both entities. There is an intermediate signal intensity on T2 within the mandible and in the soft tissues surrounding the mandible (*arrows*). On DWI, there is restriction of diffusivity (*arrows*) within the mandible but the area with restricted diffusivity does not show enhancement on F (*arrow*). This aspect strongly suggests osteoradionecrosis of the mandible. The soft tissues surrounding the mandible have an increased diffusivity and strong enhancement (*green asterisks on E and F*). They correspond to inflammation. The patient underwent hyperbaric oxygen therapy and 1 year later, there is still no evidence of recurrent SCC.

Studies evaluating the diagnostic performance of PET and PET/CT for the follow-up of HNSCC found that the sensitivity and NPV of PET and PET/CT for detecting residual/recurrent HNSCC at the primary site were very high, however—due to posttreatment inflammatory changes—the specificity and PPV were limited—especially on the baseline scan at 12 weeks after radiotherapy.[98–100] Several investigators have reported a high sensitivity and specificity with DWIMR imaging to detect posttreatment HNSCC recurrence; however, the PPV and NPV varied significantly among the different studies.[101–103] These discrepant DWIMR imaging results can be explained by the fact that different MR imaging criteria and different DWI protocols with different combinations of b values were used. As recently shown, different combinations of b values have a direct impact on ADC values and even on the ability of DWI to distinguish between HPV-positive and HPV-negative HNSCC.[104,105] Nevertheless, the

combination of precise morphologic MR imaging criteria with DWI and PET characteristics enables reliable distinction between edema, fibrosis, and recurrent/residual HNSCC on PET/DWIMR imaging.[6] Inflammatory edema can have a variable FDG uptake on PET images and variable contrast enhancement on MR imaging. On T2W images, poorly delineated areas with a high signal intensity are seen, and on DWI, there is no restricted diffusivity; therefore, ADC values are high (T2 shine through effect)[6,103,106] (**Fig. 14**). Fibrosis can display variable FDG uptake and variable contrast enhancement; however, a very low signal intensity on T2W images and a low ADC.[13,103] Because late fibrosis is mainly composed of densely packed collagen, ADCs tend to be low because of the T2 blackout effect (**Fig. 15**). Finally, recurrent HNSCC typically displays a strong FDG uptake, moderate contrast enhancement, an intermediate signal intensity on T2W images and restricted diffusivity[6] (**Figs. 16** and **17**). By combining these criteria, we reported a high diagnostic performance with PET/DWIMR imaging for the detection of recurrent/residual disease after radiotherapy in a prospective study including 74 patients.[6] The standard of reference was histopathology of the resected specimen in 62% and a mean follow-up of 34 months in 38% of patients. Sensitivity, specificity, PPV, and NPV of PET/DWIMR imaging were 97%, 92%, 92.5%, and 97% per patient and 93.0%, 93.5%, 91%, and 95% per lesion, respectively. Agreement between imaging-based and pathologic T stage of resected tumors was excellent (kappa = 0.84, $P < .001$).

The interpretation of multiparametric data is challenging, especially if morphologic MR imaging, DWI, and PET findings are discrepant. On the one hand, this diagnostic uncertainty can lead to unnecessary biopsy in irradiated tissues; on the other hand, it can lead to delay in diagnosis if a "wait and see" policy is adopted. Our study may show a way to manage concordant/discordant readings as positive concordant results with PET, DWI, and MR imaging corresponded to recurrent tumors in 97.5% of cases and discordant results corresponded to benign lesions in 87% of cases, respectively[6] (Fig. 18). This approach could also be applied in indeterminate/suspicious FDG-PET/CT readings in which case a high ADC revealed by DWIMR imaging or the typical aspect of fibrosis on T2W and DWI images would lead to a wait and see policy instead of biopsy (Fig. 19). Moreover, based on a series of 69 HNSCC posttreatment patients, Ashour and colleagues have recently reported that the addition of DWI features and T2 signal to the American College of Radiology (ACR) Neck Imaging Reporting and Data System (NI-RADS) criteria for the primary tumor site enhanced specificity, sensitivity, PPV, NPV, and NI-RADS accuracy.[107]

Applying the NI-RADS criteria[16] to PET/MR imaging in a retrospective study including 46 patients, Patel and colleagues reported that PET/MR imaging scores showed a strong association with treatment failure for the primary site, neck lymph nodes, and combined sites, and the AUCs of PET/MR imaging scores versus treatment failure were 0.864 to 0.987, $P < .001$.[108] The investigators, therefore, concluded that PET/MR imaging has an excellent discriminatory performance for treatment outcomes of HNSCC when NI-RADS is applied.

An increasing number of studies using PET, DWI, DCE perfusion, and MR imaging parameters have recently investigated which imaging-based biomarkers could predict disease-free survival and overall survival in HNSCC patients.[109–112] A detailed discussion is beyond the scope of this article. Nevertheless, the published results suggest that models based on combined imaging biomarkers and clinical characteristics (eg, plasma EBV or HPV status) are very promising and may aid in planning the optimal personalized treatment strategy.

SUMMARY

Although the published research regarding the use of PET/MR imaging in HNSCC is relatively sparse, it seems that PET/MR imaging has at least a similar diagnostic performance as PET/CT for locoregional tumor staging with advantages in certain scenarios. Such scenarios include the assessment of tumor invasion in anatomic areas, which affect resectability, for example, the prevertebral space or PNS. As in most publications, the MR imaging part of PET/MR imaging has been mainly used for anatomic orientation, the full potential of PET/MR imaging has not been used, and only very few studies have incorporated multiparametric information so far. Nevertheless, multiparametric FDG PET/MR imaging with DWI has been shown to have a high diagnostic accuracy for the detection of residual/recurrent HNSCC after radiotherapy with an excellent agreement between imaging-based and pathologic T stage. FDG PET/MR imaging also has an excellent and similar diagnostic performance as FDG PET/CT for detecting distant metastases and distant second primary cancers in HNSCC patients. Imaging biomarkers derived from multiparametric PET/MR imaging with diffusion and perfusion sequences hold promise in predicting patient outcome and, therefore, in planning the optimal personalized treatment strategy. DL-based automatic tumor segmentation using PET data has become a reality, and PET/MR imaging may facilitate DL-based segmentation tasks incorporating multimodality information.

CLINICS CARE POINTS

- Both primary and recurrent head and neck squamous cell carcinoma (HNSCC) have characteristic PET/diffusion-weighted imaging (DWI) MR imaging features, which include the following: an intermediate signal intensity on T1W, T2W, or fat-saturated T2W sequences, and moderate enhancement after IV administration of contrast material; restricted diffusivity with apparent diffusion coefficient (ADC) values less than 1.2 to 1.3 × 10 to 3 mm²/s; increased FDG uptake with SUVmax values most often greater than 3.

- MR imaging reliably detects perineural spread (PNS). Findings on MR imaging scans include thickening, nodularity, nerve enhancement and fat pad obliteration, and denervation of muscles. PNS can be detected on FDG PET if tumors are FDG avid or in the presence of extensive PNS; nevertheless, correlation with MR imaging improves its assessment.

- The combination of morphologic MR imaging, DWI, and PET criteria allows improved detection of posttreatment recurrent HNSCC and distinction from inflammatory edema and fibrosis. Inflammatory edema can have variable FDG uptake and variable enhancement after IV administration of contrast material. On T2W images, inflammatory edema has a high signal intensity, and diffusivity is increased on DWI; therefore, ADC values are high. Fibrosis (scar tissue) can display variable FDG uptake and variable enhancement after IV administration of contrast material. Fibrosis has a very low signal intensity on T2W images and a low ADC.

- In HNSCC, both PET/MR imaging and PET/CT have a similar diagnostic performance for the detection of distant metastases and distant second primary cancers. Both benign and malignant lesions can show FDG uptake; however, SUVmean and SUVmax values are significantly higher in malignant lesions. As high FDG uptake can also cause false positive assessments, especially in the mediastinum, biopsy is necessary in certain situations.

DISCLOSURE

This review was part of a clinical research project funded by the Swiss National Science Foundation (SNSF) under grants No 320030_173091/1 and 320030_176052.

REFERENCES

1. Becker M, Zaidi H. Imaging in head and neck squamous cell carcinoma: the potential role of PET/MRI. Br J Radiol 2014;87(1036):20130677.
2. Zaidi H, Becker M. The promise of hybrid PET/MRI: Technical advances and clinical applications. IEEE Signal Proc Mag 2016;33(3):67–85.
3. Bülbül HM, Bülbül O, Sarıoğlu S, et al. Relationships Between DCE-MRI, DWI, and ^{18}F-FDG PET/CT Parameters with Tumor Grade and Stage in Patients with Head and Neck Squamous Cell Carcinoma. Mol Imaging Radionucl Ther 2021;30(3):177–86.
4. Zhang L, Song T, Meng Z, et al. Correlation between apparent diffusion coefficients and metabolic parameters in hypopharyngeal squamous cell carcinoma: A prospective study with integrated PET/MRI. Eur J Radiol 2020;129:109070.
5. Chan SC, Yeh CH, Ng SH, et al. Prospective Investigation of ^{18}FDG-PET/MRI with Intravoxel Incoherent Motion Diffusion-Weighted Imaging to Assess Survival in Patients with Oropharyngeal or Hypopharyngeal Carcinoma. Cancers 2022;14(24):6104.
6. Becker M, Varoquaux AD, Combescure C, et al. Local recurrence of squamous cell carcinoma of the head and neck after radio(chemo)therapy: Diagnostic performance of FDG-PET/MRI with diffusion-weighted sequences. Eur Radiol 2018; 28(2):651–63.
7. Varoquaux A, Rager O, Dulguerov P, et al. Diffusion-weighted and PET/MR Imaging after Radiation Therapy for Malignant Head and Neck Tumors. Radiographics 2015;35(5):1502–27.
8. Purohit BS, Ailianou A, Dulguerov N, et al. FDG-PET/CT pitfalls in oncological head and neck imaging. Insights Imaging 2014;5(5):585–602.
9. Albertson M, Chandra S, Sayed Z, et al. PET/CT Evaluation of Head and Neck Cancer of Unknown Primary. Semin Ultrasound CT MR 2019;40(5):414–23.
10. Noij DP, Martens RM, Zwezerijnen B, et al. Diagnostic value of diffusion-weighted imaging and ^{18}F-FDG-PET/CT for the detection of unknown primary head and neck cancer in patients presenting with cervical metastasis. Eur J Radiol 2018;107:20–5.
11. Johnson DE, Burtness B, Leemans CR, et al. Head and neck squamous cell carcinoma. Nat Rev Dis Primers 2020;6:92.
12. Pisani P, Airoldi M, Allais A, et al. Metastatic disease in head & neck oncology. Acta Otorhinolaryngol Ital 2020;40(SUPPL. 1):S1–86.
13. Becker M, De Vito C, Monnier Y. Imaging of laryngeal and hypopharyngeal cancer. Magn Reson Imag Clin N Am 2022;30(Issue 1):53–72.
14. Ng SP, Pollard C 3rd, Berends J, et al. Usefulness of surveillance imaging in patients with head and neck cancer who are treated with definitive radiotherapy. Cancer 2019;125(11):1823–9.
15. Galgano SJ, Marshall RV, Middlebrooks EH, et al. PET/MR Imaging in Head and Neck Cancer: Current Applications and Future Directions. Magn Reson Imaging Clin N Am 2018;26(1):167–78.
16. Mukherjee S, Fischbein NJ, Baugnon KL, et al. Contemporary Imaging and Reporting Strategies for Head and Neck Cancer: MRI, FDG PET/MRI, NI-RADS, and Carcinoma of Unknown Primary-AJR Expert Panel Narrative Review. AJR Am J Roentgenol 2023;220(2):160–72.
17. Eiber M, Souvatzoglou M, Pickhard A, et al. Simulation of a MR-PET protocol for staging of head-and-neck cancer including Dixon MR for attenuation correction. Eur J Radiol 2012;81:2658–65.
18. Vargas MI, Becker M, Garibotto V, et al. Approaches for the optimization of MR protocols in

clinical hybrid PET/MRI studies. Magma 2013;26: 57–69.

19. Varoquaux A, Rager O, Poncet A, et al. Detection and quantification of focal uptake in head and neck tumours: (18)F-FDG PET/MR versus PET/CT. Eur J Nucl Med Mol Imaging 2014;41(3):462–75.

20. von Schulthess GK, Kuhn FP, Kaufmann P, et al. Clinical positron emission tomography/magnetic resonance imaging applications. Semin Nucl Med 2013;43(1):3–10.

21. Queiroz MA, Huellner MW. PET/MR in cancers of the head and neck. Semin Nucl Med 2015;45(3): 248–65.

22. Platzek I. 18)F-Fluorodeoxyglucose PET/MR Imaging in Head and Neck Cancer. Pet Clin 2016; 11(4):375–86.

23. Huellner MW. PET/MR in Head and Neck Cancer - An Update. Semin Nucl Med 2021 Jan;51(1): 26–38.

24. Katirtzidou E, Rager O, Varoquaux AD, et al. Detection of distant metastases and distant second primary cancers in head and neck squamous cell carcinoma: comparison of [18F]FDG PET/MRI and [18F]FDG PET/CT. Insights Imaging 2022 Jul 28; 13(1):121.

25. Seifert R, Kersting D, Rischpler C, et al. Clinical Use of PET/MR in Oncology: An Update. Semin Nucl Med 2022 May;52(3):356–64.

26. Drzezga A, Souvatzoglou M, Eiber M, et al. First clinical experience with integrated whole-body PET/MR: comparison to PET/CT in patients with oncologic diagnoses. J Nucl Med 2012 Jun;53(6): 845–55.

27. Wiesmüller M, Quick HH, Navalpakkam B, et al. Comparison of lesion detection and quantitation of tracer uptake between PET from a simultaneously acquiring whole-body PET/MR hybrid scanner and PET from PET/CT. Eur J Nucl Med Mol Imaging 2013 Jan;40(1):12–21.

28. Bini J, Izquierdo-Garcia D, Mateo J, et al. Preclinical evaluation of MR attenuation correction versus CT attenuation correction on a sequential whole-body MR/PET scanner. Invest Radiol 2013 May; 48(5):313–22.

29. Arabi H, Rager O, Alem A, et al. Clinical assessment of MR-guided 3-class and 4-class attenuation correction in PET/MR. Mol Imaging Biol 2015;17(2): 264–76.

30. Varoquaux A, Rager O, Lovblad KO, et al. Functional imaging of head and neck squamous cell carcinoma with diffusion-weighted MRI and FDG PET/CT: quantitative analysis of ADC and SUV. Eur J Nucl Med Mol Imaging 2013 Jun;40(6): 842–52.

31. Freihat O, Zoltán T, Pinter T, et al. Correlation between Tissue Cellularity and Metabolism Represented by Diffusion-Weighted Imaging (DWI) and

18F-FDG PET/MRI in Head and Neck Cancer (HNC). Cancers 2022 Feb 8;14(3):847.

32. Fruehwald-Pallamar J, Czerny C, Mayerhoefer ME, et al. Functional imaging in head and neck squamous cell carcinoma: Correlation of PET/CT and diffusion-weighted imaging at 3 Tesla. Eur J Pediatr 2011;38:1009–19.

33. Min M, Lee MT, Lin P, et al. Assessment of serial multi-parametric functional MRI (diffusion-weighted imaging and R2*) with18F-FDG-PET in patients with head and neck cancer treated with radiation therapy. Br J Radiol 2016;89:20150530.

34. Rasmussen JH, Nørgaard M, Hansen AE, et al. Feasibility of Multiparametric Imaging with PET/MR in Head and Neck Squamous Cell Carcinoma. J Nucl Med 2017;58:69–74.

35. Covello M, Cavaliere C, Aiello M, et al. Simultaneous PET/MR head–neck cancer imaging: Preliminary clinical experience and multiparametric evaluation. Eur J Radiol 2015;84:1269–76.

36. Cheng Y, Bai L, Shang J, et al. Preliminary clinical results for PET/MR compared with PET/CT in patients with nasopharyngeal carcinoma. Oncol Rep 2020;43(1):177–87.

37. Nakajo M, Nakajo M, Kajiya Y, et al. FDG PET/CT and diffusion-weighted imaging of head and neck squamous cell carcinoma: Comparison of prognostic significance between primary tumour standardized uptake value and apparent diffusion coefficient. Clin Nucl Med 2012;37:475–80.

38. Han M, Kim SY, Lee SJ, et al. The Correlations Between MRI Perfusion, Diffusion Parameters, and 18F-FDG PET Metabolic Parameters in Primary Head-and-Neck Cancer. Medicine 2015;94:e2141.

39. Schaarschmidt BM, Heusch P, Buchbender C, et al. Locoregional tumour evaluation of squamous cell carcinoma in the head and neck area: a comparison between MRI, PET/CT and integrated PET/MRI. Eur J Nucl Med Mol Imaging 2016; 43(1):92–102.

40. Huang C, Song T, Mukherji SK, et al. Comparative Study Between Integrated Positron Emission Tomography/Magnetic Resonance and Positron Emission Tomography/Computed Tomography in the T and N Staging of Hypopharyngeal Cancer: An Initial Result. J Comput Assist Tomogr 2020; 44(4):540–5.

41. Sekine T a, de Galiza Barbosa F, Kuhn FP, et al. PET+MR versus PET/CT in the initial staging of head and neck cancer, using a trimodality PET/CT+MR system. Clin Imaging 2017;42:232–9.

42. Samolyk-Kogaczewska N, Sierko E, Dziemianczyk-Pakiela D, et al. Usefulness of Hybrid PET/MRI in Clinical Evaluation of Head and Neck Cancer Patients. Cancers 2020;12(2):511.

43. Flygare L, Erdogan ST, Söderkvist K. PET/MR versus PET/CT for locoregional staging of oropharyngeal

squamous cell cancer. Acta Radiol 2023;64(5): 1865–72.

44. Chan SC, Yeh CH, Yen TC, et al. Clinical utility of simultaneous whole-body ^{18}F-FDG PET/MRI as a single-step imaging modality in the staging of primary nasopharyngeal carcinoma. Eur J Nucl Med Mol Imaging 2018;45(8):1297–308.

45. Kuhn FP, Hüllner M, Mader CE, et al. Contrast-enhanced PET/MR imaging versus contrast-enhanced PET/CT in head and neck cancer: how much MR information is needed? J Nucl Med 2014;55(4):551–8.

46. Meerwein CM, Pizzuto DA, Vital D, et al. Use of MRI and FDG-PET/CT to predict fixation of advanced hypopharyngeal squamous cell carcinoma to prevertebral space. Head Neck 2019;41(2):503–10.

47. Sekine T b, Barbosa FG, Delso G, et al. Local resectability assessment of head and neck cancer: Positron emission tomography/MRI versus positron emission tomography/CT. Head Neck 2017;39(8): 1550–8.

48. Medvedev O, Hedesiu M, Ciurea A, et al. Perineural spread in head and neck malignancies: imaging findings - an updated literature review. Bosn J Basic Med Sci 2022;22(1):22–38.

49. Lee H, Lazor JW, Assadsangabi R, et al. An Imager's Guide to Perineural Tumor Spread in Head and Neck Cancers: Radiologic Footprints on ^{18}F-FDG PET, with CT and MRI Correlates. J Nucl Med 2019;60(3):304–11.

50. Abdelaziz TT, Abdel Razek AAK. Magnetic Resonance Imaging of Perineural Spread of Head and Neck Cancer. Magn Reson Imaging Clin N Am 2022;30(1):95–108.

51. Cao C, Xu Y, Huang S, et al. Locoregional Extension Patterns of Nasopharyngeal Carcinoma Detected by FDG PET/MR. Front Oncol 2021;11:763114.

52. Nie X, Zhou J, Zeng J, et al. Does PET scan have any role in the diagnosis of perineural spread associated with the head and neck tumors? Adv Clin Exp Med 2022;31(8):827–35.

53. Audet N, Beasley NJ, MacMillan C, et al. Lymphatic vessel density, nodal metastases, and prognosis in patients with head and neck cancer. Arch Otolaryngol Head Neck Surg 2005;131:1065–70.

54. Platzek I, Beuthien-Baumann B, Schneider M, et al. FDG PET/MR for lymph node staging in head and neck cancer. Eur J Radiol 2014;83(7):1163–8.

55. Cebeci S, Aydos U, Yeniceri A, et al. Diagnostic performance of FDG PET/MRI for cervical lymph node metastasis in patients with clinically N0 head and neck cancer. Eur Rev Med Pharmacol Sci 2023;27(10):4528–35.

56. Crimì F, Borsetto D, Stramare R, et al. [^{18}F]FDG PET/MRI versus contrast-enhanced MRI in detecting regional HNSCC metastases. Ann Nucl Med 2021;35(2):260–9.

57. Mundada P, Varoquaux AD, Lenoir V, et al. Utility of MRI with morphologic and diffusion weighted imaging in the detection of post-treatment nodal disease in head and neck squamous cell carcinoma. Eur J Radiol 2018;101:162–9.

58. Vandecaveye V, De Keyzer F, Vander Poorten V, et al. Head and neck squamous cell carcinoma: value of diffusion-weighted MR imaging for nodal staging. Radiology 2009;251(1):134–46.

59. de Bondt RB, Hoeberigs MC, Nelemans PJ, et al. Diagnostic accuracy and additional value of diffusion-weighted imaging for discrimination of malignant cervical lymph nodes in head and neck squamous cell carcinoma. Neuroradiology 2009; 51(3):183–92.

60. Dirix P, Vandecaveye V, De Keyzer F, et al. Diffusion-weighted MRI for nodal staging of head and neck squamous cell carcinoma: impact on radiotherapy planning. Int J Radiat Oncol Biol Phys 2010 Mar 1;76(3):761–6.

61. Driessen JP, van Kempen PM, van der Heijden GJ, et al. Diffusion-weighted imaging in head and neck squamous cell carcinomas: a systematic review. Head Neck 2015;37(3):440–8.

62. Belfiore MP, Gallo L, Reginelli A, et al. Quantitative Evaluation of the Lymph Node Metastases in the Head and Neck Malignancies Using Diffusion-Weighted Imaging and Apparent Diffusion Coefficient Mapping: A Bicentric Study. Magnetochemistry 2023;9(5):124.

63. Chen J, Hagiwara M, Givi B, et al. Assessment of metastatic lymph nodes in head and neck squamous cell carcinomas using simultaneous ^{18}F-FDG-PET and MRI. Sci Rep 2020;10(1):20764.

64. Freihat O, Pinter T, Kedves A, et al. Diffusion-Weighted Imaging (DWI) derived from PET/MRI for lymph node assessment in patients with Head and Neck Squamous Cell Carcinoma (HNSCC). Cancer Imag 2020;20(1):56.

65. Gao S, Li S, Yang X, et al. 18FDG PET-CT for distant metastases in patients with recurrent head and neck cancer after definitive treatment. A meta-analysis. Oral Oncol 2014;50(3):163–7.

66. Yeh CH, Chan SC, Lin CY, et al. Comparison of ^{18}F-FDG PET/MRI, MRI, and ^{18}F-FDG PET/CT for the detection of synchronous cancers and distant metastases in patients with oropharyngeal and hypopharyngeal squamous cell carcinoma. Eur J Nucl Med Mol Imaging 2020;47(1):94–104.

67. de Bree R, Senft A, Coca-Pelaz A, et al. Detection of Distant Metastases in Head and Neck Cancer: Changing Landscape. Adv Ther 2018;35(2): 161–72.

68. Chandarana H, Heacock L, Rakheja R, et al. Pulmonary nodules in patients with primary malignancy: comparison of hybrid PET/MR and PET/CT imaging. Radiology 2013;268(3):874–81.

69. Lee KH, Park CM, Lee SM, et al. Pulmonary Nodule Detection in Patients with a Primary Malignancy Using Hybrid PET/MRI: Is There Value in Adding Contrast-Enhanced MR Imaging? PLoS One 2015;10(6):e0129660.

70. Zhang C, Liang Z, Liu W, et al. Comparison of whole-body 18F-FDG PET/CT and PET/MRI for distant metastases in patients with malignant tumors: a meta-analysis. BMC Cancer 2023;23(1):37.

71. Botsikas D, Bagetakos I, Picarra M, et al. What is the diagnostic performance of 18-FDG-PET/MR compared to PET/CT for the N- and M- staging of breast cancer? Eur Radiol 2019;29(4):1787–98.

72. Schwenzer NF, Schraml C, Müller M, et al. Pulmonary lesion assessment: comparison of whole-body hybrid MR/PET and PET/CT imaging–pilot study. Radiology 2012;264(2):551–8.

73. van Weert S, Hendrickx JJ, Leemans CR. Carcinoma of Unknown Primary: Diagnostics and the Potential of Transoral Surgery. In: Vermorken JB, Budach V, Leemans CR, et al, editors. Critical issues in head and neck oncology. Cham: Springer; 2023.

74. Brierley JD, Gospodarowicz MK, Wittekind C, et al, editors. UICC TNM classification of malignant tumours. 8th edition. Hoboken, New Jersey: Wiley Blackwell: Union for International Cancer Control; 2017.

75. Kalavacherla S, Sanghvi P, Lin GY, et al. Updates in the management of unknown primary of the head and neck. Front Oncol 2022;12:991838.

76. Chen B, Zhang H, Liu D, et al. Diagnostic performance of 18F-FDG PET/CT for the detection of occult primary tumors in squamous cell carcinoma of unknown primary in the head and neck: a single-center retrospective study. Nucl Med Commun 2021;42(5):523–7.

77. Rudmik L, Lau HY, Matthews TW, et al. Clinical utility of PET/CT in the evaluation of head and neck squamous cell carcinoma with an unknown primary: a prospective clinical trial. Head Neck 2011;33:935–40.

78. Ruhlmann V, Ruhlmann M, Bellendorf A, et al. Hybrid imaging for detection of carcinoma of unknown primary: a preliminary comparison trial of whole-body PET/MRI versus PET/CT. Eur J Radiol 2016;85(11):1941–7.

79. Decazes P, Hinault P, Veresezan O, et al. Trimodality PET/CT/MRI and Radiotherapy: A Mini-Review. Front Oncol 2021;10:614008.

80. Terzidis E, Friborg J, Vogelius IR, et al. Tumor volume definitions in head and neck squamous cell carcinoma - Comparing PET/MRI and histopathology. Radiother Oncol 2023;180:109484.

81. Adjogatse D, Petkar I, Reis Ferreira M, et al. The Impact of Interactive MRI-Based Radiologist Review on Radiotherapy Target Volume Delineation in Head and Neck Cancer. AJNR Am J Neuroradiol 2023;44(2):192–8.

82. Shiri I, Vafaei Sadr A, Amini M, et al. Decentralized Distributed Multi-institutional PET Image Segmentation Using a Federated Deep Learning Framework. Clin Nucl Med 2022;47(7):606–17.

83. Arslan S, Abakay CD, Sen F, et al. Role of PET/CT in treatment planning for head and neck cancer patients undergoing definitive radiotherapy. Asian Pac J Cancer Prev 2014;15(24):10899–903.

84. Newbold K, Powell C. PET/CT in Radiotherapy Planning for Head and Neck Cancer. Front Oncol 2012;2:189.

85. Nicolay NH, Wiedenmann N, Mix M, et al. Correlative analyses between tissue-based hypoxia biomarkers and hypoxia PET imaging in head and neck cancer patients during radiochemotherapy-results from a prospective trial. Eur J Nucl Med Mol Imaging 2020;47(5):1046–55.

86. Santos Armentia E, Martín Noguerol T, Suárez Vega V. Advanced magnetic resonance imaging techniques for tumors of the head and neck. Radiologia (Engl Ed) 2019;61(3):191–203.

87. Winter RM, Leibfarth S, Schmidt H, et al. Assessment of image quality of a radiotherapy-specific hardware solution for PET/MRI in head and neck cancer patients. Radiother Oncol 2018;128(3):485–91.

88. Wang K, Mullins BT, Falchook AD, et al. Evaluation of PET/MRI for Tumor Volume Delineation for Head and Neck Cancer. Front Oncol 2017;7:8.

89. Samołyk-Kogaczewska N, Sierko E, Zuzda K, et al. PET/MRI-guided GTV delineation during radiotherapy planning in patients with squamous cell carcinoma of the tongue. Strahlenther Onkol 2019;195(9):780–91.

90. Bird D, Scarsbrook AF, Sykes J, et al. Multimodality imaging with CT, MR and FDG-PET for radiotherapy target volume delineation in oropharyngeal squamous cell carcinoma. BMC Cancer 2015;15:844.

91. Braunstein S, Glastonbury CM, Chen J, et al. Impact of Neuroradiology-Based Peer Review on Head and Neck Radiotherapy Target Delineation. AJNR Am J Neuroradiol 2017 Jan;38(1):146–53.

92. Chiu K, Hoskin P, Gupta A, et al. The quantitative impact of joint peer review with a specialist radiologist in head and neck cancer radiotherapy planning. Br J Radiol 2022;95(1130):20211219.

93. Illimoottil M, Ginat D. Recent Advances in Deep Learning and Medical Imaging for Head and Neck Cancer Treatment: MRI, CT, and PET Scans. Cancers 2023;15(13):3267.

94. Arabi H, Shiri I, Jenabi E, et al. Deep Learning-based Automated Delineation of Head and Neck Malignant Lesions from PET Images. IEEE 2020. https://doi.org/10.1109/NSS/MIC42677.2020.9507977.

95. Shiri I, Arabi H, Sanaat A, et al. Fully Automated Gross Tumor Volume Delineation from PET in Head and Neck Cancer using deep learning algorithms. Clin Nucl Med 2021;46(11):872–83.

96. Shiri I, Amini M, Yousefirizi F, et al. Information fusion for fully automated segmentation of head and neck tumors from PET and CT images. Med Phys 2023. https://doi.org/10.1002/mp.16615.

97. Kaissis GA, Makowski MR, Ruckert D, et al. Secure, privacy-preserving and federated machine learning in medical imaging. Nat Mach Intell 2020; 2:305–11.

98. Sheikhbahaei S, Taghipour M, Ahmad R, et al. Diagnostic Accuracy of Follow-Up FDG PET or PET/CT in Patients With Head and Neck Cancer After Definitive Treatment: A Systematic Review and Meta-Analysis. AJR Am J Roentgenol 2015; 205(3):629–39.

99. Cheung PK, Chin RY, Eslick GD. Detecting Residual/Recurrent Head Neck Squamous Cell Carcinomas Using PET or PET/CT: Systematic Review and Meta-analysis. Otolaryngol Head Neck Surg 2016;154(3):421–32.

100. Gupta T, Master Z, Kannan S, et al. Diagnostic performance of post-treatment FDG PET or FDG PET/CT imaging in head and neck cancer: a systematic review and meta-analysis. Eur J Nucl Med Mol Imaging 2011;38:2083–95.

101. Abdel Razek AA, Kandeel AY, Soliman N, et al. Role of diffusion-weighted echo-planar MR imaging in differentiation of residual or recurrent head and neck tumors and posttreatment changes. AJNR Am J Neuroradiol 2007;28(6):1146–52.

102. Vandecaveye V, De Keyzer F, Nuyts S, et al. Detection of head and neck squamous cell carcinoma with diffusion weighted MRI after (chemo)radiotherapy: correlation between radiologic and histopathologic findings. Int J Radiat Oncol Biol Phys 2007;67(4):960–71.

103. Ailianou A, Mundada P, De Perrot T, et al. MRI with DWI for the Detection of Posttreatment Head and Neck Squamous Cell Carcinoma: Why Morphologic MRI Criteria Matter. AJNR Am J Neuroradiol 2018 Apr;39(4):748–55.

104. Lenoir V, Delattre BMA, M'RaD Y, et al. Diffusion-Weighted Imaging to Assess HPV-Positive versus HPV-Negative Oropharyngeal Squamous Cell Carcinoma: The Importance of b-Values. AJNR Am J Neuroradiol 2022;43(6):905–12.

105. de Perrot T, Lenoir V, Domingo Ayllón M, et al. Apparent Diffusion Coefficient Histograms of Human Papillomavirus-Positive and Human Papillomavirus-Negative Head and Neck Squamous Cell Carcinoma: Assessment of Tumor Heterogeneity and Comparison with Histopathology. AJNR Am J Neuroradiol 2017;38(11):2153–60.

106. King AD, Keung CK, Yu KH, et al. T2-weighted MR imaging early after chemoradiotherapy to evaluate treatment response in head and neck squamous cell carcinoma. AJNR Am J Neuroradiol 2013;34: 1237–41.

107. Ashour MM, Darwish EAF, Fahiem RM, et al. MRI Posttreatment Surveillance for Head and Neck Squamous Cell Carcinoma: Proposed MR NI-RADS Criteria. AJNR Am J Neuroradiol 2021; 42(6):1123–9.

108. Patel LD, Bridgham K, Ciriello J, et al. PET/MR Imaging in Evaluating Treatment Failure of Head and Neck Malignancies: A Neck Imaging Reporting and Data System-Based Study. AJNR Am J Neuroradiol 2022;43(3):435–41.

109. Martens RM, Noij DP, Koopman T, et al. Predictive value of quantitative diffusion-weighted imaging and 18-F-FDG-PET in head and neck squamous cell carcinoma treated by (chemo)radiotherapy. Eur J Radiol 2019;113:39–50.

110. Pace L, Nicolai E, Cavaliere C, et al. Prognostic value of 18F-FDG PET/MRI in patients with advanced oropharyngeal and hypopharyngeal squamous cell carcinoma. Ann Nucl Med 2021 Apr;35(4):479–84.

111. Chan SC, Yeh CH, Chang JT, et al. Combing MRI Perfusion and 18F-FDG PET/CT Metabolic Biomarkers Helps Predict Survival in Advanced Nasopharyngeal Carcinoma: A Prospective Multimodal Imaging Study. Cancers 2021;13(7):1550.

112. Connor S, Sit C, Anjari M, et al. The ability of postchemoradiotherapy DWI ADC$_{mean}$ and 18F-FDG SUV$_{max}$ to predict treatment outcomes in head and neck cancer: impact of human papilloma virus oropharyngeal cancer status. J Cancer Res Clin Oncol 2021;147(8):2323–36.

The Clinical Added Value of Breast Cancer Imaging Using Hybrid PET/MR Imaging

Ismini C. Mainta, MD[a,*], Ilektra Sfakianaki, MD[b], Isaac Shiri, PhD[a],
Diomidis Botsikas, MD[b], Valentina Garibotto, MD[a,c]

KEYWORDS

• PET/MR imaging • Breast cancer • Multiparametric • Correlation

KEY POINTS

- For T stage, dedicated-breast 18F-fluorodeoxyglucose (18F-FDG) PET/MR imaging is superior to whole-body acquisition with the MR imaging component being prominent for the diagnosis.
- For N stage, the high sensitivity of 18F-FDG PET/MR imaging can be combined with the high specificity of axillary ultrasound.
- For M stage, whole-body 18F-FDG PET/MR imaging has high diagnostic performance, with reduced radiation dose compared with 18F-FDG PET/computed tomography (CT).
- PET-metabolic and MR imaging-pharmacokinetic parameters, associated to histopathological characteristics of breast cancer, bear a predictive potential as proven on a research level, which could be further improved through radiomics and artificial intelligence.
- 18F-FDG PET/MR imaging can lead in change in treatment management in 14% to 33% of patients compared with conventional staging with mammography, ultrasound, and MR imaging and in 12% compared with 18F-FDG PET/CT.

INTRODUCTION

Breast cancer is the most commonly diagnosed cancer in women, partly because of the increased detection through widespread adoption of screening protocols, and it remains one of the leading cancer-related causes of death.[1,2] Imaging has a central role in breast cancer from the detection and diagnosis to staging and treatment guidance, with mammography (MMG), ultrasound (US), and MR imaging being the standard for locoregional evaluation. For advanced or stage II breast cancer with higher risk factors (large tumors, nodal involvement, aggressive biology, and clinical or biological suspicion of distant metastases), additional whole-body evaluation with computed tomography (CT) and bone scintigraphy is proposed. PET/CT remains optional in case of equivocal lesions on standard staging and may replace conventional imaging in high-risk patients, according to the current guidelines.[3–5] With the increasing availability of hybrid PET/MR imaging systems nowadays, the lower dose related to the MR imaging coupling of PET instead of the CT, the higher tissue contrast and the functional sequences of MR imaging compared with CT, PET/MR imaging could represent an attractive alternative to PET/CT and conventional imaging altogether for staging purposes.

This review summarizes current evidence on the diagnostic performance of hybrid PET/MR imaging for the assessment of the primary tumor, nodal staging and the detection of distant metastases of breast cancer, as well as treatment response

[a] Department of Nuclear Medicine and Molecular Imaging, Geneva University Hospitals, Rue Gabrielle-Perret-Gentil 4, Geneva 1205, Switzerland; [b] Department of Radiology, Geneva University Hospitals, Rue Gabrielle-Perret-Gentil 4, Geneva 1205, Switzerland; [c] Faculty of Medicine, University of Geneva, Rue Michel Servet 1, Geneva 1211, Switzerland
* Corresponding author.
E-mail address: isminicharis.mainta@hcuge.ch

Magn Reson Imaging Clin N Am 31 (2023) 565–577
https://doi.org/10.1016/j.mric.2023.06.007
1064-9689/23/© 2023 Elsevier Inc. All rights reserved.

assessment and restaging. The correlations between PET/MR imaging parameters and histopathological factors are also briefly summarized, highlighting the role PET/MR imaging could have in the development of potential new biomarkers. Finally, we present the preliminary results of artificial intelligence and radiomics studies, paving the way for new opportunities in the diagnostic and predictive value of hybrid PET/MR imaging.

PROTOCOL

Depending on the camera system, MR imaging and PET acquisitions are simultaneous[6] or sequential,[7] with a clear advantage of the first one concerning mainly the duration of the PET scan and consequently the whole examination. Traditionally, for oncologic purposes, PET scans are acquired in a whole-body manner in the supine position. For breast cancer, an additional dedicated-breast PET/MR imaging acquisition can be acquired in the prone position, including a T2-weighted, diffusion-weighted images (DWI), and dynamic contrast enhancement (DCE) nonfat suppressed T1-weighted sequence (Table 1).

Primary Tumor

For the evaluation of the primary breast lesion, the addition of dedicated-breast PET/MR imaging to the whole-body acquisition improves the detectability and characterization of lesions. In a prospective study of 38 patients by Kirchner and colleagues, dedicated-breast 18-fluorodeoxyglucose (18F-FDG) PET/MR imaging correctly identified 97% of patients with breast cancer compared with 87% for whole-body 18F-FDG PET/MR imaging. All multifocal and multicentric breast cancers were correctly detected by dedicated-breast PET/MR imaging, whereas whole-body 18F-FDG PET/MR imaging missed 2 of 6 multifocal and 1 of 4 multicentric cancers. An interesting point to remember is that tumor size was smaller in the supine position probably due to position-dependent deformation mostly in less solid, necrotic lesions.[6] All 100 lesions in 94 patients were visually detectable on PET and DWI images on dedicated 18F-FDG PET/MR imaging in a retrospective study by Sasaki and colleagues, contrary to whole body imaging, where DWI missed 13% of lesions and PET 7% of lesions.[8] Similarly, Kong and colleagues, in a retrospective study of 42 patients, demonstrated that dedicated PET/MR imaging allows a better analysis of lesions greater than 1 cm compared with whole-body 18F-FDG PET/MR imaging and improves the detectability of smaller breast lesions. The overall sensitivity was 100% for dedicated PET/MR imaging and 87.5% for whole-body PET/MR imaging.[9]

For the definition of the T-stage, dedicated 18F-FDG PET/MR imaging and breast MR imaging perform equally well and are significantly superior compared with clinical evaluation/conventional imaging, including MMG and US[7,10,11] and compared with 18F-FDG PET/CT,[12] with all lesions being detected by the MR imaging component and no additional lesion detected by PET.[7,10,12,13] Nevertheless, even if all index lesions were detected by both MR imaging and PET, in a retrospective analysis of 36 patients by Taneja and colleagues, PET/MR imaging was associated with higher diagnostic confidence. However, PET alone was inferior to dedicated MR imaging and PET/MR imaging for the detection of multifocal/multicentric cancer by identifying 48.9% of satellite lesions seen on MR imaging, probably in relation with the partial volume effect.[13] Grueneisen

Table 1			
Protocol of PET/MR imaging acquisition			
Dedicated Breast PET/MR Imaging			
MR imaging	Magnetic resonance attenuation correction (MRAC)	PET	Simultaneous PET/MR imaging acquisition 8–20 min[6,8,9,12,24]
	T2-weighted		
	DWI		Sequential PET/MR imaging acquisition
	T1W DCE		3 min/bed[7,32]
Whole-body PET/MR imaging			
MR imaging	MRAC	PET	Simultaneous PET/MR imaging acquisition 3–5 min/bed[6,8,9,13,24,42]
	T2-weighted in breath-hold		
	DWI		Sequential PET/MR imaging acquisition
	T1W postcontrast in breath-hold		1.5 min/bed[7,32]

and colleagues, in a prospective study of 49 patients, reported that PET/MR imaging and MR imaging improved the diagnostic performance compared with PET/CT both on patient-level and lesion-level analyses, although the differences were not significant and both had a tendency to overestimate the T stage contrary to PET/CT that tended to underestimate it.[12] In a retrospective analysis of 58 patients, Botsikas and colleagues showed that the area under the curve (AUC) was slightly superior for MR imaging than PET/MR imaging, with a trend toward significance; in the preoperative setting where the negative predictive value (NPV) is of particular interest, MR imaging outperformed 18F-FDG PET and PET/MR imaging.[7] In a prospective study of 40 patients, Goorts and colleagues reported that dedicated PET/MR imaging, due to its MR imaging component found more multifocal cancers than MMG and US and that tumor size was larger on MR imaging (37 mm vs 33 mm for MMG and US).[10] In a prospective study of 82 patients, Hashimoto and colleagues found that US and MR imaging had the highest overall sensitivity (98.8% and 98.6%, respectively) for the detection of primary tumors, compared with 86.9% for whole-body PET/MR imaging, 89.2% for dedicated-breast PET system, and 81.2% for MMG.[14] In a meta-analysis of 7 studies including 536 patients, the pooled sensitivity of 18F-FDG PET/MR imaging for the diagnosis of breast cancer T stage was 91% (95% CI: 84%–96%), the pooled specificity 91% (95% CI: 81%–96%), with an accuracy of 0.96 (95% CI: 0.94–0.98).[15]

Quantification, Correlations, and Prognosis

PET/MR imaging offers the advantage of simultaneous multiparametric imaging combining functional and morphologic parameters derived from both modalities. Tumor metabolism is usually measured as the maximum standardized uptake value by administered activity normalized by body weight (SUV_{max}) and less frequently as the mean or peak value over a given region (SUV_{mean} and SUV_{peak}) and can be normalized by lean body mass (denoted as SUL). Metabolic tumor volume (MTV) and total lesion glycolysis (TLG), which is a combination of the intensity of the activity as measured by the SUV_{mean} and the size of the metabolic tumor, are used as summary index for metabolic activity. The apparent diffusion coefficient (ADC) as a surrogate measure of cellular density represents the restricted water diffusion in the interstitial space in case of tumors with high cellularity. Finally, MR imaging pharmacokinetic parameters derived by the Tofts model allow a more thorough analysis of tumoral perfusion, most commonly through Ktrans and Kep. Due to the complexity of the technique and the need of a longer acquisition to obtain them, their use in clinical practice is limited. However, in a prospective study of 98 patients, Jena and colleagues demonstrated that it is feasible to obtain reliable pharmacokinetic parameters by incorporating a high temporal resolution sequence, 60 seconds short, in the routine DCE MR imaging using the 3T MR imaging of a hybrid PET/MR imaging camera.[16]

Compared with PET/CT, a significant and strong correlation has been demonstrated for PET parameters, such as SUV_{max}, SUV_{mean}, and MTV, between the 2 modalities.[17,18] However, significant differences have been found in quantification. In one study by Pace and colleagues, both SUV_{max} and SUV_{mean} of lesions (primary, nodal, and distant metastases) were significantly higher on PET/MR imaging than on PET/CT, and MTVs were 4% lower on PET/MR imaging than on PET/CT but this difference was not significant.[17] However, Pujara and colleagues showed that PET/MR-derived SUVs were not significantly compared with the PET/CT-derived SUVs in bone and nonaxillary lymph nodes metastases but were significantly lower in liver metastases.[18]

In hybrid PET/MR imaging studies, PET metabolic and MR imaging pharmacokinetic parameters have been found to be positively associated to each other.[19,20] In contrast, correlation was neither revealed between ADC and SUV in 2 studies[8,19] nor revealed between ADC and pharmacokinetic parameters,[19] whereas a significant inverse correlation was found between ADC and SUV in one study.[21] Both PET-metabolic and MR imaging-derived perfusion metrics are reportedly correlated to histopathological characteristics of breast cancer, such as ER, HER2, Ki67, and nuclear grade; whereas for ADC, the results are controversial (Table 2).[8,14,20–24] Furthermore, multivariate models combining different parameters derived from PET/MR imaging (SUV_{max}/ADC_{mean}/Kep_{mean} or $Ktrans_{max}$/SUV_{max}) have shown promising results, on a research level, to correctly predict the molecular phenotype of breast cancer.[22,23]

Nowadays, it is recognized that tumor microenvironment (TME) has an important role on tumor development.[25] One of the main cellular types of TME is tumor-infiltrating lymphocytes (TILs).[26] The presence of TILs has been found to be a positive predictive factor for the 2 most aggressive types of breast cancer, HER2-positive and Triple Negative Breast Cancer (TNBC), because they are associated with higher rates of pathologic complete

Table 2
Correlation of PET/MR imaging-derived and histopathological parameters

	Sasaki et al[8] 2018	Morawitz et al[21] 2021	Hashimoto et al[14] 2022	Jena et al[24] 2017	Catalano et al[22] 2017	Incoronato et al[23] 2018	Jena et al[20] 2017
Type (n°)	R (94 patients)	P (56 patients)	P (82 patients)	R (69 patients)	R (21 patients)	P (50 patients)	R (41 patients)
Parameters analyzed	SUV_{max}, ADC_{mean}	SUV_{max}, SUV_{mean}, ADC_{mean}, ADC_{min}	SUV_{max}	SUV_{max}, SUV_{mean}, TLG	ADC_{mean}, $Ktrans_{mean}$, Kep_{mean}, Ve_{mean}, iAUC, SUV_{max}	ADC_{mean}, $Ktrans_{mean}$, $Ktrans_{max}$, Kep_{mean}, Kep_{max}, Ve_{mean}, iAUC, SUV_{mean}, SUL, MTV, TLG	$Ktrans_{mean}$, Kep_{mean}, Ve_{mean}, iAUC, Ve/iAUC, SUV_{max}, SUV_{mean}, SUV_{peak}, TLG
Parameters presenting significant association on each study							
Estrogen receptors		SUV_{max} ($\rho = -0.45$), SUV_{mean} ($\rho = -0.45$)	SUV_{max}	SUV_{max} ($\rho = -0.397$), SUV_{mean} ($\rho = -0.384$), TLG ($\rho = -0.289$)	SUV_{max}, Kep_{mean}	$Ktrans_{mean}$, $Ktrans_{max}$, Kep_{mean}, Kep_{max}, SUV_{max}, SUV_{mean}, SUL	$Ktrans_{mean}$ ($\rho = -0.318$), SUV_{max} ($\rho = -0.527$), SUV_{mean} ($\rho = -0.492$), SUV_{peak} ($\rho = -0.527$), TLG ($\rho = -0.461$)
Progesterone receptors				SUV_{max} ($\rho = -0.407$), SUV_{mean} ($\rho = -0.392$)		$Ktrans_{max}$, Kep_{mean}, Kep_{max}, ADC_{mean}, SUL (weak)	SUV_{max} ($\rho = -0.494$), SUV_{mean} ($\rho = -0.463$), SUV_{peak} ($\rho = -0.450$)
HER2	SUV_{max}	ADC_{mean} ($\rho = -0.30$), ADC_{min} ($\rho = -0.23$)			SUV_{max}, ADC_{mean}, Kep_{mean}	$Ktrans_{max}$, Kep_{mean}, Kep_{max}	
Ki-67	SUV_{max}	SUV_{max} ($\rho = 0.41$), SUV_{mean} ($\rho = 0.28$)	SUV_{max}	SUV_{max} ($\rho = 0.340$), SUV_{mean} ($\rho = 0.346$), TLG ($\rho = 0.353$)	ADC_{mean} (964 for Ki67 $\leq$ 14% vs 1252 for Ki67 > 14%)	Kep_{max}, SUV_{max}, SUV_{mean}, SUL	

Nuclear grade	SUV$_{max}$, ADC$_{mean}$	SUV$_{max}$ (ρ = 0.30), SUV$_{mean}$ (ρ = 0.28)	SUV$_{max}$	SUV$_{max}$ (ρ = 0.455), SUV$_{mean}$ (ρ = 0.452), TLG (ρ = 0.440)	SUV$_{max}$, Kep$_{mean}$	Kep$_{max}$, ADC$_{mean}$	Ktrans$_{mean}$ (ρ = 0.358), Ve$_{mean}$ (ρ = 0.389), SUV$_{max}$ (ρ = 0.471), SUV$_{mean}$ (ρ = 0.475), SUV$_{peak}$ (ρ = 0.472), TLG (ρ = 0.458)
Tumor size/T stage		SUV$_{max}$		SUV$_{max}$ (ρ = 0.424), SUV$_{mean}$ (ρ = 0.401), TLG (ρ = 0.661)		SUV$_{max}$, SUV$_{mean}$, SUL, MTV, TLG	Ktrans$_{mean}$ (ρ = 0.436), SUV$_{max}$ (ρ = 0.428), SUV$_{mean}$ (ρ = 0.406), SUV$_{peak}$ (ρ = 0.603), TLG (ρ = 0.587)
Molecular subtype		SUV$_{max}$ (ρ = 0.52), SUV$_{mean}$ (ρ = 0.41)		SUV$_{max}$[a,b], SUV$_{mean}$[a,b], TLG[b]		Ktrans$_{max}$[c], Kep$_{max}$[c,d], SUV$_{max}$[c,d], SUV$_{mean}$[c,d], SUL[c,d], ADC$_{mean}$[e]	

Abbreviations: P, prospective; R, retrospective.

[a] HER2 > luminal.
[b] TNBC > luminal.
[c] Nonluminal from luminal A.
[d] Luminal B from luminal A.
[e] Nonluminal from luminal B.

response (pCR) after neoadjuvant chemotherapy.[27] Murakami and colleagues showed that tumors with high or intermediate TILs level had significantly higher median SUV_{max} compared with low TILs tumors (8.36 and 5.03, respectively, $P = .013$) and additionally in the low TILs group, higher SUV_{max} was noted in the presence of peritumoral edema as seen on MR imaging.[28]

Multiparametric PET/MR imaging could shed light in complex phenomena such as tumor hypoxia, a factor of poor prognosis, related to aggressive phenotypes and treatment resistance. Carmona and colleagues found an inverse correlation between tumor hypoxia (hypoxic fractions and Ki) on dynamic 18F-fluoromisonidazole (18F-FMISO) PET and perfusion (Ktrans) on DCE MR imaging in a prospective study of 29 patients with histologically confirmed breast cancer. Additionally, there was a marked intratumoral heterogeneity with both hypoperfused and hyperperfused areas presenting hypoxia. Interestingly, hypoxia and Kep were weakly associated, suggesting that hypoxia depends more on the vascular flow and less on vascular permeability.[29]

Finally, multiparametric functional imaging with PET/MR imaging could help in the development and validation of potential new biomarkers, such as circulating microRNAs. In a prospective study of 77 patients with treatment naïve breast cancer and 78 healthy controls, Incoronato and colleagues found that the expression of circulating miR-143-3p was strongly and significantly correlated to the SUV_{max}, the MR imaging perfusion parameters, $iAUC_{mean}$ and Kep_{mean}, potentially representing a biomarker of aggressiveness of the disease. However, miR-125b-5p was inversely associated to $Ktrans_{mean}$ and Ki67, representing a potential biomarker of better prognosis.[30]

LYMPH NODES METASTASES

Concerning the evaluation of the N stage (Fig. 1), a meta-analysis of 4 studies has shown a pooled sensitivity of 18F-FDG PET/MR imaging of 94% (95% CI: 83%–98%), a specificity 90% (95% CI: 81%–95%), and an AUC of 0.96 (95% CI: 0.94–0.97).[15] The addition of a dedicated-breast PET/MR imaging to the standard whole-body acquisition did not present any added value in one prospective study of 38 patients, both had the same performance, correctly rating the N stage in 94% of patients, with 93% sensitivity, 95% specificity, and an accuracy of 94%.[6] However, van Nijnatten in a feasibility study of 12 patients, showed that dedicated-axillary PET/MR imaging may improve the diagnostic performance with 40% change in the N staging compared with US and contrast-enhanced MR imaging and 22% compared with PET/CT.[31]

Comparison with other modalities has shown variable results, with some studies showing equal performance and others the superiority of 18F-FDG PET/MR imaging for the detection of lymph node metastases. In a prospective study of 49 patients, Grueneisen and colleagues found a comparable performance among prone PET/MR imaging, prone MR imaging, and supine PET/CT, classifying correctly the N stage in 86% of patients for PET/MR imaging, 80% for MR imaging, and 88% for PET/CT. The corresponding sensitivity, specificity, and accuracy were 78%, 90%, and 86% for PET/MR imaging; 67%, 87%, and 80% for MR imaging; and 78%, 94%, and 88% for PET/CT. The differences were not statistically significant.[12] In a retrospective analysis of 58 patients, Botsikas and colleagues reported a slightly higher diagnostic performance of MR imaging for the evaluation of axillary, supraclavicular and internal mammary lymph nodes, although statistically not significantly different from PET alone and PET/MR imaging.[7] In a study from the same group with 80 patients, prospectively included and retrospectively analyzed, supine PET/MR imaging and supine PET/CT demonstrated a similar performance for the detection of axillary (85% vs 81% sensitivity, respectively, $P = .157$; specificity 89% vs 92%, $P = .257$) and internal mammary lymph node metastases.[32] In a prospective study of 56 patients by Kirchner and colleagues, 18F-FDG PET/MR imaging correctly classified the N stage in 57% of patients compared with 66% for conventional imaging, consisting of MMG and US; this difference was not significant.[11]

In contrast, in 2 prospective studies of 80 and 104 patients, comparing PET/MR imaging to contrast-enhanced CT in the first one and to MR imaging alone in the second one, Bruckmann and colleagues found a significant improvement in sensitivity with PET/MR imaging and comparable specificities in both studies. PET/MR imaging correctly classified the N stage in more patients than CT and MR imaging alone, with a significantly higher overall diagnostic confidence facilitating the diagnostic assessment.[33,34] Compared with CT in particular, PET/MR imaging was able to detect all patients with N3 stage, whereas CT understaged 2 patients, with direct clinical impact on the extent of the radiation field.[33] Morawitz and colleagues, in a prospective study of 182 patients, showed that PET/MR imaging outperforms both CT and MR imaging in the detection of nodal involvement on patient-based and lesion-based analyses. Additionally, in a subgroup analysis of the different lymph node stations (axillary levels I–III,

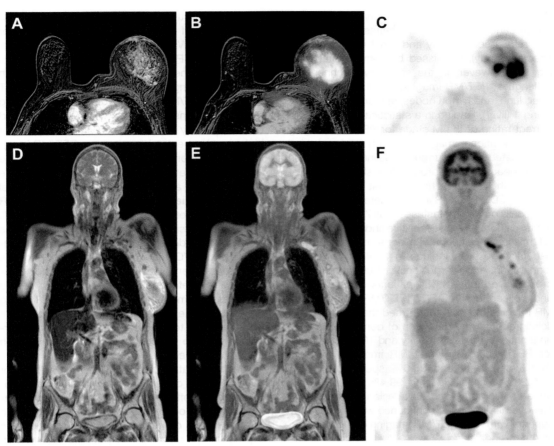

Fig. 1. Dedicated breast prone (axial arterial phase e-Thrive MR imaging (*A*), PET/MR imaging (*B*) and PET (*C*)) showing a T4b stage tumor of the left breast. Whole-body acquisition (coronal 3D T2W TSE MR imaging (*D*), PET/MR imaging (*E*), and PET (*F*)) revealing multiple ipsilateral axillary (level I–III) nodal metastases and no distant lesion.

supraclavicular, and internal mammary), PET/MR imaging detected significantly more lymph node metastases than MR imaging and CT in all locations, whereas MR imaging was superior to CT only in level I axillary lymph nodes.[35] In a retrospective analysis of 36 patients, Taneja and colleagues reported that MR imaging outperformed conventional assessment (clinical evaluation and axillary US) and PET alone for the detection of axillary nodal metastases; however, combined PET/MR imaging increased the diagnostic confidence compared with MR imaging and PET alone. Furthermore, extra-axillary lymph nodes (internal mammary and supraclavicular) were missed by conventional staging, whereas 8 were detected by MR imaging and 7 by PET.[13] Compared with dedicated breast MR imaging, thoracic MR imaging and axillary sonography, in a prospective study of 112 patients, Morawitz and colleagues, demonstrated that supine PET/MR imaging had the highest sensitivity (81.8%), accuracy (90.18%), and

AUC (0.892) in detecting the axillary lymph node metastases, significantly superior to all other 3 modalities, whereas axillary sonography had the highest specificity (98.5%).[36] Finally, in a prospective study of 40 patients by Goorts and colleagues, dedicated PET/MR imaging changed the N stage in 6 patients by confirming the suspicion in 3 patients, avoiding thus further workup and by detecting additional nodal metastases in 2 and reducing the number of suspicious lymph nodes in one patient.[10]

Distant Metastases

For the definition of the M stage, in a meta-analysis of 5 studies, 18F-FDG PET/MR imaging had a pooled sensitivity of 98% (95% CI: 96%–99%), 96% (95% CI: 83%–99%) specificity, and an AUC of 0.99 (95% CI: 0.98–1.00).[15] Compared with conventional imaging, including only abdominal US, chest radiography, and bone scintigraphy,

PET/MR imaging detected additional patients with breast cancer with distant metastases (8 out of 36 in a retrospective study and 2 out of 56 in a prospective study), all missed by conventional staging.[11,13] However, in the study by Kirchner and colleagues, PET/MR imaging had 4 false positives (liver, lung, and lymph nodes) and conventional imaging 1 (liver), leading in a statistically comparable correct rating of the M stage for PET/MR imaging and conventional imaging.[11] Using CT for staging as indicated by the current guidelines, Bruckmann and colleagues, in a prospective study of 80 patients with treatment naïve breast cancer, found that 18F-FDG PET/MR imaging detected all 36 histologically proven metastases in all 7 metastatic patients, without any false-positive findings. However, CT missed 3 patients with bone metastases and had false-positive findings in another 3 patients (bone, lung, and liver lesions).[33] Furthermore, in a prospective study of 154 patients by Bruckmann and colleagues, 18F-FDG PET/MR imaging and MR imaging alone outperformed the CT and bone scintigraphy in the detection of bone lesions both on a patient (100% sensitivity and 100% specificity for PET/MR imaging and MR imaging alone vs 71.4% sensitivity and 98.6% specificity for CT and 28.6% sensitivity and 99.4% specificity for bone scintigraphy) and on a lesion-level analysis. The overall diagnostic confidence was significantly superior with FDG PET/MR imaging compared with all other modalities.[33,37]

Compared with MR imaging in particular, in a prospective study of 104 patients with newly diagnosed breast cancer by Bruckmann and colleagues, both whole-body MR imaging and PET/MR imaging performed equally, identifying all 7 patients with distant metastases, correctly rating the M stage in 96.2% of patients, with a sensitivity of 100% (95% CI 59.0–100.0) and a specificity of 95.9% (95% CI 90.4–98.9). On a lesion level, 18F-FDG PET/MR imaging significantly increased the diagnostic confidence for the characterization of lesions compared with MR imaging alone and detected all 31 distant metastases (28 to the bone, 2 in the lungs, and 1 hilar lymph node), whereas MR imaging missed 5 bone metastases and the hilar lymph node.[34] In a prospective study of 40 patients by Goorts and colleagues, 2 had a bone metastasis in the field-of-view and PET/MR imaging proved to be of added value compared with MR imaging by confirming the diagnosis in one, avoiding thus additional examinations and by increasing the detectability of a subtle lesion in the second one, which went unrecognized in the first MR imaging reading.[10] In a retrospective study of 51 patients with untreated invasive ductal carcinoma by Catalano and colleagues, PET/MR

imaging correctly determined the stage of the disease in 98% of patients, compared with 84% for whole-body DWI and 75% for PET/CT. The difference between PET/MR imaging and PET/CT was significant, whereas the differences between PET/MR imaging and DWI and DWI and PET/CT were not. PET/MR imaging detected more lung and liver lesions compared with DWI and ruled out malignancy in T2 shine-through retention of high signal in benign bone lesions. PET/MR imaging was superior to PET/CT in detecting lytic bone and subcentimetric liver lesions.[38] In 2 prospective studies of 51[39] and 80 patients,[32] on patient-level analysis, the diagnostic performance of PET/MR imaging was not significantly superior to PET/CT. However, on lesion-level analysis, multiple studies show that the difference between PET/MR imaging and PET/CT becomes significant and is organ-dependent, with PET/MR imaging being superior in the detection of liver,[39] bone,[32,39,40] and cerebrospinal metastases[39,41] and PET/CT being superior in the detection of lung lesions,[39,41] whereas both techniques have a similar performance for the detection of mediastinal lymph node metastases.[32]

The combination of 18F-FDG and 18F-NaF for PET imaging is of particular interest in breast cancer imaging, offering the advantage of simultaneous evaluation of metabolic and osteoblastic activity. In this context, Sonni and colleagues, in a prospective study of 74 patients (23 women with breast cancer and 51 men with prostate cancer) showed that 18F-FDG/18F-NaF PET/MR imaging detected more lesions (140) in more patients (45) than bone scintigraphy (81 lesions in 37 patients), revealing additionally extraskeletal lesions in 19 patients.[42]

Response Evaluation

Although PET can be used for evaluation of treatment response in metastatic breast cancer, its use for residual disease evaluation at the end of neoadjuvant chemotherapy is not currently recommended , whereas early response assessment during neoadjuvant chemotherapy remains on a research level.[43] The accuracy and thus the predictive performance could be improved with the combination of functional and morphologic parameters of 18F-FDG PET/MR imaging.

Concerning treatment evaluation, Jena and colleagues reported that metabolic and MR imaging pharmacokinetic parameters derived from dedicated breast PET/MR imaging predicted treatment response (as defined by the RECIST criteria) in 9 out of the 11 lesions in 9 patients after chemotherapy, with reduction of both MR (65% for Ktrans) and

PET parameters (90% for SUV_{peak} and 76% for TLG).[20] Considering the histopathological characteristics of tumors, HR-positive tumors are lower cellularity tumors with a patchy pattern of shrinkage as response to treatment, whereas HR-negative tumors have higher cellularity and a centripetal pattern of shrinkage. As a result, Sekine and colleagues in a retrospective study of 74 patients with stage II and III breast cancer, reported that preoperative 18F-FDG PET/MR imaging has an excellent sensitivity in predicting pathologic complete response (pCR) to neo-adjuvant chemotherapy (NAC) for HR-positive tumors and an excellent specificity for HR-negative tumors. The overall sensitivity and specificity were 72.2% and 78.6%, respectively, with the accuracy depending more on the MR imaging component than the PET.[44]

For early response assessment, there are positive preliminary results but further research is needed. In a prospective study including 26 patients, a 44.7% reduction in TLG on PET and a 32.5% reduction in signal enhancement ratio on MR imaging after the first cycle of NAC were effective in the prediction of pCP. Their combination yielded a 100% sensitivity and 71.4% specificity. No other PET (SUV_{max}, MTV) or MR imaging (tumor size, volume, washout, edema, Breast Imaging-Reporting and Data System (BI-RADS)) parameter could distinguish responders from nonresponders. Additionally, a reduction in size and SUV_{max} was noted for axillary lymph nodes after 1 cycle of NAC but without any difference between the responders and residual tumor group.[45]

RECURRENCE

Suspected or confirmed recurrence of breast cancer is another clinical indication where 18F-FDG PET/MR imaging can prove of added value. In a prospective study of 21 patients, the authors compared PET/MR imaging, PET/CT, MR imaging, and CT for the detection of breast cancer recurrence. PET/MR imaging, PET/CT, and MR imaging detected all 17 out of 21 patients with clinically suspected recurrence, whereas CT missed 2 patients. On a lesion level, PET/MR imaging detected all lesions confirmed by the reference standard. PET/CT detected 97%, MR imaging 96.2%, and CT 74.6%. 18F FDG PET/MR imaging correctly classified 98.5% of lesions, 18F-FDG PET/CT 94.8%, MR imaging 88.1%, and CT 57.5%. The interobserver agreement was substantial in PET/MR imaging and PET/CT, moderate in MR imaging, and fair in CT evaluation.[46] In a prospective study of 36 patients with suspected recurrence of breast cancer, PET/MR imaging demonstrated a significantly higher diagnostic accuracy and confidence for the detection of breast cancer lesions compared with MR imaging alone. The accuracy was comparable between the different PET/MR sequences but the diagnostic confidence significantly increased with the inclusion of contrast-enhanced T1-weighted VIBE (Volumetric Interpolated Breathhold Examination).[47]

Clinical Impact

Published data showed that 18F-FDG PET/MR imaging led in change in treatment management in 14% up to 33% of patients, compared with conventional staging with MMG, US, and MR imaging[10,11,13] and in 12% compared with contrast-enhanced 18F-FDG PET/CT.[40] This included modification of the surgical approach most commonly, initiation of neoadjuvant chemotherapy, initiation of radiation therapy or extension of the radiotherapy field in most cases in order to include additional lesions (eg, the internal mammary chain) or less often its reduction, change of hormone treatment, avoidance of surgery, and chemotherapy initiation in patients with distant metastases.

Radiation Dose

Although there is no limit for patients' cumulative dose, as long as the risk–benefit balance justifies the additional dose to which the patient is exposed, it is common sense that a dose reduction is desirable. In hybrid PET/MR imaging cameras, we can achieve a mean dose reduction of 50% (range: 18.9%–64.3%), corresponding to a mean reduction of 8.3 mSv (CI 95%: 7.4–9.16) compared with PET/CT.[39] In addition, due to the advances of PET detectors technology, with improved sensitivity, this dose can further be decreased. In a prospective study of 26 patients, Sah and colleagues demonstrated that a simulated reduction of up to 90% of the standard activity of 18F-FDG (3MBq/kg) in dedicated-breast PET/MR imaging resulted in clinically acceptable PET images in terms of image quality and lesion detectability. For 10% of the injected activity, the estimated effective dose would have been 0.5 ± 0.1 mSv (range: 0.4–0.7 mSv), comparable to a digital MMG.[48]

RADIOMICS AND ARTIFICIAL INTELLIGENCE

With radiomics, the medical image is converted into a high-dimensional dataset from which valuable information could be mined, such as diagnosis, prognosis, and response to treatment; it could even be used to unravel genomic phenotypes of disease, otherwise known as radiogenomics.[49,50] Radiomics requires multiple steps, including feature extraction, feature selection, classifier/regression/time-to-event and evaluation,[49,50] constituting a rather laborious task. During the past decades, artificial intelligence has continued to evolve and with the development of machine learning (ML), an algorithm could do this task for us without explicit programming, whereas with deep learning (DL), a subcategory of ML, different ML algorithm steps combined in one package could perform even higher demand tasks just by feeding the input and the desired target to the DL algorithm.[50,51]

In a pilot radiomics study by Castaldo and colleagues, features from MR imaging (ADC, T2W, and T1W contrast-enhanced) and PET imaging were used for tumor grade, Ki-67 index, and molecular subtype's prediction through different ML algorithms, achieving an Area under the curve "Receiver Operating Characteristic" (AUCROC) of 0.74, 0.81, and 0.75, respectively.[52] Schiano and colleagues reported promising results from the combination of imaging 18F-FDG PET/MR imaging parameters and circulating Yin Yang 1 mRNAs for the prediction of synchronous metastatic disease in patients with breast cancer.[53] Using least absolute shrinkage and selection operator and support vector machine as feature selection and classifiers for different combinations of imaging features, respectively, Romeo and colleagues studied the performance of multiparametric 18F-FDG PET/MR imaging radiomics in 86 patients with 98 lesions and achieved an AUCROC of 0.88 for noninvasive discrimination of triple-negative breast cancer from other subtypes using combined ADC and PET image radiomics features.[54] Moreover, in another study with 102 patients (101 malignant and 19 benign lesions), Romeo and colleagues found that an integrated model combining mean transit time from DCE and mean ADC from DW with radiomics features extracted from PET and ADC achieved a very high accuracy (AUC 0.983) for the diagnosis of breast cancer, although not significantly different from that of an expert reader (AUC 0.868) ($P = .508$).[55] Umutlu and colleagues used multiparametric 18F-FDG PET/MR imaging radiomics features for breast cancer phenotype decoding, proving high performance. An AUCROC of 0.98 was achieved by MR imaging for differentiation between luminal A and B. For ER, PR, Ki-67, nodal and distant metastases, an AUCROC of 0.87, 0.88, 0.99, 0.81, and 0.99, respectively, was reached using all MR imaging and PET features.[56] In another study by Umutlu and colleagues, multiparametric 18F-FDG PET/MR imaging radiomics features-based models were used for pCR

prediction in neoadjuvant chemotherapy of patients with breast cancer. A combination of all MR imaging sequences and PET radiomics features yielded the best performance with an AUCROC of 0.8 in the entire cohort, 0.94 in HR+/HER2− and 0.92 in TN/HER2+ subgroup.[57]

Nevertheless, different challenges should be addressed in radiomics before translation into the clinical practice.[50,58] These challenges include the repeatability/reproducibility of features in various image acquisition, reconstruction, and segmentation settings and the robustness/generalizability of developed models across different centers.[50,58–60] Furthermore, sharing data between centers due to legal and ethical issue poses another challenge during model development and imbalance classes result in bias in radiomics models.[50,58–60]

CLINICS CARE POINTS

- 18F-FDG PET/MR imaging has high diagnostic performance in staging breast cancer with a high AUC of 0.99 both on patient and lesion-level analysis,[61] with half the radiation dose compared with PET/CT.[39]
- For preoperative evaluation of the primary tumor, a dedicated-breast acquisition should be regularly added to the whole-body PET/MR imaging.[6,8,9] The MR imaging component of dedicated-breast PET/MR imaging is superior in the detection and characterization of lesions.[7,10,12,13] PET-metabolic and MR imaging-pharmacokinetic parameters are reportedly inversely correlated to ER status and directly to HER2, Ki67, and nuclear grade. Beware of the different patterns of response to neoadjuvant treatment in HR-positive (infiltrative lesions with patchy shrinking) and HR-negative tumors (nodular lesions with centripetal shrinking), affecting the accuracy of the evaluation by PET/MR imaging.[44]
- For the evaluation of axillary nodal involvement, the diagnostic performance of dedicated-breast and whole-body PET/MR imaging is similar.[6] The sensitivity of PET/MR imaging is excellent but be careful of false positives in case of biopsy[36] or silicone-granulomas in patients with breast implants.[62,63] A silicone-specific MR sequence can be helpful in the second scenario.[64,65] Second look axillary US should be proposed to confirm the diagnosis because it is more specific.[36] For extra-axillary lymph node metastases (supraclavicular and internal mammary), PET/MR imaging is superior to CT,[33,35] comparable to PET/CT[12,32] and equal[7,12,13] or superior to MR imaging.[35]

- For distant metastases, 18F-FDG PET/MR imaging is superior to CT[33,37] and bone scintigraphy,[37] with a reserve concerning lung lesions. Compared with whole-body MR imaging and PET/CT, PET/MR imaging has an equal performance on a patient-based analysis[32,34,38,39] but on a lesion level, PET/MR imaging detects more lesions and increases the diagnostic confidence compared with MR imaging[10,34] and is superior to PET/CT for the detection of bone,[32,39,40] liver,[39] and brain metastases,[39,41] whereas PET/CT is superior for the detection of lung metastases.[39,41] Beware of PET false positives in case of inflammatory/infectious processes and consider further workup in order to confirm, if it changes the patient's treatment management.[11] Caution on DWI bone false positives because of a T2 shine-through retention of high signal, malignancy can be ruled out based on PET/MR imaging metabolic and morphologic parameters.[38]

DISCLOSURE

The authors have nothing to disclose.

REFERENCES

1. ECIS - European Cancer Information System https://ecis.jrc.ec.europa.eu © European Union, 2023.
2. Siegel R.L., MIller K.D., Fuchs H.E., et al., Cancer statistics, 2022, CA Cancer J Clin, 72 (1), 2022, 7–33.
3. Cardoso F., Kyriakides S., Ohno S., et al., Early breast cancer: ESMO Clinical Practice Guidelines for diagnosis, treatment and follow-updagger, Ann Oncol, 30 (8), 2019, 1194–1220.
4. Gennari A., André F., Barrios C.H., et al., ESMO Clinical Practice Guideline for the diagnosis, staging and treatment of patients with metastatic breast cancer, Ann Oncol, 32 (12), 2021, 1475–1495.
5. Gradishar W.J., Moran M.S., Abraham J., et al., Breast Cancer, Version 3.2022, NCCN Clinical Practice Guidelines in Oncology, J Natl Compr Canc Netw, 20 (6), 2022, 691–722.
6. Kirchner J., Grueneisen J., Martin O., et al., Local and whole-body staging in patients with primary breast cancer: a comparison of one-step to two-step staging utilizing (18)F-FDG-PET/MRI, Eur J Nucl Med Mol Imaging, 45 (13), 2018, 2328–2337.
7. Botsikas D, Kalovidouri A, Becker M, et al. Clinical utility of 18F-FDG-PET/MR for preoperative breast cancer staging. Eur Radiol 2016;26(7):2297–307.
8. Sasaki M., Tozaki M., Kubota K., et al., Simultaneous whole-body and breast 18F-FDG PET/MRI examinations in patients with breast cancer: a comparison of apparent diffusion coefficients and maximum standardized uptake values, Jpn J Radiol, 36 (2), 2018, 122–133.
9. Kong EJ, Chun KA, Bom HS, et al. Initial experience of integrated PET/MR mammography in patients with invasive ductal carcinoma. Hell J Nucl Med 2014;17(3):171–6.
10. Goorts B, Vöö S, van Nijnatten TJA, et al. Hybrid (18)F-FDG PET/MRI might improve locoregional staging of breast cancer patients prior to neoadjuvant chemotherapy. Eur J Nucl Med Mol Imaging 2017; 44(11):1796–805.
11. Kirchner J, Martin O, Umutlu L, et al. Impact of (18)F-FDG PET/MR on therapeutic management in high risk primary breast cancer patients - A prospective evaluation of staging algorithms. Eur J Radiol 2020;128:108975.
12. Grueneisen J., Nagarajah J., Buchbender C., et al., Positron Emission Tomography/Magnetic Resonance Imaging for Local Tumor Staging in Patients With Primary Breast Cancer: A Comparison With Positron Emission Tomography/Computed Tomography and Magnetic Resonance Imaging, Invest Radiol, 50 (8), 2015, 505–513.
13. Taneja S., Jena A., Goel R., et al., Simultaneous whole-body (1)(8)F-FDG PET-MRI in primary staging of breast cancer: a pilot study, Eur J Radiol, 83 (12), 2014, 2231–2239.
14. Hashimoto R., Akashi-Tanaka S., Watanabe C., et al., Diagnostic performance of dedicated breast positron emission tomography, Breast Cancer, 29 (6), 2022, 1013–1021.
15. Lu X.R., Qu M.M., Zhai Y.N., et al., Diagnostic role of 18F-FDG PET/MRI in the TNM staging of breast cancer: a systematic review and meta-analysis, Ann Palliat Med, 10 (4), 2021, 4328–4337.
16. Jena A, Taneja S, Singh A, et al. Role of pharmacokinetic parameters derived with high temporal resolution DCE MRI using simultaneous PET/MRI system in breast cancer: A feasibility study. Eur J Radiol 2017;86:261–6.
17. Pace L., Nicolai E., Luongo A., et al., Comparison of whole-body PET/CT and PET/MRI in breast cancer patients: lesion detection and quantitation of 18F-deoxyglucose uptake in lesions and in normal organ tissues, Eur J Radiol, 83 (2), 2014, 289–296.
18. Pujara AC, Raad RA, Ponzo F, et al. Standardized Uptake Values from PET/MRI in Metastatic Breast Cancer: An Organ-based Comparison With PET/CT. Breast J 2016;22(3):264–73.
19. Inglese M., Cavaliere C., Monti S., et al., A multi-parametric PET/MRI study of breast cancer: Evaluation of DCE-MRI pharmacokinetic models and correlation with diffusion and functional parameters, NMR Biomed, 32 (1), 2019, e4026.
20. Jena A, Taneja S, Singh A, et al. Association of pharmacokinetic and metabolic parameters derived

using simultaneous PET/MRI: Initial findings and impact on response evaluation in breast cancer. Eur J Radiol 2017;92:30–6.

21. Morawitz J., Kirchner J., Martin O., et al., Prospective Correlation of Prognostic Immunohistochemical Markers With SUV and ADC Derived From Dedicated Hybrid Breast 18F-FDG PET/MRI in Women With Newly Diagnosed Breast Cancer, *Clin Nucl Med*, 46 (3), 2021, 201–205.

22. Catalano OA, Horn GL, Signore A, et al. PET/MR in invasive ductal breast cancer: correlation between imaging markers and histological phenotype. Br J Cancer 2017;116(7):893–902.

23. Incoronato M., Grimaldi A.M., Cavaliere C., et al., Relationship between functional imaging and immunohistochemical markers and prediction of breast cancer subtype: a PET/MRI study, *Eur J Nucl Med Mol Imaging*, 45 (10), 2018, 1680–1693.

24. Jena A, Taneja S, Singh A, et al. Reliability of (18)F-FDG PET Metabolic Parameters Derived Using Simultaneous PET/MRI and Correlation With Prognostic Factors of Invasive Ductal Carcinoma: A Feasibility Study. AJR Am J Roentgenol 2017; 209(3):662–70.

25. Mao Y, Keller ET, Garfield DH, et al. Stromal cells in tumor microenvironment and breast cancer. Cancer Metastasis Rev 2013;32(1–2):303–15.

26. Shiao SL, Ganesan AP, Rugo HS, et al. Immune microenvironments in solid tumors: new targets for therapy. *Genes Dev* 2011;25(24):2559–72.

27. Solinas C, Carbognin L, De Silva P, et al. Tumor-infiltrating lymphocytes in breast cancer according to tumor subtype. Current state of the art, *Breast* 2017;35:142–50.

28. Murakami W, Tozaki M, Sasaki M, et al. Correlation between (18)F-FDG uptake on PET/MRI and the level of tumor-infiltrating lymphocytes (TILs) in triple-negative and HER2-positive breast cancer. *Eur J Radiol* 2020;123:108773.

29. Carmona-Bozo J.C., Manavaki R., Woitek R., et al., Hypoxia and perfusion in breast cancer: simultaneous assessment using PET/MR imaging, *Eur Radiol*, 31 (1), 2021, 333–344.

30. Incoronato M., Grimaldi A.M., Mirabelli P., et al., Circulating miRNAs in Untreated Breast Cancer: An Exploratory Multimodality Morpho-Functional Study, *Cancers*, 11 (6), 2019, 876.

31. van Nijnatten T.J.A., Goorts B., Vöö S., et al., Added value of dedicated axillary hybrid 18F-FDG PET/MRI for improved axillary nodal staging in clinically node-positive breast cancer patients: a feasibility study, *Eur J Nucl Med Mol Imaging*, 45 (2), 2018, 179–186.

32. Botsikas D., Bagetakos I., Picarra M., et al., What is the diagnostic performance of 18-FDG-PET/MR compared to PET/CT for the N- and M- staging of breast cancer?, *Eur Radiol*, 29 (4), 2019, 1787–1798.

33. Bruckmann N.M., Kirchner J., Morawitz J., et al., Prospective comparison of CT and 18F-FDG PET/MRI in N and M staging of primary breast cancer patients: Initial results, *PLoS One*, 16 (12), 2021, e0260804.

34. Bruckmann N.M., Sawicki L.M., Kirchner J., et al., Prospective evaluation of whole-body MRI and (18)F-FDG PET/MRI in N and M staging of primary breast cancer patients, *Eur J Nucl Med Mol Imaging*, 47 (12), 2020, 2816–2825.

35. Morawitz J., Bruckmann N.M., Dietzel F., et al., Comparison of nodal staging between CT, MRI, and [(18)F]-FDG PET/MRI in patients with newly diagnosed breast cancer, *Eur J Nucl Med Mol Imaging*, 49 (3), 2022, 992–1001.

36. Morawitz J., Bruckmann N.M., Dietzel F., et al., Determining the axillary nodal status with four current imaging modalities including (18)F-FDG PET/MRI in newly diagnosed breast cancer: A comparative study using histopathology as reference standard, *J Nucl Med*, 62 (12), 2021, 1677–1683.

37. Bruckmann N.M., Kirchner J., Umutlu L., et al., Prospective comparison of the diagnostic accuracy of 18F-FDG PET/MRI, MRI, CT, and bone scintigraphy for the detection of bone metastases in the initial staging of primary breast cancer patients, *Eur Radiol*, 31 (11), 2021, 8714–8724.

38. Catalano O.A., Daye D., Signore A., et al., Staging performance of whole-body DWI, PET/CT and PET/MRI in invasive ductal carcinoma of the breast, *Int J Oncol*, 51 (1), 2017, 281–288.

39. Melsaether AN, Raad RA, Pujara A, et al. Comparison of Whole-Body (18)F FDG PET/MR Imaging and Whole-Body (18)F FDG PET/CT in Terms of Lesion Detection and Radiation Dose in Patients with Breast Cancer. Radiology 2016;281(1): 193–202.

40. Catalano OA, Nicolai E, Rosen BR, et al. Comparison of CE-FDG-PET/CT with CE-FDG-PET/MR in the evaluation of osseous metastases in breast cancer patients. Br J Cancer 2015;112(9):1452–60.

41. Ishii S, Shimao D, Hara T, et al. Comparison of integrated whole-body PET/MR and PET/CT: Is PET/MR alternative to PET/CT in routine clinical oncology? Ann Nucl Med 2016;30(3):225–33.

42. Sonni I., Minamimoto R., Baratto L., et al., Simultaneous PET/MRI in the Evaluation of Breast and Prostate Cancer Using Combined Na[(18)F] F and [(18)F]FDG: a Focus on Skeletal Lesions, *Mol Imaging Biol*, 22 (2), 2020, 397–406.

43. Salaun P.Y., Abgral R., Malard O., et al., Good clinical practice recommendations for the use of PET/CT in oncology. Eur J Nucl Med Mol Imaging, 47 (1), 2020, 28–50.

44. Sekine C., Uchiyama N., Watase C., et al., Preliminary experiences of PET/MRI in predicting complete response in patients with breast cancer treated with

neoadjuvant chemotherapy, *Mol Clin Oncol*, 16 (2), 2022, 50.

45. Cho N., Im S.A., Cheon G.J., et al., Integrated (18)F-FDG PET/MRI in breast cancer: early prediction of response to neoadjuvant chemotherapy, *Eur J Nucl Med Mol Imaging*, 45 (3), 2018, 328–339.

46. Sawicki LM, Grueneisen J, Schaarschmidt BM, et al. Evaluation of (1)(8)F-FDG PET/MRI, (1)(8)F-FDG PET/CT, MRI, and CT in whole-body staging of recurrent breast cancer. Eur J Radiol 2016;85(2):459–65.

47. Grueneisen J, Sawicki LM, Wetter A, et al. Evaluation of PET and MR datasets in integrated 18F-FDG PET/MRI: A comparison of different MR sequences for whole-body restaging of breast cancer patients. Eur J Radiol 2017;89:14–9.

48. Sah B.R., Ghafoor S., Burger I.A., et al., Feasibility of (18)F-FDG Dose Reductions in Breast Cancer PET/MRI, *J Nucl Med*, 59 (12), 2018, 1817–1822.

49. LeCun Y, Bengio Y, Hinton G. Deep learning. Nature 2015;521(7553):436–44.

50. Manafi-Farid R., Askari E., Shiri I., et al., [(18)F]FDG-PET/CT Radiomics and Artificial Intelligence in Lung Cancer: Technical Aspects and Potential Clinical Applications, *Semin Nucl Med*, 52 (6), 2022, 759–780.

51. Gillies RJ, Kinahan PE, Hricak H. Radiomics: Images Are More than Pictures, They Are Data. Radiology 2016;278(2):563–77.

52. Castaldo R., Garbino N., Cavaliere C., et al., A Complex Radiomic Signature in Luminal Breast Cancer from a Weighted Statistical Framework: A Pilot Study, *Diagnostics*, 12 (2), 2022, 499.

53. Schiano C., Franzese M., Pane K., et al., Hybrid (18)F-FDG-PET/MRI Measurement of Standardized Uptake Value Coupled with Yin Yang 1 Signature in Metastatic Breast Cancer. A Preliminary Study, *Cancers*, 11 (10), 2019, 1444.

54. Romeo V., Kapetas P., Clauser P., et al., A Simultaneous Multiparametric (18)F-FDG PET/MRI Radiomics Model for the Diagnosis of Triple Negative Breast Cancer, *Cancers*, 14 (16), 2022, 3944.

55. Romeo V., Clauser P., Rasul S., et al., AI-enhanced simultaneous multiparametric (18)F-FDG PET/MRI for accurate breast cancer diagnosis, *Eur J Nucl Med Mol Imaging*, 49 (2), 2022, 596–608.

56. Umutlu L., Kirchner J., Bruckmann N.M., et al., Multiparametric Integrated (18)F-FDG PET/MRI-Based Radiomics for Breast Cancer Phenotyping and Tumor Decoding, *Cancers*, 13 (12), 2021, 2928.

57. Umutlu L., Kirchner J., Bruckmann N.M., et al., Multiparametric (18)F-FDG PET/MRI-Based Radiomics for Prediction of Pathological Complete Response to Neoadjuvant Chemotherapy in Breast Cancer, *Cancers*, 14 (7), 2022, 1727.

58. Lambin P, Leijenaar RTH, Deist TM, et al. Radiomics: the bridge between medical imaging and personalized medicine. Nat Rev Clin Oncol 2017;14(12):749–62.

59. Saboury B, Rahmim A, Siegel E. PET and AI Trajectories Finally Coming into Alignment. Pet Clin 2021;16(4):xv–xvi.

60. Zwanenburg A., Vallières M., Abdalah M.A., et al., The Image Biomarker Standardization Initiative: Standardized Quantitative Radiomics for High-Throughput Image-based Phenotyping, *Radiology*, 295 (2), 2020, 328–338.

61. Lin CY, Lin CL, Kao CH. Staging/restaging performance of F18-fluorodeoxyglucose positron emission tomography/magnetic resonance imaging in breast cancer: A review and meta-analysis. Eur J Radiol 2018;107:158–65.

62. Adejolu M., Huo L., Rohren E., et al., False-positive lesions mimicking breast cancer on FDG PET and PET/CT, *AJR Am J Roentgenol*, 198 (3), 2012, W304–W314.

63. Fernandes Vieira V., Dubruc E., Raffoul W., et al., Bilateral Silicone Granulomas Mimicking Breast Cancer Recurrence on 18F-FDG PET/CT, *Clin Nucl Med*, 46 (2), 2021, 140–141.

64. de Faria Castro Fleury E, Gianini AC, Ayres V, et al. Breast magnetic resonance imaging: tips for the diagnosis of silicone-induced granuloma of a breast implant capsule (SIGBIC). Insights Imaging 2017;8(4):439–46.

65. Ma J, Choi H, Stafford RJ, et al. Silicone-specific imaging using an inversion-recovery-prepared fast three-point Dixon technique. J Magn Reson Imaging 2004;19(3):298–302.

Abdominal Positron Emission Tomography/ Magnetic Resonance Imaging

Álvaro Badenes Romero, MD[a,b,c], Felipe S. Furtado, MD[a,b],
Madaleine Sertic, MD[a], Reece J. Goiffon, MD, PhD[a], Umar Mahmood, MD[a],
Onofrio A. Catalano, MD[a,b],*

KEYWORDS

- Fluorodeoxyglucose F18 • Positron-emission tomography • Magnetic resonance imaging
- Radiation • Ionizing • Perfusion imaging • Liver neoplasms • Lymphadenopathy

KEY POINTS

- PET/MRI combines superb soft tissue contrast and highly sensitive molecular information resulting in a one-stop-shop assessment for abdominal cancers.
- While most cancers in the abdomen present elevated [18F]FDG uptake, some cancers, for example, neuroendocrine tumors and hepatocellular carcinomas, are better evaluated with somatostatin receptor ligands and FAPI, respectively.
- In inflammatory bowel disease, PET/MRI quantifies disease activity and determines the nature of strictures, which may have management implications.

INTRODUCTION

Multimodal information is increasingly necessary for clinical care, providing data related to anatomy, physiology, or metabolism through a combination of diagnostic tests such as computed tomography (CT), magnetic resonance imaging (MRI), and positron emission tomography (PET).[1] PET/CT has become the gold standard technique for managing various neoplasms.[2] Meanwhile, the development of PET/MRI was historically more difficult due to technological and methodological challenges.[3–5] However, PET/MRI has been commercially available since 2011,[6] and its applications have been tested in several fields ranging from oncology to inflammatory and degenerative diseases.[7,8]

Simultaneously acquired PET/MRI has unparalleled potential in oncologic imaging, for example, by accurately discriminating malignant from benign lesions, improving locoregional and distant metastatic evaluation, and allowing the investigation of tumor heterogeneity, genetic profiles and phenotypes.[9–16] Imaging biomarkers extracted from PET/MRI such as the apparent diffusion coefficient (ADC), reverse efflux volume transfer constant (Kep_{mean}) and maximum standardized uptake value (SUV_{max}) have been correlated with in-vivo tumor markers such as circulating miR-NAs,[13] tumor histology and phenotype,[15,17,18] and prognosis,[19] highlighting the biological basis of those metrics and potential applications in precision medicine. Moreover, obviating the additional radiation exposure from CT becomes relevant for pediatric patients or those who need continuous follow-up.[20–22] Lastly, performing the best non-invasive diagnostic tests in a single session could improve health care efficiency. Avoiding multiple visits may result in shorter diagnostic workups[23,24] and improved patient comfort.

a Department of Radiology, Massachusetts General Hospital, Harvard Medical School, Boston, MA, USA;
b Athinoula A Martinos Center for Biomedical Imaging, Harvard Medical School, Charlestown, MA, USA;
c Department of Nuclear Medicine, Joan XXIII Hospital, Tarragona, Spain
* Corresponding author. Department of Radiology, Massachusetts General Hospital, Harvard Medical School, Boston, MA.
E-mail address: onofriocatalano@yahoo.it

Magn Reson Imaging Clin N Am 31 (2023) 579–589
https://doi.org/10.1016/j.mric.2023.06.003
1064-9689/23/

The theoretical advantages of [18F]FDG PET/ MRI have been demonstrated by initial clinical research and address critical deficiencies of PET/CT, such as poor soft tissue contrast resolution, increased radiation exposure, suboptimal image registration, and lack of motion correction capabilities. [18F]FDG PET/MRI shows improved staging that might lead to management changes in abdominal neoplasms.[10,25–28] Additional evidence demonstrates a higher detection of adenopathy, liver metastases, and bone metastases by [18F]FDG PET/MRI compared to [18F]FDG PET/CT.[28,29] This review aims to detail the particularities of abdominal imaging and current applications of PET/MRI in abdominal diseases.

NORMAL ANATOMY AND IMAGING TECHNIQUE

Abdominal imaging has peculiarities that must be considered when formulating imaging protocols. The proximity to the diaphragm implies breathing motion artifacts in the upper abdomen, whereas the lower abdomen houses hollow organs with active peristalsis that make acquiring consistent and sharp images challenging. For PET/MRI, this means that PET images should be motion-corrected to avoid lesion volume overestimation and SUV underestimation.[29,30] The MRI portion should include fast sequences with high temporal resolution to alleviate the effect of motion. Finally, it is essential to note that unlike PET/CT, where the electron density is inferred from the attenuation coefficients for CT, in PET/MRI, the attenuation correction is commonly performed through a combination of body tissue segmentation and atlas-based approaches.[31] Traditionally, a two-point Dixon sequence is used to segment the body into air, lung, fat, soft tissue, and bones.[32] These may result in pitfalls, especially in lesions adjacent to cortical bone[33] or in the presence of prosthesis or other foreign bodies.[5,34]

PROTOCOLS
Magnetic Resonance Imaging Sequences

For most PET/MRI indications in the abdomen, both whole-body non-contrast-enhanced images and gadolinium contrast-enhanced images should be acquired. Contrast-enhanced MRI improves the detection and characterization of peritoneal and hepatic lesions.[12,35,36]

The whole-body examination should cover the base of the neck to the mid-thighs. The primary sequences are as follows: 1) two-point Dixon for attenuation correction, 2) axial T2-weighted half-Fourier acquisition single-shot turbo spin-echo (HASTE/

SSFSE) to enable high temporal resolution images with sufficient soft tissue contrast for diagnostic evaluation, 3) diffusion-weighted imaging, preferably using parallel imaging techniques such as simultaneous multislice imaging to reduce scan time.[37]

Ideally, additional upper abdomen coronal precontrast T2-weighted HASTE images should be acquired, as well as axial fat-suppressed breath-triggered or navigated T2-weighted fast-spin echo (FSE) and gadolinium dynamic contrast-enhanced (CE) sequences. 3D or 2D magnetic resonance cholangiopancreatography (MRCP) can be included for pathologies involving the biliary tract or pancreas.

The above protocol lasts 45 to 60 minutes, and PET images are co-acquired and co-registered, overlaying the PET data onto the MRI images. While PET images are always obtained in free breathing mode, MRI images can be differently acquired, especially in breath hold or free breathing modalities through breath-triggered or navigated approcahes. Additionally, specific MRI sequences can be acquired continuously, using free breathing motion correction techniques, along with free breathing PET; after acquisition both MRI and PET undergo plastic deformation, rebinning, and reconstruction according to the calculated motion vector fields to allow motion corrected reconstructions in specific frames of respiration. This approach, although time consuming, given the large amount of computational power, allows ideal motion correction and therefore superb correspondence of MRI data with PET events. Motion corrected PET/MRI improves lesion conspicuity, SUV_{max} estimation and metabolic tumor volume calculation.[29,30,38–41]

Overall, the registration process allows fusion of MRI and PET data regardless of the specific kind of MRI breathing acquisition mode. Obviously, free breathing simultaneously acquired motion corrected MRI and PET data further improve the localization of metabolic events over morphologic correlates. After this process, the fused images can be continuously scrolled through.

Radiopharmaceuticals

[18F]FDG remains the mainstay of abdominal PET/ MRI. [18F]FDG is a suitable radiopharmaceutical for most abdominal neoplasms presenting increased glycolytic metabolism.[42–44] Unfortunately, several non-neoplastic conditions also result in increased glucose metabolism. Examples include active inflammation, brown fat tissue, and muscular and neuronal activities, which might be confounders.

Novel alternatives for non-[18F]FDG-avid tumors are radiolabeled fibroblast activation protein inhibitors (FAPI). FAPI ligands have been evaluated in various abdominal cancers, including gastric, duodenal, pancreatic, colorectal, and hepatocellular carcinoma (HCC), with reported sensitivities ranging from 85.7% to100%.[45–49]

For well-differentiated neuroendocrine tumors, radiolabeled somatostatin receptor ligands, such as [68Ga]Ga-DOTATOC or [68Ga]Ga-DOTATATE, have higher detection rates when compared to [18F]FDG.[50–52] However, for poorly differentiated neuroendocrine neoplasms [18F]FDG is still the best option.

CLINICAL APPLICATIONS
Esophageal Cancer

Based on the limited literature available, the assessment of the T and N staging in esophageal cancer is improved with [18F]FDG PET/MRI compared to CT or [18F]FDG PET/CT.[53] PET/MRI enables the differentiation of the esophageal wall layers and the measurement of longitudinal and transmural tumor extension due to its better soft tissue resolution. The co-acquired [18F]FDG PET further improves its sensitivity. On MRI, tumors appear as poorly defined low-to-intermediate T2w signal lesions. For N staging, diagnostic performance is enhanced by resolving pathological lymph nodes that might otherwise be obscured due to spillover effect from intense primary tumor [18F]FDG uptake. PET/MRI assessment of lymphadenopathy is based on a combination of size, morphologic (blurred or irregular margins, internal heterogeneity, round shape), and metabolic criteria, which outperform size, stand-alone morphologic criteria and stand-alone assessment of radiopharmaceutical avidity.[28]

On the other hand, endoscopic ultrasound (EUS) remains superior for evaluating T and N staging, being preferred for locoregional staging when available.[54] For example, in one study, primary tumors were correctly staged in 66.7% of the cases by PET/MRI, in 33.3% by CT, and in 86.7% by EUS. For lymph node staging, the accuracy was 83.3% with PET/MRI, 50% with CT, and 75% with EUS. However, it is indispensable to associate cross-sectional imaging to identify distant metastases.[53]

Prognosis
[18F]FDG PET provides semi-quantitative biomarkers in patients undergoing neoadjuvant chemotherapy (NAC), which may help estimate survival and select surgical candidates. Although this can be done with [18F]FDG PET/CT, PET/MRI combines SUV and apparent diffusion coefficient (ADC). Increased SUV or decreased ADC values after NAC denote worse prognosis.[55]

Gastric Cancer

EUS, CT, or [18F]FDG PET/CT are used in the staging of gastric cancer.[56] [18F]FDG PET/MRI may be superior to [18F]FDG PET/CT for T and N staging and to CT for M staging.[57] For example, in one study, T staging accuracy, leveraging on high-resolution T2 weighted sequences, was 76.9% for [18F]FDG PET/MRI and 57.7% for [18F]FDG PET/CT, while for N staging, the accuracy was 53.9% and 34%, respectively.[57] However, these differences were not statistically significant.

Colorectal Cancer

Regarding T staging in rectal and colon cancers, [18F]FDG PET/MRI has the best of both worlds. The intrinsic high resolution of MRI, especially with T2-weighted images, enables the discrimination of the rectal wall layers, the components of the anal sphincter, and allows refined assessment of the mesorectal fascia and lymph nodes. This is combined with the high sensitivity of PET, which is further boosted by the longer acquisition time of up to 15 minutes, considering the time needed to coaquire the simultaneous MRI sequences.

In fact, one study demonstrated the superiority of [18F]FDG PET/MRI over [18F]FDG PET/CT, with the latter erroneously understaging colorectal cancers in 27% of the cases.[58] For primary tumor evaluation, PET data may offer relevant information in lower rectal cancers that threaten the sphincter complex, for example, by assessing the involvement of the external sphincter, which is key to disease management.[28]

For N staging, PET and MRI are complementary. PET increases sensitivity compared to stand-alone MRI, while MRI, with better soft tissue contrast resolution and the use of DWI, can detect lesions that might be false negative on [18F]FDG PET/CT or CT.[22] Lastly, for M staging [18F]FDG PET/MRI is superior to the current standard of care using CT for whole-body staging with a sensitivity of 98% vs. 73%.[23] This improved sensitivity is especially relevant for liver metastases, the most common site of metastatic spread in colorectal cancer.[59] In the subset of patients with oligometastatic tumors, PET/MRI might change management in up to 19% of the cases when compared to standard of care imaging.[60] Moreover, gains in diagnostic yield contribute to the cost-effectiveness of [18F]FDG PET/MRI in rectal cancer, which incentivizes the adoption of PET/MRI as a replacement for separate pelvic MRI and CT for rectal cancer or CT for colon cancer.[61]

Cholangiocarcinoma

PET/MRI may overcome some inherent limitations of PET/CT, with the simultaneous acquisition of PET, and especially the use of T2-weighted sequences, including 3D magnetic resonance cholangiopancreatography (MRCP). Contrast-enhanced sequences enable the evaluation of bile duct morphology and vascular involvement, providing a surgical roadmap and facilitating the differentiation between inflammation or tumors. On the other hand, [18F]FDG PET can help detect the primary tumor and metastases and differentiate between benign and malignant biliary strictures. One study evaluated patients with untreated mass-forming intrahepatic cholangiocarcinoma, showing that [18F]FDG PET/MRI impacted clinical management in 29.7% of the cases due to more precise tumor extension assessment and ruling out distant metastases, when compared to conventional imaging–defined either as both a CT and an MRI or a combination of PET/CT ± dedicated CT ± MRI.[26]

Pancreatic adenocarcinoma

Staging

For pancreatic tumor characterization, diagnosis, staging, and preoperative assessment of resectability, preliminary studies showed that [18F]FDG PET/MRI was superior or equal to [18F]FDG PET/CT.[62] The MRI component might provide anatomic correlates for areas of increased metabolic activity that on CT might be isodense to normal parenchyma, and even more so to surrounding atrophic regions or inflammatory changes. On the other hand, diffusion restriction and the superior contrast-to-noise ratio of CE-MRI might help detect non-[18F]FDG-avid lesions. In addition, dynamic CE-MRI allows the assessment of vascular involvement similarly to CE-CT (Fig. 1).

In one study, the evaluation of patients with pancreatic ductal adenocarcinoma (PDAC) with [18F]FDG PET/MRI resulted in management changes in 49% of the cases compared to standard-of-care imaging (CT, PET/CT, and MRI).[27] In PDAC, [18F]FDG PET/MRI might improve diagnostic accuracy over [18F]FDG PET/CT and has a high specificity in detecting locoregional lymph nodes. Moreover, for metastatic disease evaluation, [18F]FDG PET/MRI complements conventional imaging.[63]

Treatment Response Evaluation

[18F]FDG PET/MRI leverages the combination of metabolic and functional parameters such as SUV values and ADC, which are independent surrogate biomarkers for tumor response assessment[64,65] and can become helpful because of the limitation of Response Evaluation Criteria in Solid Tumors (RECIST). [18F]FDG-PET/MRI biomarkers such as ADC_{min} and total lesion glycolysis demonstrated a relationship with overall survival in PDAC.[65]

PANCREATIC NEUROENDOCRINE NEOPLASMS

Somatostatin receptor (SSTR) ligands have been widely adopted for imaging neuroendocrine neoplasms (NEN). However, SSTRs are not expressed exclusively by NEN but also by other benign and malignant lesions, including inflammatory tissue, lymphomas, head and neck tumors, uterine myomas, and meningiomas. Moreover, the physiologic biodistribution of SSTR analogs in the liver and the uncinate process of the pancreas may lead to false positive findings.[66] Sometimes, these findings cannot be resolved by the CT component of PET/CT because of the insufficient soft-tissue resolution.

Alternatively, PET/MRI's superior soft tissue resolution and contrast-to-noise ratio help overcome these limitations, leading to the correct diagnosis. For example, pre and post-dynamic contrast assessment T1-weighted fat-saturated sequences and the simultaneously acquired PET can detect and characterize small lesions as well as differentiate physiologic uptake from actual neuroendocrine

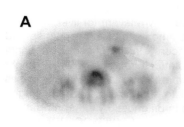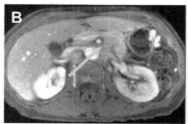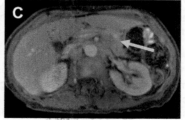

Fig. 1. Role of [18F]FDG-PET/MRI in local pancreatic adenocarcinoma staging. PET (A), contrast-enhanced T1-weighted MRI (B), fused PET/MRI (C). FDG uptake highlights a tumor in the body of the pancreas (arrows in A, C). The contrast-enhanced MRI also shows minimally FDG-avid extra-pancreatic tumor extension which presents as hypointense on contrast enhanced T1w imaging (arrow in B).

lesions in the uncinate process.[67] In fact, pancreatic tumors will present as sharply defined lesions on T1-weighted images before contrast, become markedly hyperintense during arterial phase imaging, show high T2-weighted and DWI signal. In the case of G1-G2 neuroendocrine tumors (NET), the lesions will also show SSTR ligand avidity, meanwhile, poorly differentiated NENs and neuroendocrine carcinomas (NEC) will demonstrate variable SSTR ligand avidity; NEC and high grade NET may exhibit increased FDG uptake. On the other hand, physiologic uptake in the uncinate process will lack any corresponding morphologic correlate.

Adrenal Tumors

Adrenal incidentalomas found on staging are common,[68,69] and most of them will be benign adenomas. PET/MRI may help distinguish adenomas from malignant lesions through a combination of FDG avidity evaluation and chemical shift MRI imaging, which identifies intracellular fat.[70,71] In a cohort of 173 patients, only 4.25% of the incidentalomas identified with [18F]FDG PET/MRI were deemed indeterminate, versus 22.36% for [18F]FDG PET/

CT.[70] Fig. 2 shows a case where PET/MRI helped identify an adrenal metastasis thanks to the combination of in and out of phase sequences and PET. In pheochromocytoma, [68Ga]-DOTATATE PET/MRI with DWI can improve sensitivity compared to PET alone.[72]

Liver Metastases

PET/MRI with dynamic contrast-enhanced sequences (DCE) and DWI or hepatobiliary phase imaging demonstrated better diagnostic accuracy than contrast-enhanced PET/CT.[35,73] A recent multicentric study in the assessment of liver metastases showed PET/MRI had a sensitivity of 95% and a specificity of 97%,[73] being capable of characterizing 80% of hepatic lesions that were indeterminate on MRI alone and 91% of hepatic lesions indeterminate by PET alone (Figs. 3 and 4). PET/MRI can also assist in delineating the relationship of liver lesions to adjacent structures and ensure that such lesions are properly localized.[74] The characterization of lesions previously considered indeterminate into benign or malignant is one of the PET/MRI's main advantages,[75] and may

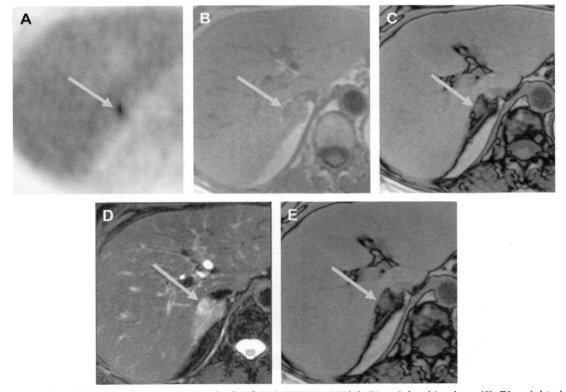

Fig. 2. Adrenal incidentaloma evaluation by [18F] FDG-PET/MRI: PET(*A*), T1-weighted in phase (*B*), T1-weighted out of phase (*C*), T2-weighted fat suppressed FSE (*D*), fused PET/MRI (*E*). A metastasis (*arrows*) within an adrenal adenoma demonstrates signal retention on out of phase imaging, hyperintensity on T2-weighted imaging, and moderate FDG uptake, allowing discrimination from the coexistent adenoma.

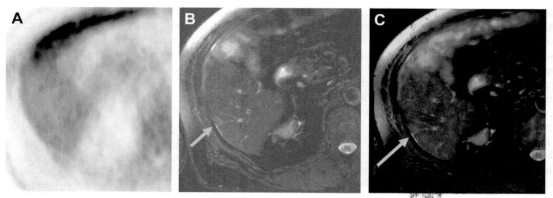

Fig. 3. Complementarity of PET and MRI in liver metastasis evaluation. [18F]FDG-PET/MRI: PET(*A*), T2-weighted FSE MRI (*B*), fused PET/MRI (*C*). A focus (*arrow* in *B*) of low T2-weighted signal with a faint rim of T2-weighted hyperintensity, adjacent to the liver capsule in segment VI, does not demonstrate increased FDG uptake (*arrow* in *C*). This corresponds to a metabolically inactive lesion, in keeping with a treated, non-viable liver metastasis.

change the management in 30–49% of patients.[26,27,76] This can be achieved through the improved co-registration and fusion of PET and MRI images to interrogate FDG uptake and enhancement patterns in each lesion (**Fig. 5**). A correct assessment is vital because hepatic metastasectomy in patients with oligometastatic disease can improve survival and even lead to cure-defining progression-free stretches.[77–79]

INFLAMMATORY BOWEL DISEASE

PET/MRI is a promising non-invasive imaging methodology in patients with inflammatory bowel disease, especially in Crohn disease.[80–82] The co-acquisition of PET and MRI images lead to

high-quality images and reduces misregistration due to bowel peristalsis. PET/MRI may also be performed with MRI enterography.

In Crohn disease, PET/MRI has the potential to serve as a high-quality, non-invasive alternative for assessment and therapy monitoring.[80] Possible roles involve detecting and quantifying disease activity and complications, as well as discriminating fibrotic strictures from inflammatory and mixed strictures.[83] In fact, PET/MRI can leverage on the picomolar sensitivity of PET to detect possible candidates for active disease; those candidate areas can be more definitively characterized as active disease in the case MRI detects wall thickening, edema, and increased vascularity, ruling out potential false-positive FDG uptake. This point is critical

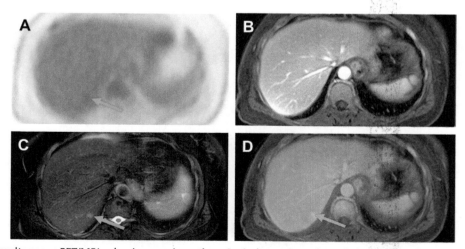

Fig. 4. Simultaneous PET/MRI value in assessing otherwise indeterminate hepatic lesions. [18F] FDG-PET/MRI: PET (*A*), T1-weighted contrast-enhanced MRI (*B*), T2-weighted FSE MRI (*C*), fused PET/MRI (*D*). One small metastasis, invisible on the contrast-enhanced MRI (*B*), demonstrates mild T2-weighted hyperintensity and mildly FDG avidity (*arrow*). The combined information from MR and PET allows both lesion detection and characterization. This lesion would be indeterminate on either PET alone or MRI alone.

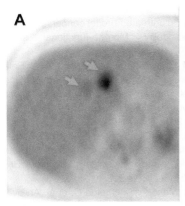 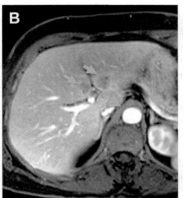 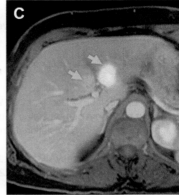

Fig. 5. MRI adding value to PET in PET/MRI. [18F]FDG-PET/MRI: PET(*A*), T1-weighted contrast-enhanced MRI (*B*), fused PET/MRI (*C*). Three liver metastases are seen. However, only two are demonstrated on PET (*arrows*) The third, smaller lesion is not FDG-avid likely to small size but is still detected on the contrast-enhanced MRI (*arrowhead*).

to guide management: inflammatory strictures are treated with medical therapy, whereas fibrotic strictures are treated with surgical resection or dilatation. A study demonstrated that a hybrid biomarker combining ADC and SUV_{max} is better than either modality alone.[83]

COST-EFFECTIVENESS

While PET/MRI can be almost 50% more expensive than PET/CT on a per-scan basis[84] (holding radiopharmaceutical costs constant), in most clinical scenarios a separate dedicated MRI would also be billed for. Depending on the specific protocol, the added cost of MRI and PET/CT might match or even surpass PET/MRI's cost. Additionally, single-session scanning reduces transportation and lodging costs, diminishes ionizing radiation exposure (vs. PET/CT),[22] and increases time savings. Moreover, according to a study conducted in Europe, PET/MRI's increased accuracy over PET/CT, coupled with frequent management changes, results in incremental cost-effectiveness ratios of €14.26 per percent of diagnostic accuracy, and €23.88 per percent of correctly managed patients.[84]

An other preliminary study comparing PET/MRI head-to-head with other modalities found a favorable cost-to-benefit ratio. In the M staging of rectal cancer, whole-body 18F FDG PET/MRI is a cost-effective diagnostic alternative to standard of care imaging (defined as pelvic MRI + chest and abdominopelvic CT), with a slightly higher cost but comparable effectiveness, yielding an incremental cost-effectiveness ratio of $70,291 per QALY.[61]

In conclusion, when evaluating the cost-effectiveness of PET/MRI for abdominal imaging, it is clear that, despite its higher per-scan cost, PET/MRI is generally a cost-efficient choice in most clinical situations. The benefits of conducting the scan in a single session and its better diagnostic profile are reflected in the observed incremental cost-effectiveness ratios. However, further studies are needed to confirm the cost-effectiveness of PET/MRI in specific application areas.

SUMMARY

PET/MRI provides anatomical, functional, and metabolic tissue information with a single scan. Moreover, the high soft tissue contrast resolution and multiparametric sequences such as DWI increase the accuracy of the diagnosis. PET/MRI has demonstrated its equality or superiority in multiple cancers compared with standard-of-care imaging studies. With increased adoption and mounting evidence on cost-effectiveness, its role is likely to expand in oncologic and non-oncologic applications.

CLINICS CARE POINTS

- PET/MRI combines the superb soft-tissue contrast of MRI and the picomolar sensitivity of PET to provide a one-stop-shop assessment of several abdominal cancers
- PET/MRI is of particular utility in the evaluation of distant lymphadenopathy and liver metastases
- PET/MRI enables whole-body assessment with a lower radiation exposure than PET/CT
- PET/MRI is an emerging tool to guide the management of inflammatory bowel disease and differentiate between inflammatory and fibrotic strictures

DISCLOSURE

The authors declare that they have no conflict of interest.

REFERENCES

1. Pace L, Nicolai E, Aiello M, et al. Whole-body PET/MRI in oncology: current status and clinical applications. Clinical and Translational Imaging 2013;1(1):31–44.
2. Townsend DW, Carney JPJ, Yap JT, et al. PET/CT today and tomorrow. J Nucl Med 2004;45(1 suppl):4S–14S.
3. Carreras-Delgado JL, Pérez-Dueñas V, Riola-Parada C, et al. PET/MRI: a luxury or a necessity? Rev Española Med Nucl Imagen Mol 2016;35(5):313–20.
4. Catana C, Guimaraes AR, Rosen BR. PET and MR imaging: the odd couple or a match made in heaven? J Nucl Med 2013;54(5):815–24.
5. Attenberger U, Catana C, Chandarana H, et al. Whole-body FDG PET-MR oncologic imaging: pitfalls in clinical interpretation related to inaccurate MR-based attenuation correction. Abdom Imaging 2015;40(6):1374–86.
6. Delso G, Fürst S, Jakoby B, et al. Performance measurements of the Siemens mMR integrated whole-body PET/MR scanner. J Nucl Med 2011;52(12):1914–22.
7. Li Y, Beiderwellen K, Nensa F, et al. [18F]FDG PET/MR enterography for the assessment of inflammatory activity in Crohn's disease: comparison of different MRI and PET parameters. Eur J Nucl Med Mol Imaging 2018;45(8):1382–93.
8. Fernández-Friera L, Fuster V, López-Melgar B, et al. Vascular inflammation in subclinical atherosclerosis detected by hybrid PET/MRI. J Am Coll Cardiol 2019;73(12):1371–82.
9. Catalano OA, Nicolai E, Rosen BR, et al. Comparison of CE-FDG-PET/CT with CE-FDG-PET/MR in the evaluation of osseous metastases in breast cancer patients. Br J Cancer 2015;112(9):1452–60.
10. Catalano OA, Rosen BR, Sahani DV, et al. Clinical impact of PET/MR imaging in patients with cancer undergoing same-day PET/CT: initial experience in 134 patients–a hypothesis-generating exploratory study. Radiology 2013;269(3):857–69.
11. Zhang C, O'Shea A, Parente CA, et al. Evaluation of the diagnostic performance of positron emission tomography/magnetic resonance for the diagnosis of liver metastases. Invest Radiol 2021;56(10):621–8.
12. Furtado FS, Wu MZ, Esfahani SA, et al. Positron emission tomography/magnetic resonance imaging versus the standard of care imaging in the diagnosis of peritoneal carcinomatosis. Ann Surg 2022. https://doi.org/10.1097/SLA.0000000000005418.
13. Incoronato M, Grimaldi AM, Mirabelli P, et al. Circulating miRNAs in untreated breast cancer: an exploratory multimodality Morpho-functional study. Cancers 2019;11(6):876.
14. Incoronato M, Grimaldi AM, Cavaliere C, et al. Relationship between functional imaging and immunohistochemical markers and prediction of breast cancer subtype: a PET/MRI study. Eur J Nucl Med Mol Imaging 2018;45(10):1680–93.
15. Catalano OA, Horn GL, Signore A, et al. PET/MR in invasive ductal breast cancer: correlation between imaging markers and histological phenotype. Br J Cancer 2017;116(7):893–902.
16. Catalano OA, Masch WR, Catana C, et al. An overview of PET/MR, focused on clinical applications. Abdom Radiol (NY) 2017;42(2):631–44.
17. Jena A, Taneja S, Singh A, et al. Reliability of 18F-FDG PET metabolic parameters derived using simultaneous PET/MRI and correlation with prognostic factors of invasive ductal carcinoma: a feasibility study. AJR Am J Roentgenol 2017;209(3):662–70.
18. Morawitz J, Kirchner J, Martin O, et al. Prospective correlation of prognostic immunohistochemical markers with SUV and ADC derived from dedicated hybrid breast 18F-FDG PET/MRI in women with newly diagnosed breast cancer. Clin Nucl Med 2021;46(3):201–5.
19. Huang SY, Franc BL, Harnish RJ, et al. Exploration of PET and MRI radiomic features for decoding breast cancer phenotypes and prognosis. NPJ Breast Cancer 2018;4:24.
20. Ramalho M, AlObaidy M, Catalano OA, et al. MR-PET of the body: early experience and insights. Eur J Radiol Open 2014;1:28–39.
21. Martin O, Schaarschmidt BM, Kirchner J, et al. PET/MRI versus PET/CT for whole-body staging: results from a single-center observational study on 1,003 sequential examinations. J Nucl Med 2020;61(8):1131–6.
22. Atkinson W, Catana C, Abramson JS, et al. Hybrid FDG-PET/MR compared to FDG-PET/CT in adult lymphoma patients. Abdom Radiol (NY) 2016;41(7):1338–48.
23. Yoon JH, Lee JM, Chang W, et al. Initial M staging of rectal cancer: FDG PET/MRI with a hepatocyte-specific contrast agent versus contrast-enhanced CT. Radiology 2020;294(2):310–9.
24. Lee SI, Catalano OA, Dehdashti F. Evaluation of gynecologic cancer with MR imaging, 18F-FDG PET/CT, and PET/MR imaging. J Nucl Med 2015;56(3):436–43.
25. Amorim BJ, Hong TS, Blaszkowsky LS, et al. Clinical impact of PET/MR in treated colorectal cancer patients. Eur J Nucl Med Mol Imaging 2019;46(11):2260–9.
26. Ferrone C, Goyal L, Qadan M, et al. Management implications of fluorodeoxyglucose positron emission

tomography/magnetic resonance in untreated intrahepatic cholangiocarcinoma. Eur J Nucl Med Mol Imaging 2020;47(8):1871–84.

27. Furtado FS, Ferrone CR, Lee SI, et al. Impact of PET/MRI in the treatment of pancreatic adenocarcinoma: a retrospective cohort study. Mol Imaging Biol 2021; 23(3):456–66.

28. Catalano OA, Lee SI, Parente C, et al. Improving staging of rectal cancer in the pelvis: the role of PET/MRI. Eur J Nucl Med Mol Imaging 2021;48(4): 1235–45.

29. Fuin N, Catalano OA, Scipioni M, et al. Concurrent respiratory motion correction of abdominal PET and dynamic contrast-enhanced-MRI using a compressed sensing approach. J Nucl Med 2018; 59(9):1474–9.

30. Catalano OA, Umutlu L, Fuin N, et al. Comparison of the clinical performance of upper abdominal PET/DCE-MRI with and without concurrent respiratory motion correction (MoCo). Eur J Nucl Med Mol Imaging 2018;45(12):2147–54.

31. Chen Y, An H. Attenuation correction of PET/MR imaging. Magn Reson Imaging Clin N Am 2017;25(2): 245–55.

32. Berker Y, Franke J, Salomon A, et al. MRI-based attenuation correction for hybrid PET/MRI systems: a 4-class tissue segmentation technique using a combined ultrashort-echo-time/Dixon MRI sequence. J Nucl Med 2012;53(5):796–804.

33. Aznar MC, Sersar R, Saabye J, et al. Whole-body PET/MRI: the effect of bone attenuation during MR-based attenuation correction in oncology imaging. Eur J Radiol 2014;83(7):1177–83.

34. Fuin N, Pedemonte S, Catalano OA, et al. PET/MRI in the presence of metal implants: completion of the attenuation map from PET emission data. J Nucl Med 2017;58(5):840–5.

35. Choi SH, Kim SY, Park SH, et al. Diagnostic performance of CT, gadoxetate disodium-enhanced MRI, and PET/CT for the diagnosis of colorectal liver metastasis: Systematic review and meta-analysis. J Magn Reson Imaging 2018;47(5): 1237–50.

36. Vilgrain V, Esvan M, Ronot M, et al. A meta-analysis of diffusion-weighted and gadoxetic acid-enhanced MR imaging for the detection of liver metastases. Eur Radiol 2016;26(12):4595–615.

37. Furtado FS, Mercaldo ND, Vahle T, et al. Simultaneous multislice diffusion-weighted imaging versus standard diffusion-weighted imaging in whole-body PET/MRI. Eur Radiol 2022. https://doi.org/10.1007/s00330-022-09275-4.

38. Polycarpou I, Tsoumpas C, King AP, et al. Impact of respiratory motion correction and spatial resolution on lesion detection in PET: a simulation study based on real MR dynamic data. Phys Med Biol 2014;59(3): 697–713.

39. Li G, Schmidtlein CR, Burger IA, et al. Assessing and accounting for the impact of respiratory motion on FDG uptake and viable volume for liver lesions in free-breathing PET using respiration-suspended PET images as reference. Med Phys 2014;41.

40. Liu C, Pierce LA, Alessio AM, et al. The impact of respiratory motion on tumor quantification and delineation in static PET/CT imaging. Phys Med Biol 2009;54:7345–62.

41. Callahan J, Kron T, Siva S, et al. Geographic miss of lung tumours due to respiratory motion: a comparison of 3D vs 4D PET/CT defined target volumes. Radiat Oncol 2014;9(1):291.

42. Vander Heiden MG, Cantley LC, Thompson CB. Understanding the warburg effect: the metabolic requirements of cell proliferation. Science 2009; 324(5930):1029–33.

43. Buck AK, Reske SN. Cellular origin and molecular mechanisms of 18F-FDG uptake: is there a contribution of the endothelium? J Nucl Med 2004;45(3): 461e463.

44. Wadsak W, Mitterhauser M. Basics and principles of radiopharmaceuticals for PET/CT. Eur J Radiol 2010; 73(3):461–9.

45. Wang H, Zhu W, Ren S, et al. 68Ga-FAPI-04 versus 18F-FDG PET/CT in the detection of hepatocellular carcinoma. Front Oncol 2021;11:693640.

46. Guo W, Pang Y, Yao L, et al. Imaging fibroblast activation protein in liver cancer: a single-center post hoc retrospective analysis to compare [68Ga]Ga-FAPI-04 PET/CT versus MRI and [18F]-FDG PET/CT. Eur J Nucl Med Mol Imaging 2021;48(5):1604–17.

47. Pang Y, Zhao L, Luo Z, et al. Comparison of 68Ga-FAPI and 18F-FDG uptake in gastric, duodenal, and colorectal cancers. Radiology 2021;298(2):393–402.

48. Kuten J, Levine C, Shamni O, et al. Head-to-head comparison of [68Ga]Ga-FAPI-04 and [18F]-FDG PET/CT in evaluating the extent of disease in gastric adenocarcinoma. Eur J Nucl Med Mol Imaging 2022;49(2):743–50.

49. Veldhuijzen van Zanten SEM, Pieterman KJ, Wijnhoven BPL, et al. FAPI PET versus FDG PET, CT or MRI for staging pancreatic-, gastric- and cholangiocarcinoma: Systematic review and head-to-head comparisons of diagnostic performances. Diagnostics 2022;12(8):1958.

50. Hennrich U, Benešová M. [68Ga]Ga-DOTA-TOC: the first FDA-Approved 68Ga-radiopharmaceutical for PET imaging. Pharmaceuticals 2020;13(3). https://doi.org/10.3390/ph13030038.

51. Kroiss A, Putzer D, Decristoforo C, et al. 68Ga-DOTA-TOC uptake in neuroendocrine tumour and healthy tissue: differentiation of physiological uptake and pathological processes in PET/CT. Eur J Nucl Med Mol Imaging 2013;40(4):514–23.

52. Han S, Suh CH, Woo S, et al. Performance of 68Ga-DOTA-conjugated somatostatin receptor-targeting

peptide PET in detection of pheochromocytoma and paraganglioma: a systematic review and metaanalysis. J Nucl Med 2019;60(3):369–76.

53. Lee G, Hoseok I, Kim SJ, et al. Clinical implication of PET/MR imaging in preoperative esophageal cancer staging: comparison with PET/CT, endoscopic ultrasonography, and CT. J Nucl Med 2014;55(8):1242–7.

54. Bruzzi JF, Munden RF, Truong MT, et al. PET/CT of esophageal cancer: its role in clinical management. Radiographics 2007;27(6):1635–52.

55. Yu CW, Chen XJ, Lin YH, et al. Prognostic value of 18F-FDG PET/MR imaging biomarkers in oesophageal squamous cell carcinoma. Eur J Radiol 2019;120(108671):108671.

56. Matthews R, Choi M. Clinical utility of positron emission tomography magnetic resonance imaging (PET-MRI) in gastrointestinal cancers. Diagnostics 2016;6(3):35.

57. Liu Y, Zheng D, Liu JJ, et al. Comparing PET/MRI with PET/CT for pretreatment staging of gastric cancer. Gastroenterol Res Pract 2019;2019:9564627.

58. Catalano OA, Coutinho AM, Sahani DV, et al. Colorectal cancer staging: comparison of whole-body PET/CT and PET/MR. Abdom Radiol (NY) 2017;42(4):1141–51.

59. Simmonds PC, Primrose JN, Colquitt JL, et al. Surgical resection of hepatic metastases from colorectal cancer: a systematic review of published studies. Br J Cancer 2006;94(7):982–99.

60. Furtado FS, Suarez-Weiss KE, Vangel M, et al. Clinical impact of PET/MRI in oligometastatic colorectal cancer. Br J Cancer 2021. https://doi.org/10.1038/s41416-021-01494-8.

61. Gassert FG, Rübenthaler J, Cyran CC, et al. 18F FDG PET/MRI with hepatocyte-specific contrast agent for M staging of rectal cancer: a primary economic evaluation. Eur J Nucl Med Mol Imaging 2021;48(10):3268–76.

62. Joo I, Lee JM, Lee DH, et al. Preoperative assessment of pancreatic cancer with FDG PET/MR imaging versus FDG PET/CT plus contrast-enhanced multidetector CT: a prospective preliminary study. Radiology 2017;282(1):149–59.

63. Yeh R, Dercle L, Garg I, et al. The role of 18F-FDG PET/CT and PET/MRI in pancreatic ductal adenocarcinoma. Abdom Radiol (NY) 2018;43(2):415–34.

64. Kittaka H, Takahashi H, Ohigashi H, et al. Role of (18)F-fluorodeoxyglucose positron emission tomography/computed tomography in predicting the pathologic response to preoperative chemoradiation therapy in patients with resectable T3 pancreatic cancer. World J Surg 2013;37(1):169–78.

65. Chen BB, Tien YW, Chang MC, et al. PET/MRI in pancreatic and periampullary cancer: correlating diffusion-weighted imaging, MR spectroscopy and glucose metabolic activity with clinical stage and prognosis. Eur J Nucl Med Mol Imaging 2016;43(10):1753–64.

66. Hofman MS, Lau WFE, Hicks RJ. Somatostatin receptor imaging with 68Ga DOTATATE PET/CT: clinical utility, normal patterns, pearls, and pitfalls in interpretation. Radiographics 2015;35(2):500–16.

67. Hope TA, Bergsland EK, Bozkurt MF, et al. Appropriate use criteria for somatostatin receptor PET imaging in neuroendocrine tumors. J Nucl Med 2018;59(1):66–74.

68. Boland GWL, Dwamena BA, Jagtiani Sangwaiya M, et al. Characterization of adrenal masses by using FDG PET: a systematic review and meta-analysis of diagnostic test performance. Radiology 2011;259(1):117–26.

69. Song JH, Chaudhry FS, Mayo-Smith WW. The incidental adrenal mass on CT: prevalence of adrenal disease in 1,049 consecutive adrenal masses in patients with no known malignancy. AJR Am J Roentgenol 2008;190(5):1163–8.

70. Schaarschmidt BM, Grueneisen J, Heusch P, et al. Does 18F-FDG PET/MRI reduce the number of indeterminate abdominal incidentalomas compared with 18F-FDG PET/CT? Nucl Med Commun 2015;36(6):588–95.

71. Blake MA, Cronin CG, Boland GW. Adrenal imaging. AJR Am J Roentgenol 2010;194(6):1450–60.

72. Xu S, Pan Y, Zhou J, et al. Integrated PET/MRI with 68Ga-DOTATATE and 18F-FDG in pheochromocytomas and paragangliomas: An initial study. Clin Nucl Med 2022;47(4):299–304.

73. Patel S, Cheek S, Osman H, et al. MRI with gadoxetate disodium for colorectal liver metastasis: is it the new "imaging modality of choice". J Gastrointest Surg 2014;18(12):2130–5.

74. Guniganti P, Kierans AS. PET/MRI of the hepatobiliary system: review of techniques and applications. Clin Imaging 2021;71:160–9.

75. Reiner CS, Stolzmann P, Husmann L, et al. Protocol requirements and diagnostic value of PET/MR imaging for liver metastasis detection. Eur J Nucl Med Mol Imaging 2014;41(4):649–58.

76. Beiderwellen K, Geraldo L, Ruhlmann V, et al. Accuracy of [18F]FDG PET/MRI for the detection of liver metastases. PLoS One 2015;10(9):e0137285.

77. Neeff H, Hörth W, Makowiec F, et al. Outcome after resection of hepatic and pulmonary metastases of colorectal cancer. J Gastrointest Surg 2009;13(10):1813–20.

78. Wei AC, Greig PD, Grant D, et al. Survival after hepatic resection for colorectal metastases: a 10-year experience. Ann Surg Oncol 2006;13(5):668–76.

79. Tomlinson JS, Jarnagin WR, DeMatteo RP, et al. Actual 10-year survival after resection of colorectal liver metastases defines cure. J Clin Oncol 2007;25(29):4575–80.

80. Le Fur M, Zhou IY, Catalano O, et al. Toward molecular imaging of intestinal pathology. Inflamm Bowel Dis 2020;26(10):1470–84.

81. Catalano OA, Wu V, Mahmood U, et al. Diagnostic performance of PET/MR in the evaluation of active inflammation in Crohn disease. Am J Nucl Med Mol Imaging 2018;8(1):62–9.

82. Pellino G, Nicolai E, Catalano OA, et al. PET/MR Versus PET/CT imaging: impact on the clinical management of small-bowel crohn's disease. J Crohns Colitis 2016;10(3):277–85.

83. Catalano OA, Gee MS, Nicolai E, et al. Evaluation of quantitative PET/MR enterography biomarkers for discrimination of inflammatory strictures from fibrotic strictures in Crohn disease. Radiology 2016;278(3): 792–800.

84. Mayerhoefer ME, Prosch H, Beer L, et al. PET/MRI versus PET/CT in oncology: a prospective single-center study of 330 examinations focusing on implications for patient management and cost considerations. Eur J Nucl Med Mol Imaging 2020; 47(1):51–60.

Clinical Value of Hybrid PET/MR Imaging
Brain Imaging Using PET/MR Imaging

Aurélie Kas, MD, PhD[a,b,*], Laura Rozenblum, MD[a,b],
Nadya Pyatigorskaya, MD, PhD[c,d]

KEYS WORDS

• Hybrid PET/MR imaging • Brain tumors • Epilepsy • Neurodegenerative dementia • Parkinsonism

KEY POINTS

- PET/MR imaging offers optimal alignment of PET and MR imaging data, synergistic integration of findings from both modalities, streamlined clinical workflow, and convenience for patients and caregivers.
- In neuro-oncology, clinical utility of PET/MR imaging is established in distinguishing between radio-necrosis and tumor progression and is increasingly recognized for defining tumor extent, assisting with grading, aiding genotype determination, guiding biopsy site selection, and evaluating patient prognosis.
- PET/MR imaging improves the diagnosis of neurodegenerative dementia, especially in cases of co-morbidities, and aids in the differential diagnosis.
- PET/MR imaging emerges as a transformative tool for diagnosing atypical parkinsonism, enhancing diagnostic precision and providing insights into disease pathophysiology.
- PET/MR imaging significantly enhances the detection of previously unidentified epileptic lesions, directly impacting treatment planning.

INTRODUCTION

Hybrid PET/magnetic resonance (MR) has emerged as a powerful tool in a wide range of neurologic applications. PET/MR offers particular advantages for brain imaging compared with PET/computed tomography (CT), as MRI is the modality of choice for assessing brain tumors, cognitive impairment, and epilepsy, which are the most prevalent indications for brain PET studies in clinical settings. With high spatial-resolution and soft tissue contrast, MR is more suitable than CT for assessing small anatomic structures, detecting subtle changes, and segmenting regions to extract quantitative parameters. It also offers a wide range of quantitative and functional information, such as water and metabolite diffusion, metabolite concentrations, regional perfusion, and activation. Furthermore, MR imaging does not expose patients to additional ionizing radiation, making it particularly beneficial in pediatric patients.[1] PET imaging has separate ability to visualize physiologic functions and neurotransmitter systems that are crucial for understanding central nervous system diseases, and new radiopharmaceuticals targeting protein aggregates have led to increasing interest in the use of PET in dementia. In clinical practice, PET has been widely adopted for the diagnosis and monitoring of neurodegenerative diseases, brain tumors, and localizing epileptic

[a] Department of Nuclear Medicine, Pitié-Salpêtrière Hospital, APHP Sorbonne Université, Paris, France;
[b] Sorbonne Université, INSERM, CNRS, Laboratoire d'Imagerie Biomédicale, LIB, Paris F-75006, France;
[c] Neuroradiology Department, Pitié-Salpêtrière Hospital, APHP Sorbonne Université, Paris, France;
[d] Sorbonne Université, UMR S 1127, CNRS UMR 722, Institut du Cerveau, Paris, France
* Corresponding author. Nuclear medicine department, 47-83 boulevard de l'Hôpital, Pitié-Salpêtrière Hospital, Paris 75013, France.
E-mail address: aurelie.kas@aphp.fr

Magn Reson Imaging Clin N Am 31 (2023) 591–604
https://doi.org/10.1016/j.mric.2023.06.004
1064-9689/23/© 2023 Elsevier Inc. All rights reserved.

focus in drug-resistant partial epilepsy. Moreover, it serves as a valuable complementary tool to MR imaging in neuroinflammatory conditions, such as autoimmune encephalitis.[2]

he most important advantage of PET/MR imaging is the integrated use of high-resolution MR imaging data with molecular data provided by PET, with optimal temporal and spatial alignment between both modalities. Although it is possible to coregister brain PET/CT images with MR imaging acquired separately, this remains time-consuming and difficult to implement for consecutive PET/CT studies in high patient flow. In addition, retrospective reviews of separate MR imaging and PET may result in discrepancies with prior reports, which then require additional effort and time to reconcile the differences. In practice, both studies are often interpreted by 2 different specialists without an opportunity for consensus, and the integration of separate conclusions is often left to the referring clinician.[3,4] With PET/MR imaging, both modalities are interpreted simultaneously, and the report is made concurrently during a single reading session; having consistent findings between PET and MR imaging enhances readers confidence and prompts them to explicitly state the imaging diagnosis in their final reports. The sequential approach also assumes that no modification in pathologic conditions has occurred between 2 imaging sessions. Hybrid PET/MR imaging inherently overcomes this limitation.

For patients and caregivers too, PET/MR imaging provides several practical benefits that should not be underestimated. The combination of both examinations in a single session is advantageous for elderly patients and others with advanced disorders who may be unable to undergo multiple imaging sessions. Mukku and colleagues[5] noted that PET/MR imaging may reduce the need for sedation in cognitively impaired patients owing to the reduced scanning time. This also benefits their caregivers, as it reduces the number of appointments to imaging centers, thereby minimizing the need for them to take time off work. The convenience of hybrid PET/MR imaging compared with separate PET and MR imaging was reported by 88% of patients and caregivers.[6]

TECHNICAL CONSIDERATIONS

PET/MR systems produce brain PET images of comparable quality to that obtained from PET/CT systems. When compared with the brain-dedicated HRRT system, one of the highest-resolution PET scanners, the PET/MR system, exhibited similar performance in terms of recovery coefficients, while also exhibiting lower voxel-level noise. The comparison of in vivo human data further confirmed the comparability of these systems.[7] Notably, because of the high sensitivity of PET (MR imaging) detectors, it is feasible to reduce the injected dose in clinical brain PET/MR imaging studies without compromising diagnostic performance or image quality.[8]

Improvements have been made in attenuation correction (AC) methods in the clinic. In addition to the single-atlas–based method, zero echo time or ultrashort echo time MR-based AC methods are now implemented to correct for bone attenuation. They provide quantitatively acceptable results compared with CT-based AC.[9] In a multicenter study comparing 11 AC methods, including vendor-implemented ones, the best performing techniques showed only slight differences of a few percent.[10] Regarding adults with normal anatomy, the AC problem in PET/MR imaging is now widely considered to be solved.

Head motion can significantly degrade image quality. To address this issue, various methods have been developed. Some methods use external tracking devices, including optical tracking, to monitor the patient's head or directly track the patient's head to correct for rigid motion.[11] Another method, known as fully data-driven motion correction, can detect and correct motion with high accuracy (<1 mm) and high-temporal resolution.[12] This approach retrospectively corrects PET data and does not require changes to the acquisition protocol or additional motion-tracking hardware. For translations up to 2 cm and rotations up to 45°, this approach provides comparable results with optical feature-recognition method.[13] Recently, Spangler-Bickell and colleagues[12] demonstrated that data-driven motion correction had a significant impact on brain PET images reconstruction, both qualitatively and quantitatively, with 80% of all data sets improved from diagnostically unacceptable to acceptable after correction. Another approach involves coregistering multicontrast MR images with PET, using dynamic MR sequences with high resolution, such as blood oxygenation level-dependent (BOLD) or Echo Planar Imaging, as image navigators. These sequences track head movements and provide high-temporal-resolution motion estimates during neuroimaging examinations.[14]

Structural MR imaging can also be used for PET images for partial volume effects[15] and can also be automatically segmented to extract regional quantitative measures from PET images. Absolute quantification of dynamic PET can be achieved without invasive arterial blood sampling, by calculating the image-derived input function (IDIF) using perfusion-MR imaging[16] or through MR-based segmentation of the internal carotid artery.[17] Another example of PET/MR synergy is the simultaneous use of 18F-fluorodeoxyglucose PET (FDG-PET) with BOLD–functional MR imaging (fMR imaging) to improve temporal resolution in FDG-PET imaging. In addition, comparing FDG-PET activation with BOLD-fMR imaging activation can enhance the understanding of the underlying physiologic processes.

CLINICAL UTILITY IN NEUROLOGIC CONDITIONS
PET/MR Imaging in Brain Tumor Management

MR imaging is the primary imaging technique for initial assessment and follow-up of gliomas.[18–20] Typically, imaging protocols include morphologic sequences with precontrast and postcontrast T1-weighted imaging (WI), fluid-attenuated inversion recovery (FLAIR), and T2WI. However, morphologic MR imaging is less reliable after surgical procedures, radiation therapy, or chemotherapy owing to increasing incidence of treatment-induced signal changes caused by inflammation, edema, or ischemia. Advanced techniques, like perfusion-weighted imaging (PWI) and diffusion-weighted imaging (DWI), have been proposed to improve diagnostic accuracy, but doubts remain in many cases. The significant role of PET using radiolabeled amino acids and FDG in managing gliomas has been endorsed in the joint European Association of Nuclear Medicine (EANM)/European Association of Neuro-Oncology (EANO)/Response Assessment in Neuro-Oncology (RANO) practice guidelines.[21,22] PET/MR imaging systems offer the combined benefits of functional and anatomic imaging, improving accuracy in various steps of patient management, including biopsies, radiation treatment planning, predicting outcomes, and guiding chemotherapy.[23]

In the first or preoperative assessment, delineation of tumor extension is important, because it affects the recurrence rate and prognosis.[24] Conventional MR imaging using contrast-enhanced T1WI and FLAIR sequences may not always provide reliable delineation of tumor extension.[25,26] Advanced techniques and the use of PET imaging have been suggested as potential solutions for this purpose. Using PET/MR imaging with DWI sequences and O-(2–18F-fluoroethyl)-L-tyrosine PET imaging (FET-PET), a greater tumor extension could be detected than that one with conventional MR imaging alone or with FET-PET alone, whereas for the low-grade tumors FLAIR-MR imaging has shown its superiority to FET-PET in delineation of tumor infiltration.[27] The same was observed with simultaneous analysis of MR perfusion relative cerebral blood volume (rCBV) and FET-PET or arterial spin labeling (ASL)-based rCBF and 6-fluoro-(18F)-L-DOPA PET (DOPA-PET).[28,29] MR-based clusters did not anatomically match areas of increased tracer uptake, indicating different underlying pathophysiological mechanisms. MR imaging enhancement suggests blood-brain barrier disruption; high DWI signal indicates hypercellularity, and increased rCBV relates to neoangiogenesis. Also, enhanced amino acid uptake in endothelial walls correlates with FET or DOPA uptake.[30]

Accurate grading of glioma is crucial but challenging owing to sampling bias and intratumoral heterogeneity. Advanced MR imaging techniques provide moderate diagnostic accuracy, but invasive biopsies are still required for definitive histologic diagnosis. Leveraging the synergy of PET/MR imaging biomarkers offers a noninvasive and comprehensive approach to tumor characterization. Recent evidence from the study by Göttler and colleagues[31] involving 30 de novo gliomas indicated that FET-PET/MR imaging could detect areas of higher biological malignancy based on FET uptake and rCBV perfusion. Likewise, a prospective study involving 38 biopsy samples, that underwent DOPA-PET/MR imaging, demonstrated that combined PET/MR imaging could detect high-grade tumor subregions with a sensitivity of 58%, compared with 42% with MR imaging alone.[32]

The World Health Organization classification updates of brain tumors emphasize the importance of molecular markers like IDH1 mutation or CDKN2A/B deletion.[20] Multimodal MR and PET imaging have been investigated for predicting genotype alterations associated with molecular markers, including IDH gene mutation, 1p/19q chromosome arm loss of heterozygosity, and MGMT promoter. MR spectroscopy (MRS) enables the assessment of metabolites such as NAA, creatine, choline, lipids, lactates, and recently, 2-hydroxyglutarate (2-HG). In high-grade gliomas, NAA and creatine are decreased along with an increase in choline, lipids, and lactate.[33] Combined PET/MR imaging studies have demonstrated that the accuracy of tumor characterization could be increased when conventional MR imaging is combined with FET-PET and single-voxel MRS.[34] The accumulation of 2-HG is caused by gene mutations encoding the enzyme isocitrate dehydrogenase (IDH). Recent studies have shown that this marker can specifically predict the IDH mutation,[23] but technique remains challenging. Bumes and colleagues[35] used FET-PET maps during simultaneous PET/MR imaging to localize the 2-HG spectroscopy to the most hypermetabolic cluster, resulting in excellent accuracy of 88.2% for predicting IDH status. This synergy is particularly interesting because the spectroscopy results directly depend on the voxel positioning. For other biomarkers, Song and colleagues[24] demonstrated that the combined use of FET-PET and CBV could accurately distinguish between IDH-mutant astrocytoma and IDH-wildtype glioblastoma (area under the curve [AUC] of 0.903) in a cohort of 52 newly diagnosed glioma patients. Cheng and colleagues[36] used tandem FET-PET and DWI-MR imaging to predict tumor grade and IDH1, TERT, and EGFR mutation statuses.

MR imaging fingerprinting allows for the quantification of T1W and T2W maps, providing access to multiple tissue properties. Combining multiparametric data, including FET-PET and fingerprinting data, with machine learning techniques has demonstrated excellent diagnostic performance in predicting various genetic markers, such as MGMT promoter methylation, IDH mutation, 1p19q codeletion, and IDH1 mutation status.[37] Deep learning algorithms improve genotype prediction and enhance PET/MR imaging synergy. FET-PET/MR imaging and textural parameters achieved diagnostic accuracy as high as 93%.[38]

Radiomics analysis improves diagnostic performance by extracting quantitative features and correlating them with tumor histology and patient outcomes. In Zhang and colleagues,[39] the clinical radiomics-integrated model using FDG-PET, 3-dimensional (3D) contrast-enhanced T1WI, and DWI information achieved promising performance in predicting the ATRX mutation status of IDH-mutant low-grade glioma. Nevertheless, further validation and standardization are needed for PET-MR–based radiomics to become a clinical decision-making tool and potentially replace the need for biopsy.

Amide proton transfer-weighted (APTw) chemical exchange saturation transfer (CEST) magnetic resonance imaging (MRI) is sensitive to protein and peptide concentrations, providing indirect access to tumor cellularity. It shows promise in tumor grading and recurrence detection and has potential when combined with PET imaging.[40] The most malignant parts of a tumor have been shown to correlate with tumor cellularity for both APTw and FET-PET, whereas rCBV, as well as FET-PET, correlates with vascularity.[40] This suggests that although both APT and FET-PET provide information on cellularity, each marker can offer complementary information. This is consistent with da Silva and colleagues,[41] who suggest that APT and FET uptake does not colocalize, shows no correlation, and therefore seems to provide different biological information. Recently, Paprottka and colleagues[42] demonstrated that using an automatic Random Forest classifier with PET-FET and multimodal MR imaging data, including DSC perfusion and APT, improved diagnostic accuracy.

Although FDG-PET is poorly used for glioma imaging owing to its low specificity, the addition of simultaneous multimodal MR imaging can improve its performance, achieving excellent diagnostic accuracy when combining morphologic imaging with ASL perfusion[43] or using rCBV, diffusion, and spectroscopy.[44] Therefore, this reliable and cost-saving tracer could serve as a practical alternative in situations where amino acid tracers are unavailable.

PET/MR imaging has a promising application in target delineation for radiation therapy, improving tumor delineation and treatment planning by combining FET-PET with MR imaging–based parameters. This enables functionally guided dose painting in high-risk recurrence areas and shows higher delineation performance compared with individual markers, including FET-PET, diffusion, spectroscopy, and rCBV[45], with the lowest input for diffusion.

Combined PET and MR imaging have shown superiority over individual modalities in differentiating between tumor progression and treatment-related necrosis in glioma lesions, with studies reporting higher diagnostic accuracy for the combined modality compared with MR imaging alone[29,46–48] (Fig. 1). Bertaux and colleagues[48] demonstrated the value of morphometabolic parameters with DOPA-PET and ASL for distinguishing true progression from treatment-related changes in a cohort of 76 patients with an accuracy of 87%. Recently, Smith and colleagues[46] demonstrated the positive impact of FET-PET/MR imaging on clinical care in a cohort of 88 patients with brain tumors. They reported an overall diagnostic accuracy for difficult diagnostic cases of 86% for the combined modality (hybrid FET-PET/MR imaging with perfusion), as opposed to 66% for MR imaging alone. Similarly, Steidl and colleagues[47] showed that the combination of amino acid PET and rCBV map improved diagnostic accuracy over each modality individually.

PET/MR imaging scans are being investigated for monitoring gliomas during chemotherapy, with studies indicating that the persistence of FET-PET uptake in tumors without contrast enhancement after bevacizumab and radiotherapy may be associated with unfavorable outcomes.[49] In addition, FET-PET/MR imaging has shown potential in complementing MR imaging–based RANO criteria for assessing response and

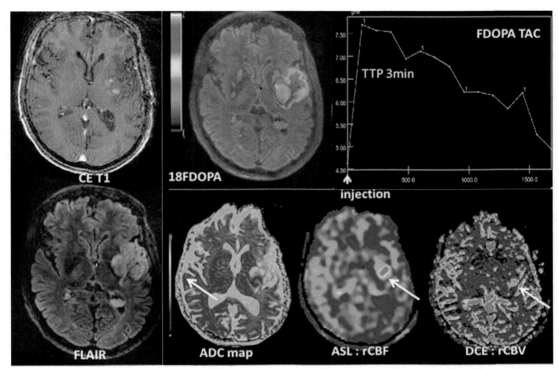

Fig. 1. DOPA-PET/MR imaging in a suspected recurrence of oligodendroglioma. Suspicion of glioma recurrence in a 35-year-old woman with previously treated grade 2 oligodendroglioma. DOPA-PET/MR imaging reveals mild postcontrast enhancement in the left lenticular region, along with a large FLAIR hypersignal and increased DOPA uptake extending to the insula. The DOPA hot spot is spatially matched with the area showing a low ADC value on DWI-MR imaging and high perfusion on PWI-MR imaging. The time activity curve of DOPA uptake demonstrates a short time to peak and rapid washout, further supporting the diagnosis of a recurrent high-grade glioma.

predicting prognosis in recurrent glioma patients receiving Lomustine-based chemotherapy or Regorafenib treatment.[50] In low-grade tumors without blood-brain barrier breakdown and lower FET-PET uptake, evaluating treatment response becomes more challenging, emphasizing the need to use all available biomarkers for better diagnostic accuracy.[30]

For other cerebral neoplasms, such as primary central nervous system lymphoma and brain metastases, the role of PET/MR imaging is primarily being explored in the context of radiomics, with the goal of improving differential diagnosis capabilities.[51]

ROLE OF PET/MR IN NEURODEGENERATIVE DISORDERS
Dementia

Dementia is a major cause of disability among the elderly, with Alzheimers disease (AD) accounting for 60% to 80% of cases. In patients with suspected dementia, MR imaging plays a crucial role in identifying potentially treatable causes and in identifying coexisting vascular lesions or post-traumatic injuries. It also assesses the volume of the hippocampus and can identify specific patterns of atrophy and signal abnormality. PET imaging is able to detect abnormalities associated with AD or other types of dementia before structural changes occur. Numerous studies have validated FDG-PET to predict progression from mild cognitive impairment (MCI) to AD and to distinguish different types of dementia, such as frontotemporal dementia (FTD), based on distinctive hypometabolism patterns. Combining FDG-PET with MR imaging has been shown to better predict conversion of MCI to AD compared with either MR imaging or PET alone.

As PET and MR are complementary, synergistic information is expected in neurodegenerative dementia from the combination of both. First, the fusion of PET with MR imaging produces high-resolution images that improve PET analysis and enable the detection of anomalies in very small structures, as illustrated Fig. 2. In Carlson and

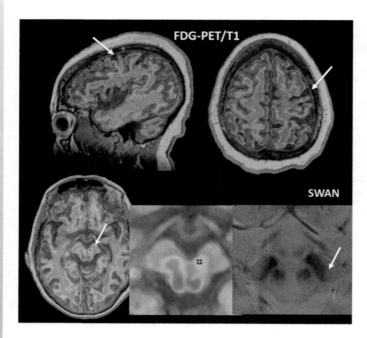

Fig. 2. FDG-PET/MR imaging in a suspected case of CBD. A 60-year-old man presents with atypical parkinsonian syndrome. FDG-PET/MR imaging identified small but spatially matched anomalies in the left precentral cortex (*white arrow*) and left midbrain (*white arrow*). Furthermore, the loss of nigral dorsolateral hypersignal on MR imaging (*swallow tail sign*) as shown by the white arrow indicates dopaminergic nigrostriatal denervation, consistent with the diagnosis of CBD. SWAN, susceptibility-weighted angiography.

colleagues,[52] the subfield analysis of hippocampus using FDG-PET/MR demonstrated structural and metabolism changes—specifically in the dentate gyrus and cornu ammonis—in AD and MCI. Others studies have demonstrated the ability of PET/MR to investigate previously unexplored regions with PET/CT, such as the mammillary bodies[53] or brainstem.[54]

FDG-PET/MR imaging holds great potential for complex diagnoses. Structural MR imaging changes are observed in advanced stages of common dementias but lack specificity in early disease stages. The presence of specific hypometabolism patterns (eg, associative parietotemporal cortex in AD, frontotemporal cortex in FTD[55]) along with subtle regional cortical volume loss can enhance reader's confidence in the imaging diagnosis for patients with mild to moderate cognitive impairment. Hippocampal atrophy, although commonly associated with AD, is not highly specific. Primary age-related tauopathy and limbic-predominant age-related TDP-43 encephalopathy, seizures with or without hippocampal sclerosis, or other conditions,[53] can also lead to hippocampal atrophy. The simultaneous visualization of FDG-PET with structural MR imaging provides valuable feedback to radiologists, potentially changing their interpretation of subtle findings. This feedback from MR imaging in FDG-PET/MR imaging can also enhance diagnostic accuracy for age-related coexisting pathologic conditions in patients with suspected dementia. It assists in identifying cortical

hypometabolism caused by stroke, microhemorrhages, or other brain injuries, thereby increasing diagnostic specificity. This capability helps differentiate between vascular and neurodegenerative dementia. In addition, it enables the study of deafferentation mechanisms in both vascular diseases and neurodegenerative conditions.[56]

Several studies have supported the role of FDG-PET/MR imaging in patients with AD, FTD, vascular dementia, Lewy body disease (LBD), and corticobasal degeneration (CBD).[57–60] The diagnosis utility of FDG-PET/MR imaging was examined in patients with MCI or dementia. In 90.5% of these patients, hypometabolism and structural atrophy were consistent with clinical diagnoses, providing valuable assistance in dementia subtyping and patient management.[5] Comparative studies evaluating the diagnostic accuracy of FDG-PET/MR versus FDG-PET/CT are scarce. In Kaltoft and colleagues,[61] hybrid FDG-PET/MR imaging detected a higher incidence of vascular pathologic condition in 35% of memory clinic patients compared with FDG-PET/CT. This resulted in a change in the interpretation of FDG-PET for 17% of patients and influenced the management of 22% of patients. In addition, reader confidence ratings for diagnostic classification were higher for PET/MR compared with PET/CT. Interestingly, these results were obtained using an abbreviated FDG-PET/MR imaging protocol that only included axial T2W and 3D T1W sequences in the MR imaging protocol.

Combining voxelwise analyses of FDG-PET/MR biomarkers can further improve dementia diagnosis compared with unimodal approaches. Classification accuracies based on multimodal voxelwise regional patterns were 77.5% for AD, 82.5% for FTD, 97.5% for semantic dementia, and 87.5% for nonfluent variant of primary progressive aphasia, compared with other syndromes.[62] Gupta and colleagues[63] successfully predicted the conversion of MCI to AD with an accuracy of nearly 94% by combining FDG-PET, structural MR imaging, cerebrospinal fluid biomarker findings, and Apolipoprotein-E genotype using machine learning techniques.

Other radiopharmaceuticals enable targeting specific pathologic processes in clinical settings, such as cortical amyloid load in AD (amyloid-PET), using 18F-florbetaben, 18F-flutemetamol, or 18F-florbetapir, or nigrostriatal dopaminergic deficit with DOPA-PET. Radiopharmaceuticals targeting neurofibrillary tangles in tauopathy are currently limited to research. In clinical practice, amyloid-PET/MR imaging can provide both amyloid load (with PET) and neuronal degeneration (with medial temporal lobe atrophy on MR imaging) in a single imaging session. The feasibility of this one-stop imaging approach was demonstrated in 100 patients with clinical diagnoses of MCI, AD dementia, and frontotemporal lobe dementia. PET/MR imaging assisted in diagnostic categorization in 67% of patients, and 82% of the referrers reported that PET/MR imaging findings had a significant impact on their final diagnosis.[6]

Advanced MR imaging techniques also allow for the measurement of brain connectivity and cerebral perfusion with ASL sequences without the need for intravenous contrast. Some studies have reported that ASL-MR imaging could provide comparable diagnostic information to FDG-PET in patients with AD[64–66] and FTD[67,68] because of the coupling of perfusion to glucose metabolism. Their respective accuracies for diagnosing FTD were compared with PET/MR imaging. ASL detected similar spatial patterns of abnormalities in individual patients compared with FDG-PET; however, its sensitivity was found to be lower.[69] Regional and quantitative anomalies with ASL were found to be similar to FDG-PET in patients with AD, but ASL performed worse than FDG-PET in patients with MCI.[70] Similarly, the direct comparison between enhanced multiplane tagging ASL and FDG-PET found that PET performed better compared with ASL in terms of sensitivity and reader confidence, as well as volume and intensity of abnormalities for the diagnosis of AD, LBD, and FTD.[71,72] However, diagnostic accuracy between both modalities was similar when performing semiquantitative analyses. ASL may still serve as a complement to neuroreceptor or protein deposition PET/MR studies in clinical practice when a single simultaneous investigation is warranted.

MR imaging is the most established modality for in vivo investigation of brain connectivity. Hybrid PET/MR enables a more comprehensive assessment of brain dysfunction in neurodegenerative disorders by optimizing the comparison between MR/PET metrics. In a single session, structural connectivity within white matter tracts and functional connectivity within the default mode network can be explored, along with measurements of glucose consumption, abnormal Tau, or amyloid deposition. This area represents a current focal point of active research in neurodegenerative dementia.

Parkinsonism

The diagnosis of parkinsonian syndrome poses challenges, particularly in the early stages of the disease. Although 123I-FP-CIT SPECT and DOPA-PET are used to assess presynaptic dopaminergic neuron loss, they are limited in differentiating between Parkinson disease (PD) and atypical parkinsonism. When PD is suspected, MR imaging in clinical practice is mostly used to withdraw differential diagnosis, including atypical parkinsonism forms. Volumetric sequences can reveal specific volume loss patterns, such as mesencephalic volume loss in progressive supranuclear palsy (PSP), putamen or pons volume loss in multiple system atrophy (MSA), or frontoparietal asymmetrical volume loss in CBD (see **Fig. 2**). Putamen and pons signal abnormalities can also be observed in MSA.[72] Nevertheless, all these aspects may be subtle, especially in the early stages of the disease. Recently, more specific presynaptic dopaminergic neuron loss biomarkers have been developed, including the loss of dorsolateral nigral hyperintensity on high-resolution 3D T2* sequence or the absence of high neuromelanin signal in the substantia nigra(SN) on spin-echo T1W sequence.[73] However, these signs cannot differentiate between parkinsonism syndromes as well as DOPA-PET. FDG-PET can be informative in atypical parkinsonism, with typical patterns of metabolism; however, its sensitivity and specificity remain moderate.[74] Consequently, combining PET with MR imaging, including structural, iron, perfusion, diffusion, or functional imaging, as well as artificial intelligence algorithms not only can increase diagnostic accuracy but also can lead to better understanding on the disease physiopathology. In this context, Shang and colleagues[75] used DOPA-PET/MR imaging to simultaneously analyze the putaminal metabolism using DOPA-PET and microstructure using diffusion tractography imaging (DTI). Significant associations between DTI metrics and motor performance were mediated by putaminal DOPA-PET depletion, suggesting that molecular degeneration mediates the microstructural disorganization and motor dysfunction in the early stages of PD. Another study on DOPA-PET MR imaging with neuromelanin and iron analysis found[76] positive correlation between dopaminergic function as observed by DOPA-PET and neuromelanin signal in lateral SN, indicating that dopaminergic function impairment progresses with depigmentation in the SN. It has been shown that quantitative analysis of DOPA-PET, especially using machine learning algorithms, was considerably improved by precise MR-based putamen segmentation.[77] In another study using dopamine transporter PET, gray matter density using voxel-based morphometry was correlated to dopaminergic degeneration, suggesting compensatory changes between clinical phenotypes and spatial patterns of neurodegeneration.[78]

PET/MR imaging can aid in the differential diagnosis between PD and MSA. Hu and colleagues[79] found an AUC of 0.96 when using the radiomics signature derived from metabolic (FDG), structural (T1WI), and susceptibility-WI provided by hybrid PET/MR imaging to distinguish between PD and MSA.

PET/MR imaging has also been used as a tool for validating MR imaging sequences, which can be beneficial when PET imaging is not accessible. In patients with PD, perfusion and metabolic covariance patterns were identified using pseudo continuous Arterial Spin Labeling (PCASL) and FDG-PET, indicating that PCASL holds promise as a potential biomarker for early PD diagnosis.[80]

To enhance specificity of differential diagnosis, radiopharmaceuticals are under development for TAU-PET. TAU-PET/MR imaging could improve imaging specificity for tauopathies, such as PSP and CBD, providing deeper insights into their pathophysiology. However, certain tracers, like 18F-AV-1451, still face challenges owing to off-target binding. New-generation tracers, such as 18F-PI-2620, in addition to structural MR imaging have shown high accuracy for early PSP diagnosis.[81]

PET/MR Imaging in Epilepsy

Epilepsy affects approximately 1% to 2% of the global population, with one-third of cases being medically refractory. Surgery is the most effective treatment for drug-resistant focal epilepsy. However, its success depends on accurately identifying the epileptogenic focus, which can be challenging, as structural lesions may be subtle or undetectable on MR imaging scans in approximately one-third of patients.[82] Temporal lobe epilepsy (TLE) has a better prognosis than extratemporal lobe epilepsy (ETLE), as they are more easily identified on presurgical imaging, increasing the likelihood of a complete lesion resection.[83]

The epileptogenic zone typically exhibits focal hypometabolism on interictal FDG-PET. FDG-PET is particularly helpful in patients with suspected focal cortical dysplasia[84] or negative MR imaging,[85] as illustrated in Fig. 3. It has good prognostic value for postsurgical outcomes,[83,85] particularly in cases where hypometabolism is limited.[86] FDG-PET demonstrates high sensitivity in TLE,[87] but its sensitivity decreases in ETLE with identification of the epileptogenic zone in 38% to 67% of cases.[88] In all instances, the correlation between MR imaging and FDG-PET is crucial in identifying initially unknown lesions.[84]

Poirier and colleagues[89] found high but similar diagnostic accuracy and sensitivity in FDG-PET/MR imaging versus FDG-PET/CT, with values of 87% versus 85% and 83% versus 83%, respectively. However, subsequent studies have shown that hybrid FDG-PET/MR imaging performed better for identifying epileptogenic lesions, compared with sequential MR imaging and PET/CT readings. In Shin and colleagues,[90] PET/MR imaging identified additional lesions in 17% of patients that were consistent with clinical symptoms, electroencephalography (EEG), and SPECT imaging. In 31 patients with hippocampal sclerosis, focal cortical dysplasia, or brain tumors, FDG-PET/MR reading had a significantly higher sensitivity (77.4%–90.3%) than PET/CT (58.1%–64.5%) or standalone MR imaging reading (45.2%–80.6%) for the detection of seizure foci in presurgical workup.[91] Similarly, in Oldan and colleagues,[92] lesion detection was increased in 10 out of 74 patients. It is worth noting that the specificity was not improved by using PET/MR imaging. This is not a significant limitation because presurgical imaging aims to identify all potential targets for potential resection, rather than confirming a single focal point that must definitively be resected. As imaging findings must always align with clinical symptoms and EEG findings, the risk of false positives leading to unnecessary surgery is minimal. Conversely, false negatives compromise resective surgery. In complex cases with negative MR imaging, FDG-PET/MR imaging also improved the lesion detection in 13% of cases (mainly focal cortical dysplasia) compared with the interpretation of FDG-PET/CT coregistered with MR imaging, resulting in an overall detection rate of 55%.[93] PET/MR imaging

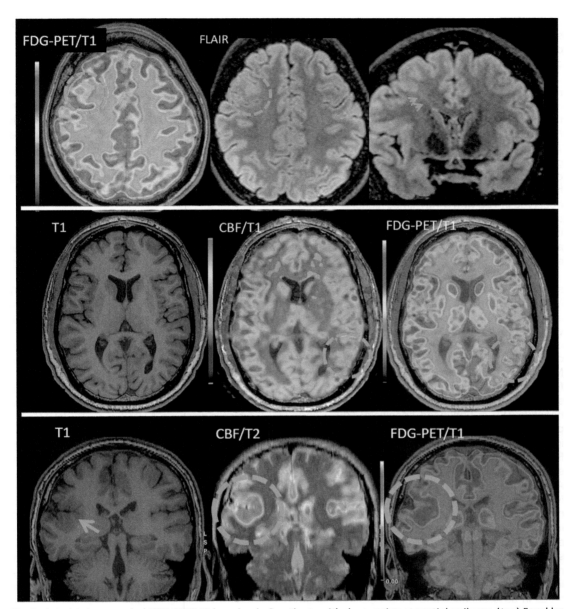

Fig. 3. Interictal presurgical FDG-PET/MR imaging in 3 patients with drug-resistant partial epilepsy. (*top*) Focal hypometabolism (*dashed circle*) was observed in the right frontal cortex (FDG-PET) leading to the further identification of a focal cortical dysplasia (TIW-MR imaging) characterized by the thickening of the right precentral gyrus (*dashed circle*), the loss of demarcation between the gray and white matter, and a transmantle sign (*arrowhead*). (*middle*) Epileptogenic location identified by a left temporal hypoperfusion with spatially matched hypometabolism on interictal FDG-PET/ASL-MR imaging (*dashed circles*) in a negative-structural MR imaging TLE. (*bottom*) Right perisylvian polymicrogyria observed on T1WI (*arrow*), exhibiting spatially matched increased perfusion and metabolism suggesting persistent infraclinical epileptiform activity (*dashed circles*). The transmantle sign is a high T2/FLAIR signal extending from the ventricle to the cortex. This is an MRI feature of focal cortical dysplasia.

also aids in determining the need for resective surgery, intracranial EEG monitoring, or additional invasive diagnostic procedures.[85,93] It helps identify nonlesional patients requiring intracranial EEG monitoring and patients deemed inoperable

necessitating alternative treatment options.[94] In the latter study, surgical decision was altered for 40% of the patients after PET/MR imaging, and 86% of those who underwent cortical resection achieved a seizure-free outcome for more than

1 year after surgery. In Tóth and colleagues,[94] presurgical FDG-PET/MR imaging findings led to a change in the initial treatment plan in 32% of cases.

As previously suggested, FDG-PET/MR imaging may contribute to the success rate of surgery. In a meta-analysis on 1292 refractory epilepsy patients, the detection of epileptic lesions with FDG-PET/MR imaging was associated with a 71% rate of good epilepsy outcome following surgery.[83] Among these patients, 65% achieved postoperative seizure-free outcomes. Notably, a higher rate of good postoperative outcomes was observed in TLE with a 1.27 times higher likelihood compared with extratemporal surgery. These findings support the integration of FDG-PET/MR imaging into the routine presurgical workup for epilepsy.

To further increase diagnostic accuracy and specificity, EEG has been used with FDG-PET/MR imaging. This innovative approach offers reliable interictal data in presurgical examination with improved efficiency, reduced bias, and decreased cost.[95] Studies have investigated the clinical utility of implementing ASL in FDG-PET/MR imaging. It increased the detection of seizure focus and enhances both sensitivity (100%) and specificity (90%) in patients with MR imaging–negative TLE.[96] Enhanced specificity (75%) and positive predictive value (75%) were also reported in children with refractory TLE but not in ETLE.[97] Boscolo and colleagues[98] further confirmed the strong concordance between FDG-PET and ASL-MR imaging findings in patients with negative MR imaging. Notably, reading z-score maps of metabolic and perfusion asymmetry indices significantly enhanced readers confidence in both TLE and ETLE. Maps of metabolic rate of glucose consumption can be generated using IDIF-MR and dynamic FDG-PET.[99] In nonlesional ETLE, it improved the localization of subtle hypometabolic areas in 53% of cases and enhanced confidence in PET interpretations in 33% of cases. In addition, this approach facilitated the identification of hypermetabolic focus associated with frequently spiking cortex, which is often overlooked in conventional readings. However, despite these findings, it did not provide substantial additional information to alter the initial clinical management decisions.

PET/MR imaging has shown promise in other conditions associated with epilepsy. It has been found to be more effective than MR imaging alone in identifying patients with limbic encephalitis with a diagnostic rate of 95% versus 80% for MR imaging alone.[2] In Rasmussen encephalitis, PET/MR imaging improves diagnostic precision by revealing congruent hypometabolism and atrophy areas, even in early stages.[100]

SUMMARY

PET/MR imaging has demonstrated its value in recent years for the management of patients with neurologic diseases. The latest challenges, such as motion attenuation or correction, are on the cusp of being solved, and accessibility is on the increase. This reinforces its position as the examination of choice for diagnosing and monitoring neurologic diseases.

REFERENCES

1. Garibotto V, Heinzer S, Vulliemoz S, et al. Clinical applications of hybrid PET/MRI in neuroimaging. Clin Nucl Med 2013;38(1):e13–8.
2. Deuschl C, Rüber T, Ernst L, et al. 18F-FDG-PET/MRI in the diagnostic work-up of limbic encephalitis. Treglia G, éditeur. PLOS ONE 2020;15(1): e0227906.
3. Suarez J, Tartaglia MC, Vitali P, et al. Characterizing radiology reports in patients with frontotemporal dementia. Neurology 2009;73(13):1073–4.
4. Lorking N, Murray AD, O'Brien JT. The use of positron emission tomography/magnetic resonance imaging in dementia: A literature review. Int J Geriatr Psychiatry 2021;36(10):1501–13.
5. Mukku SSR, Sivakumar PT, Nagaraj C, et al. Clinical utility of 18F-FDG-PET/MRI brain in dementia: Preliminary experience from a geriatric clinic in South India. Asian J Psychiatry 2019;44:99–105.
6. Schütz L, Lobsien D, Fritzsch D, et al. Feasibility and acceptance of simultaneous amyloid PET/MRI. Eur J Nucl Med Mol Imaging 2016;43(12): 2236–43.
7. Mannheim JG, Cheng JC (Kevin), Vafai N, et al. Cross-validation study between the HRRT and the PET component of the SIGNA PET/MRI system with focus on neuroimaging. EJNMMI Phys 2021; 8(1):20.
8. Soret M, Maisonobe JA, Desarnaud S, et al. Ultra-low-dose in brain 18F-FDG PET/MRI in clinical settings. Sci Rep 2022;12(1):15341.
9. Blanc-Durand P, Khalife M, Sgard B, et al. Attenuation correction using 3D deep convolutional neural network for brain 18F-FDG PET/MR: Comparison with Atlas, ZTE and CT based attenuation correction. Ginsberg SD, éditeur. PLOS ONE 2019; 14(10):e0223141.
10. Ladefoged CN, Law I, Anazodo U, et al. A multicentre evaluation of eleven clinically feasible brain PET/MRI attenuation correction techniques using a large cohort of patients. NeuroImage 2017;147: 346–59.

11. Kyme AZ, Aksoy M, Henry DL, et al. Marker-free optical stereo motion tracking for in-bore MRI and PET-MRI application. Med Phys 2020;47(8):3321–31.

12. Spangler-Bickell MG, Hurley SA, Pirasteh A, et al. Evaluation of Data-Driven Rigid Motion Correction in Clinical Brain PET Imaging. J Nucl Med 2022; 63(10):1604–10.

13. Gershenson J, Goddard J, Hong I, et al. Motion correction for PET; brain imaging case series comparisons of optical-pose and data-driven methods. J Nucl Med 2021;62(supplement 1):1142.

14. Chen Z, Jamadar SD, Li S, et al. From simultaneous to synergistic MR-PET brain imaging: A review of hybrid MR-PET imaging methodologies. Hum Brain Mapp 2018;39(12):5126–44.

15. Mehranian A, Belzunce MA, Prieto C, et al. Synergistic PET and SENSE MR Image Reconstruction Using Joint Sparsity Regularization. IEEE Trans Med Imaging 2018;37(1):20–34.

16. Ssali T, Anazodo UC, Thiessen JD, et al. A Noninvasive Method for Quantifying Cerebral Blood Flow by Hybrid PET/MRI. J Nucl Med Off Publ Soc Nucl Med 2018; 59(8):1329–34.

17. Shiyam Sundar LK, Muzik O, Rischka L, et al. Promise of Fully Integrated PET/MRI: Noninvasive Clinical Quantification of Cerebral Glucose Metabolism. J Nucl Med Off Publ Soc Nucl Med 2020; 61(2):276–84.

18. Almansory KO, Fraioli F. Combined PET/MRI in brain glioma imaging. Br J Hosp Med Lond Engl 2005 2019;80(7):380–6.

19. Davis ME. Glioblastoma: Overview of Disease and Treatment. Clin J Oncol Nurs 2016;20(5 Suppl): S2–8.

20. Louis DN, Perry A, Wesseling P, et al. The 2021 WHO Classification of Tumors of the Central Nervous System: a summary. Neuro-Oncol 2021; 23(8):1231–51.

21. Law I, Albert NL, Arbizu J, et al. Joint EANM/EANO/RANO practice guidelines/SNMMI procedure standards for imaging of gliomas using PET with radiolabelled amino acids and [18F]FDG: version 1.0. Eur J Nucl Med Mol Imag 2019;46(3):540–57.

22. Brendle C, Maier C, Bender B, et al. Impact of ^{18}F-FET PET/MR on clinical management of brain tumor patients. J Nucl Med 2021;262051. jnumed. 121.

23. Choi C, Ganji SK, DeBerardinis RJ, et al. 2-hydroxyglutarate detection by magnetic resonance spectroscopy in IDH-mutated patients with gliomas. Nat Med 2012;18(4):624–9.

24. Song S, Wang L, Yang H, et al. Static 18F-FET PET and DSC-PWI based on hybrid PET/MR for the prediction of gliomas defined by IDH and 1p/19q status. Eur Radiol 2021;31(6):4087–96.

25. Lohmann P, Werner JM, Shah NJ, et al. Combined Amino Acid Positron Emission Tomography and Advanced Magnetic Resonance Imaging in Glioma Patients. Cancers 2019;11(2):153.

26. Pirotte BJM, Levivier M, Goldman S, et al. Positron emission tomography-guided volumetric resection of supratentorial high-grade gliomas: a survival analysis in 66 consecutive patients. Neurosurgery 2009;64(3):471–81.

27. Verburg N, Koopman T, Yaqub MM, et al. Improved detection of diffuse glioma infiltration with imaging combinations: a diagnostic accuracy study. Neuro-Oncol 2020;22(3):412–22.

28. Verger A, Filss CP, Lohmann P, et al. Comparison of 18F-FET PET and perfusion-weighted MRI for glioma grading: a hybrid PET/MR study. Eur J Nucl Med Mol Imaging 2017;44(13):2257–65.

29. Pellerin A, Khalifé M, Sanson M, et al. Simultaneously acquired PET and ASL imaging biomarkers may be helpful in differentiating progression from pseudo-progression in treated gliomas. Eur Radiol 2021;31(10):7395–405.

30. Dhermain FG, Hau P, Lanfermann H, et al. Advanced MRI and PET imaging for assessment of treatment response in patients with gliomas. Lancet Neurol 2010;9(9):906–20.

31. Göttler J, Lukas M, Kluge A, et al. Intra-lesional spatial correlation of static and dynamic FET-PET parameters with MRI-based cerebral blood volume in patients with untreated glioma. Eur J Nucl Med Mol Imag 2017;44(3):392–7.

32. Girard A, Le Reste PJ, Metais A, et al. Combining 18F-DOPA PET and MRI with perfusion-weighted imaging improves delineation of high-grade subregions in enhancing and non-enhancing gliomas prior treatment: a biopsy-controlled study. J Neurooncol 2021;155(3):287–95.

33. Glunde K, Bhujwalla ZM, Ronen SM. Choline metabolism in malignant transformation. Nat Rev Cancer 2011;11(12):835–48.

34. Floeth FW, Pauleit D, Wittsack HJ, et al. Multimodal metabolic imaging of cerebral gliomas: positron emission tomography with [18F]fluoroethyl-L-tyrosine and magnetic resonance spectroscopy. J Neurosurg 2005;102(2):318–27.

35. Bumes E, Wirtz FP, Fellner C, et al. Non-Invasive Prediction of IDH Mutation in Patients with Glioma WHO II/III/IV Based on F-18-FET PET-Guided In Vivo 1H-Magnetic Resonance Spectroscopy and Machine Learning. Cancers 2020;12(11): 3406.

36. Cheng Y, Song S, Wei Y, et al. Glioma Imaging by O-(2-18F-Fluoroethyl)-L-Tyrosine PET and Diffusion-Weighted MRI and Correlation With Molecular Phenotypes, Validated by PET/MR-Guided Biopsies. Front Oncol 2021;11:743655.

37. Haubold J, Demircioglu A, Gratz M, et al. Non-invasive tumor decoding and phenotyping of cerebral gliomas utilizing multiparametric 18F-FET PET-MRI

and MR Fingerprinting. Eur J Nucl Med Mol Imaging 2020;47(6):1435–45.

38. Lohmann P, Lerche C, Bauer EK, et al. Predicting IDH genotype in gliomas using FET PET radiomics. Sci Rep 2018;8(1):13328.

39. Zhang L, Pan H, Liu Z, et al. Multicenter clinical radiomics-integrated model based on [18F]FDG PET and multi-modal MRI predict ATRX mutation status in IDH-mutant lower-grade gliomas. Eur Radiol 2023;33(2):872–83.

40. Schön S, Cabello J, Liesche-Starnecker F, et al. Imaging glioma biology: spatial comparison of amino acid PET, amide proton transfer, and perfusion-weighted MRI in newly diagnosed gliomas. Eur J Nucl Med Mol Imaging 2020;47(6):1468–75.

41. da Silva NA, Lohmann P, Fairney J, et al. Hybrid MR-PET of brain tumours using amino acid PET and chemical exchange saturation transfer MRI. Eur J Nucl Med Mol Imaging 2018;45(6):1031–40.

42. Paprottka KJ, Kleiner S, Preibisch C, et al. Fully automated analysis combining [18F]-FET-PET and multiparametric MRI including DSC perfusion and APTw imaging: a promising tool for objective evaluation of glioma progression. Eur J Nucl Med Mol Imaging. déc 2021;48(13):4445–55.

43. Pyatigorskaya N, De Laroche R, Bera G, et al. Are Gadolinium-Enhanced MR Sequences Needed in Simultaneous 18F-FDG-PET/MRI for Tumor Delineation in Head and Neck Cancer? AJNR Am J Neuroradiol 2020;41(10):1888–96.

44. Jena A, Taneja S, Jha A, et al. Multiparametric Evaluation in Differentiating Glioma Recurrence from Treatment-Induced Necrosis Using Simultaneous 18 F-FDG-PET/MRI: A Single-Institution Retrospective Study. Am J Neuroradiol 2017;38(5):899–907.

45. Pyka T, Hiob D, Preibisch C, et al. Diagnosis of glioma recurrence using multiparametric dynamic 18F-fluoroethyl-tyrosine PET-MRI. Eur J Radiol 2018;103:32–7.

46. Smith NJ, Deaton TK, Territo W, et al. Hybrid 18F-Fluoroethyltyrosine PET and MRI with Perfusion to Distinguish Disease Progression from Treatment-Related Change in Malignant Brain Tumors: The Quest to Beat the Toughest Cases. J Nucl Med Off Publ Soc Nucl Med 2023;28. jnumed.122.265149.

47. Steidl E, Langen KJ, Hmeidan SA, et al. Sequential implementation of DSC-MR perfusion and dynamic [18F]FET PET allows efficient differentiation of glioma progression from treatment-related changes. Eur J Nucl Med Mol Imaging 2021;48(6):1956–65.

48. Bertaux M, Berenbaum A, Di Stefano AL, et al. Hybrid [18F]-F-DOPA PET/MRI Interpretation Criteria and Scores for Glioma Follow-up After Radiotherapy. Clin Neuroradiol 2022;32(3):735–47.

49. Wirsching HG, Roelcke U, Weller J, et al. MRI and 18FET-PET Predict Survival Benefit from Bevacizumab Plus Radiotherapy in Patients with Isocitrate Dehydrogenase Wild-type Glioblastoma: Results from the Randomized ARTE Trial. Clin Cancer Res Off J Am Assoc Cancer Res 2021;27(1):179–88.

50. Wollring MM, Werner JM, Bauer EK, et al. Prediction of response to lomustine-based chemotherapy in glioma patients at recurrence using MRI and FET PET. Neuro-Oncol 2023;25(5):984–94.

51. Zhang S, Wang J, Wang K, et al. Differentiation of high-grade glioma and primary central nervous system lymphoma: Multiparametric imaging of the enhancing tumor and peritumoral regions based on hybrid 18F-FDG PET/MRI. Eur J Radiol 2022;150:110235.

52. Carlson ML, DiGiacomo PS, Fan AP, et al. Simultaneous FDG-PET/MRI detects hippocampal subfield metabolic differences in AD/MCI. Sci Rep 2020;10(1):12064.

53. Rozenblum L, Habert MO, Pyatigorskaya N, et al. FDG PET/MRI Findings Pointing Toward a Gayet-Wernicke Encephalopathy. Clin Nucl Med 2019;44(7). e456-e457.

54. Zanovello M, Sorarù G, Campi C, et al. Brain Stem Glucose Hypermetabolism in Amyotrophic Lateral Sclerosis/Frontotemporal Dementia and Shortened Survival: An 18F-FDG PET/MRI Study. J Nucl Med Off Publ Soc Nucl Med 2022;63(5):777–84.

55. Guedj E, Varrone A, Boellaard R, et al. EANM procedure guidelines for brain PET imaging using [18F]FDG, version 3. Eur J Nucl Med Mol Imag 2022;49(2):632–51.

56. Franceschi AM, Clifton MA, Naser-Tavakolian K, et al. FDG PET/MRI for Visual Detection of Crossed Cerebellar Diaschisis in Patients With Dementia. AJR Am J Roentgenol 2021;216(1):165–71.

57. Barthel H, Schroeter ML, Hoffmann KT, et al. PET/MR in Dementia and Other Neurodegenerative Diseases. Semin Nucl Med 2015;45(3):224–33.

58. Moodley KK, Minati L, Barnes A, et al. Simultaneous PET/MRI in frontotemporal dementia. Eur J Nucl Med Mol Imaging 2013;40(3):468–9.

59. Franceschi AM, Abballe V, Raad RA, et al. Visual detection of regional brain hypometabolism in cognitively impaired patients is independent of positron emission tomography-magnetic resonance attenuation correction method. World J Nucl Med 2018;17(3):188–94.

60. Shepherd TM, Nayak GK. Clinical Use of Integrated Positron Emission Tomography-Magnetic Resonance Imaging for Dementia Patients. Top Magn Reson Imaging TMRI 2019;28(6):299–310.

61. Kaltoft NS, Marner L, Larsen VA, et al. Hybrid FDG PET/MRI vs. FDG PET and CT in patients with suspected dementia - A comparison of diagnostic yield and propagated influence on clinical diagnosis and patient management. PLoS One 2019;14(5):e0216409.

62. Tahmasian M, Shao J, Meng C, et al. Based on the Network Degeneration Hypothesis: Separating Individual Patients with Different Neurodegenerative Syndromes in a Preliminary Hybrid PET/MR Study. J Nucl Med Off Publ Soc Nucl Med 2016;57(3):410–5.

63. Gupta Y, Lama RK, Kwon GR, Alzheimer's Disease Neuroimaging Initiative. Prediction and Classification of Alzheimer's Disease Based on Combined Features From Apolipoprotein-E Genotype, Cerebrospinal Fluid, MR, and FDG-PET Imaging Biomarkers. Front Comput Neurosci 2019;13:72.

64. Musiek ES, Chen Y, Korczykowski M, et al. Direct Comparison of FDG-PET and ASL-MRI in Alzheimer's Disease. Alzheimers Dement J Alzheimers Assoc 2012;8(1):51–9.

65. Wabik A, Trypka E, Bladowska J, et al. Comparison of dynamic susceptibility contrast enhanced MR and FDG-PET brain studies in patients with Alzheimer's disease and amnestic mild cognitive impairment. J Transl Med 2022;20(1):259.

66. Yan L, Liu CY, Wong KP, et al. Regional association of pCASL-MRI with FDG-PET and PiB-PET in people at risk for autosomal dominant Alzheimer's disease. NeuroImage Clin 2018;17:751–60.

67. Fällmar D, Haller S, Lilja J, et al. Arterial spin labeling-based Z-maps have high specificity and positive predictive value for neurodegenerative dementia compared to FDG-PET. Eur Radiol 2017;27(10):4237–46.

68. Verfaillie SCJ, Adriaanse SM, Binnewijzend MAA, et al. Cerebral perfusion and glucose metabolism in Alzheimer's disease and frontotemporal dementia: two sides of the same coin? Eur Radiol 2015;25(10):3050–9.

69. Anazodo UC, Finger E, Kwan BYM, et al. Using simultaneous PET/MRI to compare the accuracy of diagnosing frontotemporal dementia by arterial spin labelling MRI and FDG-PET. NeuroImage Clin 2018;17:405–14.

70. Riederer I, Bohn KP, Preibisch C, et al. Alzheimer Disease and Mild Cognitive Impairment: Integrated Pulsed Arterial Spin-Labeling MRI and 18 F-FDG PET. Radiology 2018;288(1):198–206.

71. Ceccarini J, Bourgeois S, Van Weehaeghe D, Goffin K, Vandenberghe R, Vandenbulcke M, et al. Direct prospective comparison of 18F-FDG PET and arterial spin labelling MR using simultaneous PET/MR in patients referred for diagnosis of dementia. Eur J Nucl Med Mol Imaging (Internet). 20 janv 2020 (cité 17 févr 2020); Disponible sur: http://link.springer.com/10.1007/s00259-020-04694-1.

72. Lehericy S, Vaillancourt DE, Seppi K, et al. The role of high-field magnetic resonance imaging in parkinsonian disorders: Pushing the boundaries forward. Mov Disord Off J Mov Disord Soc 2017;32(4):510–25.

73. Pyatigorskaya N, Magnin B, Mongin M, et al. Comparative Study of MRI Biomarkers in the Substantia Nigra to Discriminate Idiopathic Parkinson Disease. AJNR Am J Neuroradiol 2018;39(8):1460–7.

74. Meyer PT, Frings L, Rücker G, et al. 18F-FDG PET in Parkinsonism: Differential Diagnosis and Evaluation of Cognitive Impairment. J Nucl Med Off Publ Soc Nucl Med 2017;58(12):1888–98.

75. Shang S, Li D, Tian Y, et al. Hybrid PET-MRI for early detection of dopaminergic dysfunction and microstructural degradation involved in Parkinson's disease. Commun Biol 2021;4(1):1162.

76. Depierreux F, Parmentier E, Mackels L, et al. Parkinson's disease multimodal imaging: F-DOPA PET, neuromelanin-sensitive and quantitative iron-sensitive MRI. Npj Park Dis 2021;7(1):57.

77. Iep A, Chawki MB, Goldfarb L, et al. Relevance of 18F-DOPA visual and semi-quantitative PET metrics for the diagnostic of Parkinson disease in clinical practice: a machine learning-based inference study. EJNMMI Res 2023;13(1):13.

78. Choi H, Cheon GJ, Kim HJ, et al. Gray matter correlates of dopaminergic degeneration in Parkinson's disease: A hybrid PET/MR study using (18) F-FP-CIT. Hum Brain Mapp 2016;37(5):1710–21.

79. Hu X, Sun X, Hu F, et al. Multivariate radiomics models based on 18F-FDG hybrid PET/MRI for distinguishing between Parkinson's disease and multiple system atrophy. Eur J Nucl Med Mol Imag 2021;48(11):3469–81.

80. Teune LK, Renken RJ, de Jong BM, et al. Parkinson's disease-related perfusion and glucose metabolic brain patterns identified with PCASL-MRI and FDG-PET imaging. NeuroImage Clin 2014;5:240–4.

81. Messerschmidt K, Barthel H, Brendel M, et al. 18F-PI-2620 Tau PET Improves the Imaging Diagnosis of Progressive Supranuclear Palsy. J Nucl Med Off Publ Soc Nucl Med 2022;63(11):1754–60.

82. Hainc N, McAndrews MP, Valiante T, et al. Imaging in medically refractory epilepsy at 3 Tesla: a 13-year tertiary adult epilepsy center experience. Insights Imaging 2022;13(1):99.

83. Guo J, Guo M, Liu R, et al. Seizure Outcome After Surgery for Refractory Epilepsy Diagnosed by 18F-fluorodeoxyglucose positron emission tomography (18F-FDG PET/MRI): A Systematic Review and Meta-Analysis. World Neurosurg 2023;173:34–43.

84. Desarnaud S, Mellerio C, Semah F, et al. 18F-FDG PET in drug-resistant epilepsy due to focal cortical dysplasia type 2: additional value of electroclinical data and coregistration with MRI. Eur J Nucl Med Mol Imaging 2018;45(8):1449–60.

85. Steinbrenner M, Duncan JS, Dickson J, et al. Utility of 18F-fluorodeoxyglucose positron emission tomography in presurgical evaluation of patients

with epilepsy: A multicenter study. Epilepsia 2022; 63(5):1238–52.

86. Guedj E, Varrone A, Boellaard R, Albert NL, Barthel H, van Berckel B, et al. EANM procedure guidelines for brain PET imaging using (18F)FDG, version 3. Eur J Nucl Med Mol Imaging (Internet). 9 déc 2021 (cité 23 déc 2021); Disponible sur: https://link.springer.com/10.1007/s00259-021-05603-w.

87. Spencer SS. The relative contributions of MRI, SPECT, and PET imaging in epilepsy. Epilepsia 1994;35(Suppl 6):S72–89.

88. Verger A, Lagarde S, Maillard L, et al. Brain molecular imaging in pharmacoresistant focal epilepsy: Current practice and perspectives. Rev Neurol (Paris) 2018;174(1–2):16–27.

89. Poirier SE, Kwan BYM, Jurkiewicz MT, et al. An evaluation of the diagnostic equivalence of 18F-FDG-PET between hybrid PET/MRI and PET/CT in drug-resistant epilepsy: A pilot study. Epilepsy Res 2021;172:106583.

90. Shin HW, Jewells V, Sheikh A, et al. Initial experience in hybrid PET-MRI for evaluation of refractory focal onset epilepsy. Seizure 2015;31:1–4.

91. Kikuchi K, Togao O, Yamashita K, et al. Diagnostic accuracy for the epileptogenic zone detection in focal epilepsy could be higher in FDG-PET/MRI than in FDG-PET/CT. Eur Radiol 2021;31(5): 2915–22.

92. Oldan JD, Shin HW, Khandani AH, et al. Subsequent experience in hybrid PET-MRI for evaluation of refractory focal onset epilepsy. Seizure 2018; 61:128–34.

93. Flaus A, Mellerio C, Rodrigo S, et al. 18F-FDG PET/ MR in focal epilepsy: A new step for improving the detection of epileptogenic lesions. Epilepsy Res 2021;178:106819.

94. Tóth M, Barsi P, Tóth Z, et al. The role of hybrid FDG-PET/MRI on decision-making in presurgical evaluation of drug-resistant epilepsy. BMC Neurol 2021;21(1):363.

95. Grouiller F, Delattre BMA, Pittau F, et al. All-in-one interictal presurgical imaging in patients with epilepsy: single-session EEG/PET/(f)MRI. Eur J Nucl Med Mol Imaging 2015;42(7):1133–43.

96. Shang K, Wang J, Fan X, et al. Clinical Value of Hybrid TOF-PET/MR Imaging-Based Multiparametric Imaging in Localizing Seizure Focus in Patients with MRI-Negative Temporal Lobe Epilepsy. AJNR Am J Neuroradiol 2018;39(10):1791–8.

97. Khalaf AM, Nadel HR, Dahmoush HM. Simultaneously acquired MRI arterial spin-labeling and interictal FDG-PET improves diagnosis of pediatric temporal lobe epilepsy. Am J Neuroradiol 2022; 43(3):468–73.

98. Boscolo Galazzo I, Mattoli MV, Pizzini FB, et al. Cerebral metabolism and perfusion in MR-negative individuals with refractory focal epilepsy assessed by simultaneous acquisition of 18 F-FDG PET and arterial spin labeling. NeuroImage Clin 2016;11: 648–57.

99. Traub-Weidinger T, Muzik O, Sundar LKS, et al. Utility of absolute quantification in non-lesional extratemporal lobe epilepsy using FDG PET/MR imaging. Front Neurol 2020;11:54.

100. Tang C, Ren P, Ma K, et al. The correspondence between morphometric MRI and metabolic profile in Rasmussen's encephalitis. NeuroImage Clin 2022;33:102918.

Systematic Review and Metanalysis on the Role of Prostate-Specific Membrane Antigen Positron Emission Tomography/Magnetic Resonance Imaging for Intraprostatic Tumour Assessment

Paola Mapelli, MD, PhD[a,b], Samuele Ghezzo, MSc[a,b],
Alessandro Spataro, MD[c], Carolina Bezzi, MSc[a,b],
Ana Maria Samanes Gajate, MD[b], Arturo Chiti, MD[a,b],
Maria Picchio, MD[a,b,*]

KEYWORDS

- PET/MRI • Prostate cancer • Staging • Primary • 68Ga-PSMA • 18F-DCFPyL • 18F-PSMA-1007
- Accuracy

KEY POINTS

- PSMA PET/MRI provides accurate visualization of intraprostatic prostate cancer localization and is highly sensitive in detecting nodal and distant metastases.
- PSMA PET/MRI has better sensitivity and diagnostic accuracy in detecting primary PCa compared to mp-MRI and PET alone, especially in patients with PIRADS 3 PCa.
- A better characterization of primary PCa provided by PSMA PET/MRI may improve the targeted biopsies approach.

INTRODUCTION

An accurate staging of patients with primary prostate cancer (PCa) is of utmost relevance to plan the optimal treatment strategies. In this scenario, imaging modalities are essential, although no single modality is still currently able to address all the clinical needs for PCa staging and therefore patients often undergo multiple imaging prior starting treatment.[1]

Magnetic resonance imaging (MRI) is the modality of choice to define local tumour staging, including extracapsular extension (ECE) and seminal vesicle invasion (SVI), while CT is used to assess locoregional lymph nodal metastases and distant metastases, and bone scintigraphy is recommended to investigate bone localization.

In the past years, positron emission tomography (PET) with radiotracers targeting prostate-specific

[a] Vita-Salute San Raffaele University, Via Olgettina 58, Milan 20132, Italy; [b] Nuclear Medicine Department, IRCCS San Raffaele Scientific Institute, Via Olgettina 60, Milan 20132, Italy; [c] Department of Biomedical and Dental Sciences and of Morpho-Functional Imaging, Nuclear Medicine Unit, University of Messina, Piazza Pugliatti 1, Messina 98122, Italy
* Corresponding author. Nuclear Medicine Department, IRCCS San Raffaele Scientific Institute, Via Olgettina 60, Milan 20132, Italy.
E-mail address: picchio.maria@hsr.it

Magn Reson Imaging Clin N Am 31 (2023) 605–611
https://doi.org/10.1016/j.mric.2023.06.006

membrane antigen (PSMA), both labelled with ^{68}Ga or ^{18}F, has gained high value in the field of prostate cancer, in view of the higher expression of PSMA on PCa cells compared to other organs. Currently, PSMA PET has been mainly used in the restaging phase of PCa, having high sensitivity even at low prostate specific antigen (PSA) values.[1,2]

Available data suggest that PSMA PET seems to outperform conventional imaging modalities in defining N and M stages, with excellent sensitivity in the initial diagnosis of PCa.[3–5]

The relatively recent introduction of PET/MRI scanners in the last years, has improved the assessment of PCa, as this hybrid imaging technique represents a one-stop shop modality allowing an accurate visualization of local tumour by MRI and a sensitive detection of lymph nodal and distant metastases thanks to the PSMA radiotracer.[6,7] The present systematic review and metanalysis summarizes the information on diagnostic accuracy obtained with PSMA PET/MRI in patients with primary PCa patients.

MATERIALS AND METHODS
Search Strategy and Study Selection

A literature search on the papers published in the last 10 years, up to 30th November 2022 was conducted in the PubMed data-base. The terms used for the search were as follows: "PSMA" AND "prostate cancer" or "prostate" AND "PET/MRI" or "PET MRI" or "PET-MRI" or "PET-MR" AND "primary" or "staging." Additional filters including English language only, type of article (original article, research article), and subjects (humans only) were applied. The literature search and the selection of studies to be included was conducted by two reviewers (P.M. and A.S.). In case of any discrepancy, a consensus was reached among the two reviewers. Article types such as reviews, clinical reports, abstracts of meetings, and editorials were excluded.

A qualitative analysis was also performed in order to include papers meeting the following inclusion criteria: (i) a sample size of >10 patients; (ii) the presence of histological (biopsy or surgical specimen) validation of PSMA PET/MRI findings, as only studies assessing the diagnostic accuracy of PSMA PET/MRI in the primary staging of prostate cancer were considered; (iii) the article included data regarding true positive/negative and false positive/negative results, or the authors made these data available on request. Papers with both [18]F- and ^{68}Ga-PSMA radiotracers have been included for the qualitative analysis; only studies using ^{68}Ga-PSMA-11 PET/MRI were included for the metanalysis.

Statistical Analysis

Pooled sensitivity and specificity with 95% confidence intervals (CI) of PET/MRI with ^{68}Ga-PSMA-11 were calculated using random effects analysis. I^2 was used to test heterogeneity, and values of I^2 of 25%, 50%, and 75% were considered low, moderate, and high; respectively. To study whether the performance of PET/MRI with ^{68}Ga-PSMA-11 differs at the per-patient and per-lesion level, analyses were repeated calculating sensitivity and specificity considering only studies (a) investigating diagnostic accuracy at the per-patient level and (b) investigating diagnostic accuracy at the per-lesion level, separately. Meta-regression was used to compare sensitivity and specificity at the per-patient and per-lesion level; p-value < 0.05 was considered statistically significant. All statistical analyses were performed using Meta-DiSc version 2.0.[8]

RESULTS
Qualitative Results

In total, 10 studies were eligible for qualitative analysis (Fig. 1, Table 1), 3 of them had a retrospective design, while 7 were prospective.

In 7/10 papers ^{68}Ga-PSMA-11 was used as radiotracer, while the remaining 3 used fluorine-labelled PSMA (1/3 ^{18}F-PSMA-1007 and 2/3 ^{18}F-DCFPyL). In all included studies, PET and MR images were simultaneously acquired on a PET/MRI scanner and the main endpoint for all papers was the diagnostic accuracy of PSMA PET/MRI in detecting primary prostate cancer.

DISCUSSION

The present review and metanalysis is focused on a specific topic, related to the diagnostic accuracy of PSMA PET/MRI in detecting intraprostatic tumour lesion. The number of the included studies is relatively low; however, it has to be noted that we only selected those studies with PET and MRI scans acquired simultaneously and having histology as reference standard to validate imaging findings.

The qualitative analysis of the papers included in the analysis suggests that the integrated PET/MRI system demonstrated better sensitivity and in general better diagnostic accuracy in detecting primary PCa compared to multiparametric (mp) MRI[9–13] and also to PET alone.[14]

Hicks and colleagues in a cohort of 32 men reported region-specific sensitivities for ^{68}Ga-PSMA-11 PET/MRI and mp-MRI of 74% (95% confidence interval–CI: 70%, 77%) and 50% (95% CI: 45%, 54%), respectively. Region-specific specificity for ^{68}Ga-PSMA-11 PET/MRI was similar to

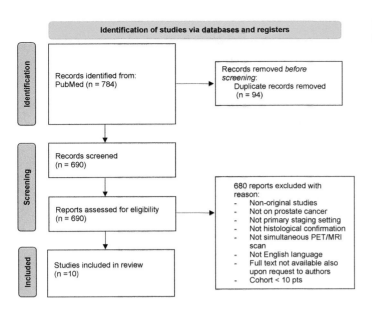

Fig. 1. PRISMA method for study selection.

that of mp-MRI (88%, CI: 85%, 91% vs 90%, CI: 87%, 92%; p = 0.99). Moreover, Authors described an association between standardized uptake value (SUV) max and a Gleason score of 7 and higher (odds ratio: 1.71, CI: 1.27, 2.31; p < 0.001).[9]

Metser and colleagues in a prospective study including 55 patients with suspicion of PCa investigated the contribution of ^{18}F-DCFPyL PET/mp-MRi in diagnosing clinically significant PCa (csPCa), compared to the sole use of mp-MRI. They found a sensitivity for ^{18}F-DCFPyL PET on lesion-level analysis higher than mp-MRI and PET/MR (86% vs 67% and 69%; p = 0.027 and 0.041, respectively]), but at a lower specificity (32% vs 85% and 86%, respectively; p < 0.001). For PET image analysis, all focal tracer accumulation greater than background activity which could not be attributed to a physiological or benign entity were recorded. Mp-MR was reported independently by a MR readers using PI-RADS v.2 criteria. After PET and mp-MR data were documented, combined PET/mp-MR data was tabulated by an independent radiologist, using the PROMISE standardized reporting framework for PSMA ligand PET (molecular imaging TNM, v. 1).

For the identification of csPCa in PIRADS ≥ 3 lesions, the area under the curve (AUC) (95% CI) for ^{18}F-DCFPyLPET PET, mp-MR, and PET/MR was 0.75 (0.65–0.86), 0.69 (0.56–0.82), and 0.78 (0.67–0.89), respectively. Notably, the AUC for PET/MR was significantly larger than that of mp-MR (p = 0.04).[10]

Zeng and colleagues assessed the diagnostic value of ^{18}F-PSMA-1007 PET/MRI in 29 patients

with suspected PCa who underwent ^{18}F-PSMA-1007 PET/MRI and subsequent targeted biopsy. ^{18}F-PSMA-1007 PET/MRI showed higher diagnostic accuracy, sensitivity, specificity, positive predictive value, and negative predictive value compared to bi-parametric MRI (bp-MRI) (0.974 versus 0.711, 94.74% versus 92.11%, 100% versus 50%, 100% versus 87.50%, and 83.33% versus 62.50%, respectively). Moreover, SUVmax showed higher accuracy compared to apparent diffusion coefficient (ADC) in PCa detection (AUC: 0.874 vs 0.776, respectively). The ISUP grade was positively associated with SUVmax, but no association was found with ADC. This study clearly demonstrated a better diagnostic value of ^{18}F-PSMA-1007 PET/MRI compared to bp-MRI in detecting PCa and an association between PET parameters and ISUP grade.[12]

In a cohort of 30 patients with suspected PCa, Bodar and colleagues demonstrated areas under the receiver operating characteristics curves (AUC), sensitivity, specificity, PPV and NPV and for the total-agreement detection (defined as the direct segmental comparison without any discrepancy) of csPCa per segment of 70%, 50.0%, 89.9%, 71.7%, and 77.9%, respectively, while for mp-MRI 75%, 54.2%, 94.2%, 82.8%, and 80.1%, respectively. This results suggested that although ^{18}F-DCFPyL PET/MRI can adequately detect csPCa, it does not still outperform mp-MRI.[11]

Margel and colleagues compared the sensitivity and specificity of ^{68}Ga-PSMA-11 PET/MRI with mp-MRI in 99 patients with suspected csPCa

Table 1
Characteristics of the selected studies

Author, Ref, Year	Prospective/ Retrospective	N. Pts	Radioligand	Scanner Type	Outcome
Eiber et al,[14] 2016	Retrospective	53	^{68}Ga-PSMA-11	Siemens Biograph mMR	^{68}Ga-PSMA-11 PET/MRI improves diagnostic accuracy for PCa localization both compared with mp-MRI and with PET imaging alone.
Hicks et al,[9] 2018	Retrospective	32	^{68}Ga-PSMA-11	Signa PET/MR, GE Healthcare	^{68}Ga-PSMA-11 PET/MRI has better sensitivity in detecting PCa compared to mp-MRI
Metser et al,[10] 2021	Prospective	55	^{18}F-DCFPyL	Siemens Biograph mMR	The performance of ^{18}F-DCFPyL PET/MR is better than mp-MR for detection of csPCa in PIRADS ≥ 3 lesions.
Margel et al,[13] 2021	Prospective	99	^{68}Ga-PSMA-11	Siemens Biograph mMR	^{68}Ga-PSMA-11 PET/MRI improves the specificity for clinically significant prostate cancer compared with mp-MRI, especially in PIRADS ≥ 3 lesions.
Ferraro et al,[15] 2021	Prospective	42	^{68}Ga-PSMA-11	Signa PET/MR, GE Healthcare	^{68}Ga-PSMA PSMA-11 PET/MRI has a high accuracy in detecting csPCa and is a promising tool to select patients with suspicion of PCa for biopsy.
Moradi et al,[17] 2022	Prospective	73	^{68}Ga-PSMA-11	Signa PET/MR, GE Healthcare	^{68}Ga-PSMA-11 PET can risk stratify patients with intermediate or high-grade prostate cancer prior to prostatectomy based on the degree of uptake in prostate and presence of metastatic disease.
Zeng et al,[12] 2022	Retrospective	29	^{18}F-PSMA-1007	Siemens Biograph mMR	The diagnostic value of ^{18}F-PSMA-1007 PET/MRI in detecting PCa is better than that of biparametric MRI; a high SUVmax may indicate a lesion with high ISUP grade.
Mapelli et al,[7] 2022	Prospective	22	^{68}Ga-PSMA-11	Signa PET/MR, GE Healthcare	^{68}Ga-PSMA-11 PET/MRI has a higher detection rate for intraprostatic PCa localization compared to ^{68}Ga-DOTA-RM2
Bodar et al,[11] 2022	Prospective	30	^{18}F-DCFPyL	Ingenuity TF PET/MRI (Philips)	^{18}F-DCFPyL PET/MRI adequately detects csPCa, but it does not outperform mp-MRI.
Ferraro et al,[16] 2022	Prospective	39	^{68}Ga-PSMA-11	Signa PET/MR, GE Healthcare	^{68}Ga-PSMA-11 PET/MRI has similar accuracy and reliability to mp-MRI in primary PCa localization. Semiquantitative parameters from PSMA PET/MRI correlate with tumour grade and are more reliable than the mp-MRI derived parameters

undergoing biopsy. ^{68}Ga-PSMA-11 PET/MRI showed higher specificity compared to mp-MRI in detecting csPCa (76%, CI: 62, 86 vs 49%, CI: 35, 63%, respectively; p < 0.001), with similar sensitivities (88%, CI: 69, 98 vs 92%, CI: 74, 99%, respectively; p > 0.99). Considering PIRADS 3 lesions, ^{68}Ga-PSMA-11 PET/MRI still showed higher specificity compared to mp-MRI: 86% (95% CI: 73, 95%) versus 59% (95% CI: 43, 74%), respectively p = 0.002). Interestingly, the decision curve analysis showed that biopsies targeted to PSMA uptake increased the net benefit of mp-MRI only in patients presenting PIRADS 3 lesions. Conversely, the net benefit of targeted biopsy was similar for PIRADS 4 and 5 lesions, regardless of PSMA uptake.[13]

Eiber and colleagues compared the diagnostic performance of ^{68}Ga-PSMA-11 PET/MRI versus mp-MRI in 53 patients with suspected PCa. Mp-MRI, PET, and PET/MRI detected cancer in 66% (35 of 53), 92% (49 of 53), and 98% (52 of 53) of patients, respectively, with PET/MRI statistically outperforming mp-MRI (AUC: 0.88 vs 0.73; p < 0.001) and PET (AUC: 0.88 vs 0.83; p = 0.002) in localizing PCa. PET was more accurate than mp-MRI (AUC: 0.83 vs 0.73; p = 0.003) and provided a high uptake ratio between malignant versus nonmalignant tissue; however, no significant correlation was observed between quantitative PET parameters and Gleason score or PSA value.[14]

Ferraro and colleagues[15] assessed the performance of ^{68}Ga-PSMA-11 PET/MRI in detecting csPCa and found a patient-based sensitivity, specificity, negative and positive predictive value

and accuracy of 96%, 81%, 93%, 89% and 90%, respectively.

The same group found similar accuracy and reliability between ^{68}Ga-PSMA-11 PET/MRI and mp-MRI in localizing primay PCa, they demonstrated how semiquantitative parameters from ^{68}Ga-PSMA-11 PET/MRI correlated with tumour grade more reliably than the ones from mp-MRI.[16]

In a study from Mapelli and colleagues[7] comparing the ability in detecting primary PCa of ^{68}Ga-PSMA-11 and ^{68}Ga-DOTA-RM2, a peptide that selectively binds to gastrin-releasing peptide receptor, ^{68}Ga-PSMA-11 PET/MRI demonstrated a higher detection rate for this imaging modality compared to ^{68}Ga-DOTA-RM2 PET/MRI.

Interestingly, Moradi and colleagues[17] in a prospective study including 73 patients with high-risk prostate cancer demonstrated the ability of ^{68}Ga-PSMA-11 PET/MRI in stratifying patients prior to prostatectomy based on degree of uptake in prostate and the presence of metastatic disease.

Regarding the qualitative analysis of the selected articles, a metanalysis was performed on 7 studies using PET/MRI with ^{68}Ga-PSMA-11 for the localization of primary PCa.[7,9,13-17] Studies using ^{18}F-PSMA were excluded as at least 5 works are required to perform a metanalysis. Pooled sensitivity and specificities were 0.954 (CI: 0.821–0.989) and 0.771 (CI: 0.515–0.915); respectively. Forest plots representing sensitivity (A) and specificity (B), as well as heterogeneity between studies are reported in **Fig. 2**. Mapelli and colleagues[7] and Eiber and colleagues[14] were excluded from specificity calculations as in those papers there were no true negatives patients.

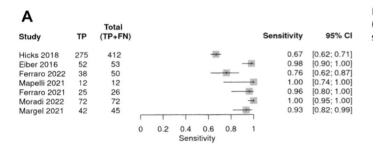

A

Study	TP	Total (TP+FN)		Sensitivity	95% CI
Hicks 2018	275	412		0.67	[0.62; 0.71]
Eiber 2016	52	53		0.98	[0.90; 1.00]
Ferraro 2022	38	50		0.76	[0.62; 0.87]
Mapelli 2021	12	12		1.00	[0.74; 1.00]
Ferraro 2021	25	26		0.96	[0.80; 1.00]
Moradi 2022	72	72		1.00	[0.95; 1.00]
Margel 2021	42	45		0.93	[0.82; 0.99]

0   0.2   0.4   0.6   0.8   1
Sensitivity

B

Study	TN	Total (TN+FP)		Specificity	95% CI
Hicks 2018	389	548		0.71	[0.67; 0.75]
Ferraro 2022	90	97		0.93	[0.86; 0.97]
Ferraro 2021	13	16		0.81	[0.54; 0.96]
Moradi 2022	1	1		1.00	[0.03; 1.00]
Margel 2021	18	33		0.55	[0.36; 0.72]

0   0.2   0.4   0.6   0.8   1
Specificity

Fig. 2. Forest plots showing sensitivity (A) and specificity (B) of the included studies.

There was a moderate heterogeneity between studies ($I^2 = 0.537$).

Subgroup analysis revealed that the pooled sensitivity and specificity of ^{68}Ga-PSMA PET/MRI at the per-patient level were 0.976 (CI: 0.943–0.991) and 0.739 (CI: 0.437–0.912); respectively. At the per-lesion level the pooled sensitivity was 0.721 (CI: 0.613–0.808) and pooled specificity = 0.838 (CI: 0.637–0.939). Meta-regression showed that there was a significantly higher pooled sensitivity at the per-patient level (p = 0.001), while specificities were comparable (p = 0.517).

PSMA PET may be complementary to mp-MRI in primary prostate cancer localization, being of particular relevance for PIRADS 3 lesions. In local tumour staging, PET/MRI seems to be superior compared to PET/CT, with major benefit related to the possibility to predict extracapsular extension in patients with MRI-occult prostate cancer. PET/MRI is very useful for local and regional disease, having almost equivalent performance in detecting bone and visceral metastases compared to PET/CT.

SUMMARY

The evidence reported in the present review is in support of the emerging and promising role of PSMA PET/MRI for intraprostatic tumour detection. The simultaneous acquisition of PET images using PSMA and mp-MRI provides metabolic, structural, and functional information regarding PCa status in a whole-body single session examination, representing an improvement in the detection and characterization of primary PCa.

In turn, a better characterization of primary PCa may lead to an improved approach for target biopsies, thus resulting in a reduced number of biopsies for men with a clinical suspicion of PCa.

CLINICS CARE POINTS

- PSMA PET/MRI is a one-stop shop modality that provides accurate visualization of local tumour by the MRI component and a sensitive detection of lymph nodal and distant metastases thanks to the PSMA radiotracer.

- PSMA PET/MRI has better sensitivity and diagnostic accuracy in detecting primary PCa compared to mp-MRI and PET alone.

- In patients with PIRADS 3 PCa, PSMA PET/MRI demonstrated a better sensitivity in detecting PCa compared to mp-MRI and PET alone.

CONFLICTS OF INTEREST

The authors have nothing to disclose. Acknowledgement to Italian Ministry of Health (Grant RF-2021-12372278), EudraCT: 2022-003905-31.

REFERENCES

1. Ling SW, de Jong AC, Schoots IG, et al. Comparison of 68Ga-labeled prostate-specific membrane antigen ligand positron emission tomography/magnetic resonance imaging and positron emission tomography/computed tomography for primary staging of prostate cancer: a systematic review and meta-analysis. Eur Urol Open Sci 2021;33:61–71.

2. Mapelli P, Picchio M. Initial prostate cancer diagnosis and disease staging—the role of choline-PET–CT. Nat Rev Urol 2015;12:510–8.

3. Corfield J, Perera M, Bolton D, et al. 68Ga-prostate specific membrane antigen (PSMA) positron emission tomography (PET) for primary staging of high-risk prostate cancer: a systematic review. World J Urol 2018;36:519–27.

4. Satapathy S, Singh H, Kumar R, et al. Diagnostic accuracy of 68 Ga-PSMA PET/CT for initial detection in patients with suspected prostate cancer: a systematic review and meta-analysis. Am J Roentgenol 2021;216:599–607.

5. von Eyben FE, Picchio M, von Eyben R, et al. 68Ga-labeled prostate-specific membrane antigen ligand positron emission tomography/computed tomography for prostate cancer: a systematic review and meta-analysis. Eur Urol Focus 2018;4:686–93.

6. Umutlu L, Beyer T, Grueneisen JS, et al. Whole-body [18F]-FDG-PET/MRI for oncology: a consensus recommendation. Nuklearmedizin 2019;58:68–76.

7. Mapelli P, Ghezzo S, Samanes Gajate AM, et al. Preliminary results of an ongoing prospective clinical trial on the use of 68Ga-PSMA and 68Ga-DOTA-RM2 PET/MRI in staging of high-risk prostate cancer patients. Diagnostics 2021;11:2068.

8. Plana MN, Arevalo-Rodriguez I, Fernández-García S, et al. Meta-DiSc 2.0: a web application for meta-analysis of diagnostic test accuracy data. BMC Med Res Methodol 2022;22:306.

9. Hicks RM, Simko JP, Westphalen AC, et al. Diagnostic accuracy of 68 Ga-PSMA-11 PET/MRI compared with multiparametric MRI in the detection of prostate cancer. Radiology 2018;289:730–7.

10. Metser U, Ortega C, Perlis N, et al. Detection of clinically significant prostate cancer with 18F-DCFPyL PET/multiparametric MR. Eur J Nucl Med Mol Imaging 2021;48:3702–11.

11. Bodar YJL, Zwezerijnen BGJC, van der Voorn PJ, et al. Prospective analysis of clinically significant prostate cancer detection with [18F]DCFPyL PET/MRI compared to multiparametric MRI: a

comparison with the histopathology in the radical prostatectomy specimen, the ProStaPET study. Eur J Nucl Med Mol Imaging 2022;49:1731–42.

12. Zeng Y, Leng X, Liao H, et al. Diagnostic value of integrated 18F-PSMA-1007 PET/MRI compared with that of biparametric MRI for the detection of prostate cancer. Prostate Int 2022;10:108–16.

13. Margel D, Bernstine H, Groshar D, et al. Diagnostic performance of 68 Ga prostate-specific membrane antigen PET/MRI compared with multiparametric MRI for detecting clinically significant prostate cancer. Radiology 2021;301:379–86.

14. Eiber M, Weirich G, Holzapfel K, et al. Simultaneous 68Ga-PSMA HBED-CC PET/MRI improves the localization of primary prostate cancer. Eur Urol 2016;70:829–36.

15. Ferraro DA, Becker AS, Kranzbühler B, et al. Diagnostic performance of 68Ga-PSMA-11 PET/MRI-guided biopsy in patients with suspected prostate cancer: a prospective single-center study. Eur J Nucl Med Mol Imaging 2021;48:3315–24.

16. Ferraro DA, Hötker AM, Becker AS, et al. 68Ga-PSMA-11 PET/MRI versus multiparametric MRI in men referred for prostate biopsy: primary tumour localization and interreader agreement. Eur J Hybrid Imaging 2022;6:14.

17. Moradi F, Duan H, Song H, et al. 68 Ga-PSMA-11 PET/MRI in patients with newly diagnosed intermediate- or high-risk prostate adenocarcinoma: PET findings correlate with outcomes after definitive treatment. J Nucl Med 2022;63:1822–8.

Hybrid PET/MR in Cardiac Imaging

Elsa Hervier, MD[a], Carl Glessgen, MD[b], René Nkoulou, MD[a], Jean François Deux, MD, PhD[b], Jean-Paul Vallee, MD, PhD[b], Dionysios Adamopoulos, PhD[c],*

KEYWORDS

- Nuclear cardiology • Cardiac MR imaging • Cardiac PET • Cardiovascular imaging
- Ischemic heart disease • Sarcoidosis

KEY POINTS

- Recent developments in PET detectors and MR imaging technology allowed the creation of truly integrated hybrid PET/MR imaging systems, readily available for research and clinical purposes.
- Over the past few years, MR imaging-based attenuation correction algorithms have been developed allowing the precise quantification of radiotracer uptake in the myocardium based on the combined PET and MR imaging images.
- The integration of highly detailed morphological, dynamic, and functional data presents a unique opportunity for a thorough investigation of cardiovascular diseases. However, the impact and clinical applicability of this approach need to be further studied.

INTRODUCTION

It was back in 2010 that a new hybrid imaging modality consisting of an integrated PET/MR imaging system was first introduced in clinical setting. Although mostly developed for oncologic applications, in 2013, innovative applications of this technology for the diagnosis of cardiovascular diseases were first described.[1] The concept is highly appealing, as this hybrid modality presents the advantage of combining strengths of both MR imaging and PET. On the one hand, the high spatial and temporal resolution of MR imaging combined with its excellent soft tissue characterization allow the anatomical and functional assessment of the myocardium including the evaluation of perfusion parameters using dynamic contrast-enhanced MR imaging acquisitions. On the other hand, PET molecular imaging can display target receptors or metabolic pathways with precise quantitative data for metabolism and perfusion.[2] The acquired information is complementary and can thereby contribute to improving the diagnostic accuracy for certain cardiovascular diseases while reducing radiation exposure compared with a conventional PET scan. The purpose of this review is to summarize from a technical and clinical point of view the advancements of hybrid cardiac PET/MR imaging as presented in the joint position statement by the European Society of Cardiovascular Radiology and the European Association of Nuclear Medicine.[3]

METHODOLOGY OF PET/MR IMAGING

From a technical point of view, conceptualizing and building PET/MR imaging systems is a challenging task. MR imaging relies on a high static magnetic field and radiofrequency pulses, which can negatively affect the function of photomultiplier tubes and electronics of the PET component. Conversely, the presence of PET detectors in the field of view (FOV) of the MR imaging scanner can also interfere with image quality and the process of image acquisition.

[a] Diagnostics Department, Nuclear Medicine and Molecular Imaging, Geneva University Hospital, Gabrielle-Perret-Gentil 4 street, 1205, Geneva, Switzerland; [b] Diagnostics Department, Radiology, Geneva University Hospital, Gabrielle-Perret-Gentil 4 street, 1205, Geneva, Switzerland; [c] Department of Medical Specialties, Cardiology, Geneva University Hospital, Gabrielle-Perret-Gentil 4 street, 1205, Geneva, Switzerland
* Corresponding author.
E-mail address: dionysios.adamopoulos@hcuge.ch

Magn Reson Imaging Clin N Am 31 (2023) 613–624
https://doi.org/10.1016/j.mric.2023.04.008

To address these difficulties, two strategies have been developed. The first approach is based on a separate or coplanar configuration for the PET and MR imaging devices which are connected via a moving table (sequential scanner).[4] This approach resolves the above-mentioned limitations as the two systems remain practically separate. The main limitation of this strategy is that simultaneous acquisition of images is not possible.

The emergence of nonconventional PET detectors robust to the electromagnetic field of MR imaging scanners, such as avalanche photodiodes or silicon photo-sensors, has allowed the development of truly integrated system, in which a PET detector ring is installed within the bore of an MR imaging scanner.[5,6] This configuration has the advantage of yielding higher sensitivity and temporal resolution as well as allowing simultaneous time-of-flight PET imaging synchronized with MR images. Then, acquisition times can be markedly reduced compared with sequential designs, leading to increased patient comfort.

The following sections are set to discuss the principal features of such integrated designs and to highlight the main challenges encountered.

Attenuation Correction

Attenuation correction (AC) is a crucial step in the processing of PET imaging data and represents an important challenge when integrating cardiac PET/MR imaging systems. This step involves the correction of photon attenuation (through absorption or scattering) by the patients' own tissues and the scanner components, after they are produced by PET radiotracers. This phenomenon causes an underestimation of tracer concentration and a reduction in image quality. In the context of cardiology applications, non-AC PET would allow for less reliable evaluation of absolute myocardial perfusion values and misregistration artifacts would lower the diagnostic performance.

In conventional PET/CT systems, attenuation maps (μ-maps) are calculated for each voxel within the volume, using the co-registered computed tomography (CT) data sampled at lower energy as base for extrapolation of the attenuation of 511 keV photons. Because MR images only provide proton density levels and do not rely on x-rays, extrapolation to obtain adequate attenuation coefficients is more challenging.[7]

The reference technique is the segmentation- or atlas-based AC. In the segmentation-based AC, the body is divided into different tissue categories with different attenuation coefficients: air, lung, fat, and soft tissue. The segmentation is performed either using a standard multipoint Dixon sequence, T1-weighted 3D turbo spin echo imaging or fat-suppressed 3D gradient echo (GRE) sequences (eg, VIBE, THRIVE, LAVA-XL, TIGRE, or 3D-QUICK, following different vendors acronyms).[8,9] These methods require breath-hold durations of 18 to 24 seconds per acquisition, which can be difficult for frail patients or patients with compromising respiratory disease. Some more recent algorithms also integrate a bone atlas using ultra-short echo time sequences to better segment cortical bone, although less suited for cardiac imaging due to smaller FOV and longer acquisition times.[10]

The segmentation-based AC has proven to be efficient with a very close agreement between PET-CT and PET/MR imaging for imaging viability with ^{18}F-fluorodeoxyglucose (18F-FDG).[11] More recently, the development of acceleration techniques allows obtaining AC images with higher resolution, which alleviate the need of additional diagnostic sequences, thus resulting in an overall reduction of the examination duration.[12]

Another important challenge for the MR imaging-based AC is the size of the FOV, which is smaller in the MR imaging scanner (because of B0 inhomogeneities and gradient nonlinearities) than in the PET scanner. This difference can lead to gaps at the edge of the attenuation map, so-called "truncation artifacts," most often seen on the arms and shoulders of patients with larger body habitus, leading to AC bias. To overcome this problem, an emission-based AC using maximum likelihood estimation of activity and attenuation is performed where non-corrected PET data are used to calculate missing parts of the attenuation map.[13] This method works well for radiotracers such as 18F-FDG but is limited when radiotracers have no or minor uptake in the truncated parts. As a solution to this problem, the B0 *homogenization using gradient* enhancement technique was proposed. This approach optimizes the readout gradient to compensate locally B0 inhomogeneities and thus reducing truncations outside the FOV of the MR imaging scanner as well as attenuation bias potentially arising in the thoracic region.[14]

Finally, in fully integrated systems, a predefined CT transmission scan-based attenuation map of the hardware components (table, radiofrequency coils (RF) coils) is added to the patient tissue attenuation map before PET reconstruction.[15]

Potential advances in obtaining optimal AC-based PET images could involve a stand-alone PET AC process using emission data which usually requires sufficient regional statistic count activity and may not be translated when using PET tracers with restricted body distribution.[16] In addition, artificial intelligence compensation methods show promising results that would enable improvement in this field.[17,18]

Artifacts and Limitations

Some of the most important intrinsic limitations encountered in PET/MR imaging applications for cardiac imaging are motion artifacts due to heartbeat and breathing, which require electrocardiographic (ECG)-gating systems and breath-hold imaging. More advanced acquisition techniques include respiratory and cardiac movement compensation using either external respiratory gating or data-driven respiratory compensation of the PET raw data.[19,20]

Artifacts generated by metallic implants can equally impair the interpretation of PET/MR imaging data. Many different devices (eg, pacemakers, stents, and defibrillators) are often present in patients undergoing cardiac imaging and the nonferromagnetic metallic components may cause susceptibility or metal artifacts that are translated into the attenuation map. This results in an underestimation of the local tracer uptake. A study including 20 patients who underwent perfusion imaging with ammonia PET/MR imaging and viability with FDG PET/MR imaging found artifacts due to sternal wires and metallic implants in 20% and 30% of cases, respectively, with maximum standardized uptake value (SUV) mean differences ranging from 11% to 196% after correction.[21]

Segmentation errors may also occur due to the use of MR imaging contrast media because of the decrease in T1 values affecting the contrast of T1-weighted MR imaging sequences used for AC segmentation. A possible solution would be to synthesize attenuation maps from MR images without relying solely on T1-weighted sequences.

An additional limitation encountered with PET/MR imaging is the fact that MR imaging data are often nonisotropic and acquired in a non-axial direction. PET data resampling can be particularly difficult if a low resolution is used in the slice direction due to time constraints. Finally, patient compliance in the setting of a lengthy examination (40 to 60 minutes) is another limiting factor.

MR imaging protocol design

In a cardiac PET/MR imaging examination, several MR imaging sequences can be used to obtain comprehensive diagnostic information. At the start of the protocol, AC is performed by acquiring one of the sequences mentioned above to generate AC maps. Indiscriminately of the clinical question, a typical cardiac MR (cMR) imagingprotocol should include T1- and T2-weighted mapping sequences

for tissue characterization and late gadolinium enhancement (LGE) to identify myocardial fibrosis and scarring. In addition, functional and wall motion assessment is provided by cine imaging, typically balanced steady-state free precession sequences, also known as TrueFISP, FIESTA, or balanced fast field echo (bFFE).

Depending on the indication, more targeted and specific sequences can be used. Phase-contrast sequences are used to evaluate blood flow and velocity across the heart valves and within the great vessels. Myocardial perfusion imaging can be performed using first-pass contrast-enhanced sequences, such as spoiled gradient-echo or turbo/fast low-angle shot (FLASH) sequences to assess myocardial blood flow and detect ischemic regions. Finally, angiographic images can be obtained by acquiring fast gradient-echo sequences after contrast media administration. A presentation of standard and specific MR imaging sequences can be found in Table 1.

PET protocol design

Depending on the investigated physiologic process, different PET radiotracers are used. For perfusion studies, two tracers are mainly used in clinical practice, that is, rubidium-82 chloride (^{82}Rb) and ^{13}N-ammonia chloride (^{13}NH$_3$). ^{82}Rb is a generator-produced (^{82}strontium/^{82}Rb) PET myocardial perfusion tracer, which acts as a potassium analog entering the myocardial cell via active transport. It is eluted from a generator by a computer-regulated elution pump and injected as a bolus directly into the patient through an intravenous (IV) infusion system. The low first-pass extraction of around 50% to 60%, decreasing with high coronary flow, in association with a high energetic positron emission, makes this radiotracer less favorable for spatial imaging resolution. ^{13}NH$_3$ is a cyclotron-produced tracer that diffuses passively or actively by transport into the myocardial cell and remains trapped through incorporation of ^{13}N into the amino acid ^{13}N-glutamine. Its excellent extraction fraction of around 80%, lower energetic positron, and good target-to-background ratio makes it one of the best available PET myocardial perfusion tracers (Fig. 1, Table 2). Unfortunately, these radiotracers have a short half-life that requires an onsite cyclotron or generator, the need to incorporate the injection module into the MR imaging environment, and the necessity of using pharmacologic (and not physiologic) stress, thus removing a powerful prognostic information.[22] Recently, a novel myocardial perfusion ^{18}F-flurpiridaz, a structural analog of the insecticide pyridaben that binds to mitochondrial complex-1, has been studied in phase-III clinical

Table 1
Overview of MR imaging sequences used in clinical cardiac MR imaging

		Purpose	Sequence Type	Sequence Names	Expected Duration (Breath-Hold)
Standard	Cine imaging	Functional assessment	SSFP	FIESTA (GE), TrueFISP (Siemens), Balanced FFE (Philips), True SSFP (Toshiba)	3–5 min for short axis stack
	T1 mapping Post-contrast T1 mapping	Tissue characterization LGE and ECV	Inversion-recovery, saturation-recovery	Look Locker imaging (MOLLI), shortened MOLLI (shMOLLI), Saturation-recovery single-shot acquisition (SASHA)	~ 1 breath-hold per slice
	T2 mapping	Tissue characterization	Single-shot balanced SSFP, gradient, and spin echo	T2p-SSFP, MESE, GraSE, FSE	~ 1 breath-hold per slice
	LGE imaging	Tissue characterization (scars/fibrosis)	IR GRE, SSFP, PSIR	IR PrepFGRE (GE), IR TurboFLASH (Siemens), IR TFE (Philips), FFESeg IR (Canon)	3–10 min depending on the method
Specific	Perfusion Imaging	Myocardial perfusion analysis	GRE, EPI	EPI-FGR-Multiphase (GE), EPI/FLASH (Siemens), TFE/EPI (Philips)	80–90 images, one per heartbeat
	Flow Imaging	Dynamic flow assessment	Velocity-encoded cine imaging	Phase contrast	~ 1 breath-hold per slice
	Angiographic Imaging	Vessel assessment	T1-weighted FSE or spoiled GRE	TRICKS, LAVA (GE), TWIST (Siemens), THRIVE (Philips)	~ 1 breath-hold per volume

Note: Standard sequences make up the core of a cardiac MR imaging protocol, whereas specific sequences are targeted toward specific indications and not systematically acquired.
Abbreviations: cMR, cardiac MR; ECV, extra-cellular volume; EPI, echo planar imaging; GRE, gradient echo imaging; IR, inversion recovery; LGE, late gadolinium enhancement; PSIR, phase-sensitive IR; PWI, perfusion-weighted image; SSFP, steady-state free precession; TSI, time–signal intensity.

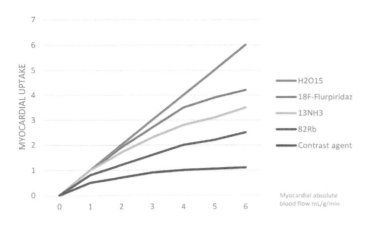

trials, showing promising results for the assessment of coronary artery disease and allowing more flexibility in protocols, because ^{18}F-flurpiridaz has a longer half-life than the tracers mentioned above, thus not requiring an on-site cyclotron and allowing injection during physical exercise with an excellent extraction fraction of around 90%.[23] Finally, $H_2^{15}O$ has also been used as a perfusion radiotracer and is considered the gold standard for the evaluation of myocardial perfusion, as it freely diffuses from blood into the myocardial cell, with a nearly 100% extraction fraction, regardless of metabolic factors and coronary flow rate.[24] Despite its success in research studies, the clinical use of $H_2^{15}O$ is still limited because image postprocessing is very demanding as the persisting circulating blood pool activity needs to be subtracted with dedicated research software; in addition, this tracer is only authorized on the European market.

For metabolic studies of the heart, the main radiotracer used is 18F-FDG. It consists of a glucose analog that is actively transported into viable cells through Glucose transporters and remains trapped within the myocytes after being phosphorylated by a hexokinase into 18F-FDG-phosphate. It can demonstrate, depending on the protocol used, either myocardial inflammation or viability.[25]

PET images are acquired in list mode imaging, which preserves all the spatiotemporal information with 3D PET mode (septa removed) allowing an improved imaging system sensitivity in association with ECG triggering. The acquisition starts briefly before radiotracer injection for perfusion application and 45 to 90 minutes after injection for viability or inflammation exploration. The total scanning session ranges between 30 and 90 minutes.

The course of typical perfusion and viability PET/MR imaging protocols is depicted in Fig. 2.

Image Analysis

Multiple software solutions are available for offline postprocessing and interpretation of PET/MR imaging images and offer semiautomatic or automated processing. Some focus on either MR imaging or PET, whereas others integrate all data, for example, OsiriX (Osirix foundation, Geneva, Switzerland), syngo.via (Siemens Healthineers, Erlangen, Germany) or Xeleris (GE Healthcare, Chicago, United States), among others. Nonetheless, software solutions for fully integrated PET/MR imaging analyses are still missing.

CLINICAL APPLICATIONS
Myocardial Perfusion

Myocardial perfusion has been evaluated for years using pure nuclear cardiology modalities, traditionally with SPECT imaging.[26] However, PET-CT has several advantages over SPECT, that is, lower radiation dose, higher spatial and temporal resolution, and the possibility to quantify the myocardial blood flow as well as the coronary flow reserve, which are valuable tools for detecting significant coronary artery disease.[27] PET-CT allows not only the visual detection of myocardial perfusion defects but also the actual, absolute quantification of the myocardial blood flow both at rest and in stress conditions, for each individual myocardial segment. It has been demonstrated that PET-CT outperforms SPECT by providing more accurate risk stratification, especially in patients with severe coronary artery disease (three vessels disease) and/or balanced ischemia.[28]

Stress MR imaging techniques offer the possibility to noninvasively quantify myocardium perfusion using IV administration of gadolinium-based contrast media. The high in-plane MR imaging resolution combined with wider MR imaging

Table 2
Cardiac PET radiotracers used in the clinical setting

Mechanism	Radionuclide	Pharmaceutical	Half-Life	Extraction Rate by Myocardial Cells	Range in Soft Tissue	Resolution and Image Quality	Production Method
Perfusion	N-13	Ammonia	10 min	70–80%	5.4 mm	++	Cyclotron
	Rb-82	Rubidium chloride	1.3 min	60%	15 mm	+	Generator
Glucose metabolism	F-18	Fluorodeoxyglucose	110 min		2.4 mm	+++	Cyclotron

availability, lack of ionizing radiation, and the combination of perfusion assessment with unparalleled tissue characterization are important advantages. Theoretically, a combination of PET and MR imaging myocardial perfusion evaluation could be used for mutual cross-validation of segmental myocardial blood flow, which could be of major clinical utility especially in case of perfusion artifacts with one or the other technique. Nonetheless, comparative studies regarding myocardial perfusion by PET and MR imaging have shown controversial results with MR imaging perfusion presenting global significant underestimation of myocardial flow.[29] This is partially explained by the fact that MR imaging signal intensity and gadolinium concentration are not related linearly, irrespectively of the deconvolution method used. Moreover, in contrast to the classic PET perfusion tracers, gadolinium is only distributed to the extracellular space and does not interact with the myocardial cells.

However, myocardial tissue characterization including infarct detection by MR imaging with an excellent spatial resolution may provide complementary information when combined with perfusion data. Especially, LGE provided by MR imaging has added prognostic value over conventional risk factors and can predict significant coronary artery disease.[30,31] Finally, the possibility of visualization of the coronary arterial tree by MR imaging can yield additional value in association with the functional and perfusion abnormalities in specific anatomical beds, with the admitted lower accuracy for non-proximal coronary segments.

Myocardial Viability Evaluation

The distinction between viable, hibernating, and nonviable myocardium is an active area of research for both therapeutic intervention (revascularization) guidance and prognosis determination. Conflicting results have recently questioned the use of viability information as guidance toward revascularization aiming at improved prognosis.[32] The concept of viability has been differently defined using different imaging modalities. The presence of hibernating myocardium induced typically by chronic ischemia, suggests underlying intact myocardial metabolism, and is associated with better outcomes when associated with targeted revascularization.[33] The accurate determination of the extent of nonviable myocardium characterized by metabolic inactivity is also of major importance, for assessing myocardial performance and prognosis, especially in patients with heart failure and/or after myocardial infarction. 18F-FDG PET has been traditionally used for the detection of myocardial viability based on basic

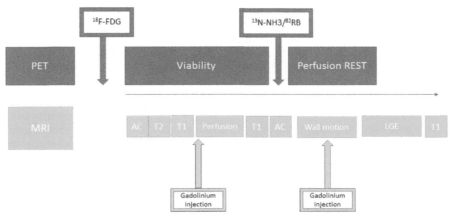

Fig. 2. Typical example of a perfusion and viability PET/MR imaging protocol.

cellular metabolic activity tracing and is considered as the gold standard.[34,35] Its utility though is limited by the required specific patient preparation to ensure that 18F-FDG is fully absorbed by the myocardium. This is achieved by the administration of glucose, the combined administration of insulin and glucose, and administration of acipimox, a niacin derivative. The 18F-FDG PET evaluation requires concomitant flow evaluation to assess myocardial metabolism in hypoperfused myocardial areas. The reduction of blood flow in dysfunctional myocardial regions with enhanced glucose utilization indicates hibernating but viable myocardium.[36] Decreased glucose utilization, though, with concomitant reduction of blood flow indicates scarred tissue. The prognostic significance is important because in patients with viable myocardium a 79.6% reduction in mortality among those who were treated with revascularization was achieved.[37]

cardiac MR (cMR) imaging is also capable of detecting nonviable myocardium. One basic approach is through the evaluation of wall thickness and contractile function on cine imaging, both being markedly reduced in case of nonviable myocardium.[38] In addition, LGE is widely used for assessing myocardial viability. Gadolinium-based contrast agents accumulate in areas of myocardial fibrosis or scarring, resulting in hyperenhancement on T1-weighted images. The extent and localization of the LGE signal can then be assessed. Sub-endocardial patterns (<25% of the wall thickness) suggest partial damage to the myocardial wall, whereas transmural enhancement ≥50% indicates higher degree of myocardial injury, which is associated with a lower likelihood of functional recovery after revascularization and reduced prognosis.[38,39] Because gadolinium enhancement is independent from cellular metabolic pathway, specific patient's preparation is not required.

Furthermore, MR imaging has the advantage of the complete absence of ionizing radiation, whereas the high spatial resolution permits the detection of even small areas of scars.

Very few studies have compared the agreement between the two methods, PET and MR imaging, in detecting nonviable myocardium, showing good agreement.[40] Further, small cohort studies have examined the additional benefit of combined PET/MR imaging over the two methods alone[41–45] in the assessment of myocardial viability with promising findings. The reclassification effect using the integrated method was reported up to 20% overall but a recent analysis demonstrated over 80% reclassification of inconclusive cases by PET or MR imaging alone.[45] In addition, scar tissue mapping by MR imaging correlated weakly with hibernation information from PET, hinting at a potential complementarity of the two imaging modalities.[40] However, the method remains investigational in the assessment of myocardial viability, and the incremental benefit of hybrid PET/MR imaging in patients with ischemic heart disease before revascularization remains to be evaluated.

Inflammation

Inflammation plays a central role in myocardial injury and healing during myocardial ischemia and can be found in cases with or without reperfusion.[46,47] Ischemic inflammation reaction is characterized by significant infiltration of the myocardium with neutrophils, monocyte-macrophages, and other inflammatory cells, which is followed by a noninflammatory subset few days later.[48] As such, inflammation has been proposed as a promising therapeutic target for myocardial healing and remodeling.

The characterization of the inflammatory process can be achieved with great precision by both PET and MR imaging scans. cMR can detect edema through T2 mapping or fluid-sensitive sequences (STIR) and hyperemia through T1 mapping. In addition, focal increases in extracellular volume as measured by pre-contrast and post-contrast T1 mapping are indirect signs of edema. Of note, T2* imaging allows to better depict hemorrhage associated with reperfusion injury.[49]

Inflammation activity can also be accurately detected by an 18F-FDG PET scan, after the suppression of the physiologic 18F-FDG uptake of the heart, which is achieved through a combination of fasting and dietary changes to switch cardiomyocyte metabolism to free fatty acid. This suppression is necessary to avoid background noise caused by normal cardiac metabolic activity which would cover potential abnormalities by taking up the glucose-mimicking 18F-FDG. Recent guidelines advise to fast 12 to 18 hours with a high-fat, low carbohydrates, protein-permitted diet and IV administration of unfractionated heparin (50 UI/Kg, 15 minutes before 18F-FDG).[50] For some patients (especially diabetics), a complete inhibition of the physiologic myocardial glucose metabolism can be hard to achieve leading to false-positive results. In this context, integrated PET/MR imaging has demonstrated an inverse correlation between 18F-FDG uptake and function outcome at 6 months, offering perspectives on the identification of at-risk patient for heart failure after myocardial infarction.

Myocarditis

The gold standard for the diagnosis of myocarditis is myocardial biopsy, an invasive procedure that may be associated with significant complications such as myocardial perforation and pericardial effusion.[51] Clinical guidelines recommend MR imaging scan as the initial evaluation of patients with suspected myocarditis, because edema, myocyte injury, and ultimately scar can be easily detected.[52] These elements are incorporated in the revised Lake Louise Criteria (LLC) for the diagnosis of myocarditis and are used in clinical practice.[53] The LLC are a set of diagnostic criteria for suspected myocarditis relying on multimodality imaging. Two criteria must be met: one T1-based criterion (increased T1 values, increased extracellular volume, or positive LGE) and one T2-based criterion (increased T2 values or increased global T2 signal intensity ratio). Although edema indicated by increased T2 values resolves within 3 to 4 weeks in uncomplicated disease, scarring can persist up to months after the initial myocarditis.[54]

In the last few years, combined 18F-FDG PET/MR imaging has been used in an increasing number of studies, showing a low sensitivity of 74% and excellent specificity of 95% as compared with the LLC alone.[55] However, 18F-FDG PET offers complementary information as compared with the MR imaging elements because it can detect and quantify the actual inflammatory activity of myocardial cells. This may be important in both long-term follow-up and evaluation of the response to immunotherapy. However, the clinical benefit in terms of treatment adaptation and prognosis of such an approach needs to be demonstrated.

Sarcoidosis

Sarcoidosis is a chronic, inflammatory, multisystem disease, characterized by noncaseating granulomas. The detection of cardiac involvement is of paramount importance because it alters prognosis and immunosuppression treatment intensity. The diagnostic approach comprises endomyocardial biopsy which is invasive in nature, associated with significant complications and a low diagnostic yield. The role of the MR imaging in the diagnostic assessment of sarcoidosis is important because it detects fibrotic tissue with precise localization and extension (typically in the basal septal and inferolateral walls), the presence of edema and extracellular volume changes (T1 and T2 mapping). It also allows the detection of regional wall abnormalities and systolic dysfunction, element with significant prognostic implications. PET imaging (both 18F-FDG and perfusion) has also a central role in staging sarcoidosis as it detects active inflammation (macrophage activity, Fig. 3). The complementary value of combining 18F-FDG PET and MR imaging for the diagnosis of cardiac sarcoidosis (CS) was studied by Vita and colleagues and showed that among the 91 patients with abnormal MR imaging (eg, LGE), 48 (45%) were reclassified as having a higher or lower likelihood of CS after the addition of PET information and most of them (80%) being correctly reclassified when compared with the final diagnosis. In such patients, positive 18F-FDG allowed higher confidence in the diagnosis of CS and identification of candidates for immunosuppressive therapy. On the other hand, eight individuals had abnormal 18F-FDG uptake without LGE, and only four of them were ultimately categorized as probable or high probability of CS. In general, 18F-FDG PET has a higher sensitivity, and MR imaging may have a slightly higher specificity in the diagnosis of CS.[56] Finally, one significant advantage of the 18F-FDG PET compared with MR imaging is the ability to quantify the degree of

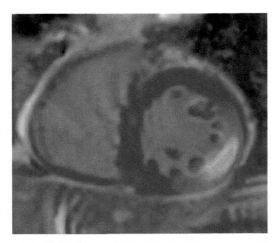

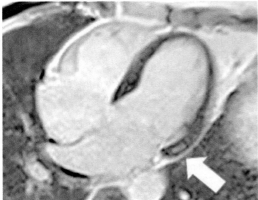

Fig. 3. Hybrid PET/MR imaging examination of a 43-year-old patient with CS. The LGE of the basal infero-lateral segment (*arrow*) corresponds to the increase in the 18F-FDG absorption seen with the PET examination.[70]

myocardial inflammation using SUVs. It can be used both for prognosis[57] and assessment response to therapy without clear benefit from the adjunction of MR imaging other than reducing radiation exposure compared with PET/CT.[58]

Cardiac masses

Cardiac masses were one of the first cardiovascular conditions investigated with PET/MR imaging with the combination of the 18F-FDG powerful oncologic tracer and the anatomic characterization with MR imaging. Both modalities have already strong diagnostic performance in the assessment of malignancy, but in some cases, the complementary information can help differentiate benign from malignant lesion as demonstrated by Yaddanapudi and colleagues.[59] In a small pilot study of 20 patients, integrated assessment of MR imaging and PET allowed to improve

the diagnostic accuracy compared with each modality alone. In this study, 18F-FDG scanning had a sensitivity and specificity of 100% and 92%, respectively. MR imaging showed similar results, but when the results from the two modalities were combined, 100% sensitivity and specificity were achieved.[60] However, considering the already strong diagnostic performance of PET and MR imaging, the high cost, and limited availability of PET/MR imaging scanners, integrated PET/MR imaging might be reserved for selected cases such as patient with complex surgery planning or treatment follow-up.

Future perspectives

A growing body of evidence recently showed that other tracers could also be of interest for specific myocardial diseases. The detection of amyloid deposition in cardiac amyloidosis with 18F-sodium fluoride (18F-NaF), a bone-seeking tracer used for skeletal imaging of bone metastasis, could be useful in diagnosing and differentiating cardiac transthyretin amyloidosis (ATTR)-amyloidosis in a similar fashion to that of 99m-Tc bone scintigraphy agents, especially in conjunction with MR imaging. Indeed, Andrews and colleagues[61] described 18F-NaF use with PET-MR imaging in 53 patients, showing its ability to accurately diagnose cardiac amyloidosis on MR imaging while on the same time differentiating ATTR from amyloid light chain (AL-amyloidosis with the tracer uptake in areas of LGE being significantly higher in ATTR-amyloidosis compared to AL-amyloidosis). Moreover, PET amyloid fluorine-labeled tracers (18F-florbetapir, 18F-florbetaben, and 18F-flutemetamol), originally developed for β-amyloid detection in Alzheimer's disease, have been acknowledged for the detection of cardiac amyloidosis. Although those PET amyloid agents bind to any type of amyloid fibrils, it has been shown that the affinity is higher for AL type and could distinguish between the two entities.[62] The quantitative nature of PET associated with the MR imaging could theoretically prevent diagnostic delay due to sequential images and potentially provide earlier diagnosis, assessment of amyloid burden, and track disease progression and/or treatment response to the array of new therapies developed for this condition.[63]

Other frequently used oncologic PET tracers have been studied for the evaluation of cardiac inflammation especially in CS. In fact, 68Ga-labeled somatostatin analogs have shown valuable results for this diagnosis as epithelioid cells, giant cells, and macrophages found in sarcoid granulomas highly expressing SSTR somatostatin receptor subtype 2 somatostatin receptor

(SSTR2).[64] Three PET tracers exist with different affinities to the different subtypes of the SSTR receptor: 68Ga-DOTANOC has a high affinity to SSTR3 and SSTR5, 68Ga-DOTATOC has mainly high affinity to SSTR5, and 68Ga-DOTATATE has a greater affinity to SSTR2.[65] The main advantages of these radiotracers are the absence of uptake in the normal heart, resulting in high signal-to-noise ratio and allowing straightforward and reproducible image interpretation[66] without rigorous preparation of the patient as needed with 18F-FDG.[67] Future studies will be necessary to provide evidence for the clinical application of SSTR2 PET/MR imaging in CS and other cardiovascular inflammation process such as vasculitis.[68]

Finally, another area of potential interest is the use of 18F-NaF for imaging vulnerable plaques in coronary disease, a tracer that accumulates in microcalcifications by chemisorption. Although this could theoretically constitute an independent predictor of cardiovascular events, the diagnostic benefit of combining PET and MR imaging in this evaluation still needs to be proven.[69]

DISCLOSURE

The Authors have nothing to disclose.

REFERENCES

1. Rischpler C, Nekolla SG, Dregely I, et al. Hybrid PET/MR imaging of the heart: potential, initial experiences, and future prospects. J Nucl Med 2013;54: 402–15.
2. Xu J, Cai F, Geng C, et al. Diagnostic performance of CMR, SPECT, and PET imaging for the identification of coronary artery disease: a meta-analysis. Front Cardiovasc Med 2021;8:621389.
3. Nensa F, Bamberg F, Rischpler C, et al. Hybrid cardiac imaging using PET/MRI: a joint position statement by the European Society of Cardiovascular Radiology (ESCR) and the European Association of Nuclear Medicine (EANM). Eur Radiol 2018;28: 4086–101.
4. Zaidi H, Ojha N, Morich M, et al. Design and performance evaluation of a whole-body Ingenuity TF PET-MRI system. Phys Med Biol 2011;56:3091–106.
5. Pichler BJ, Judenhofer MS, Catana C, et al. Performance test of an LSO-APD detector in a 7-T MRI scanner for simultaneous PET/MRI. J Nucl Med 2006;47:639–47.
6. Judenhofer MS, Wehrl HF, Newport DF, et al. Simultaneous PET-MRI: a new approach for functional and morphological imaging. Nat Med 2008;14:459–65.
7. Carney JP, Townsend DW, Rappoport V, et al. Method for transforming CT images for attenuation correction in PET/CT imaging. Med Phys 2006;33: 976–83.
8. Rausch I, Rust P, DiFranco MD, et al. Reproducibility of MRI dixon-based attenuation correction in combined PET/MR with applications for lean body mass estimation. J Nucl Med 2016;57:1096–101.
9. Schulz V, Torres-Espallardo I, Renisch S, et al. Automatic, three-segment, MR-based attenuation correction for whole-body PET/MR data. Eur J Nucl Med Mol Imaging 2011;38:138–52.
10. Keereman V, Fierens Y, Broux T, et al. MRI-based attenuation correction for PET/MRI using ultrashort echo time sequences. J Nucl Med 2010;51:812–8.
11. Lau JMC, Laforest R, Sotoudeh H, et al. Evaluation of attenuation correction in cardiac PET using PET/MR. J Nucl Cardiol 2017;24:839–46.
12. Freitag MT, Fenchel M, Baumer P, et al. Improved clinical workflow for simultaneous whole-body PET/MRI using high-resolution CAIPIRINHA-accelerated MR-based attenuation correction. Eur J Radiol 2017;96:12–20.
13. Nuyts J, Bal G, Kehren F, et al. Completion of a truncated attenuation image from the attenuated PET emission data. IEEE Trans Med Imaging 2013;32: 237–46.
14. Lindemann ME, Oehmigen M, Blumhagen JO, et al. MR-based truncation and attenuation correction in integrated PET/MR hybrid imaging using HUGE with continuous table motion. Med Phys 2017;44: 4559–72.
15. Martinez-Moller A, Souvatzoglou M, Delso G, et al. Tissue classification as a potential approach for attenuation correction in whole-body PET/MRI: evaluation with PET/CT data. J Nucl Med 2009;50:520–6.
16. Rezaei A, Defrise M, Bal G, et al. Simultaneous reconstruction of activity and attenuation in time-of-flight PET. IEEE Trans Med Imaging 2012;31: 2224–33.
17. Zaidi H, Nkoulou R. Artifact-free quantitative cardiovascular PET/MR imaging: an impossible dream? J Nucl Cardiol 2019;26:1119–21.
18. Liu F, Jang H, Kijowski R, et al. Deep learning MR imaging-based attenuation correction for PET/MR Imaging. Radiology 2018;286:676–84.
19. Villagran Asiares A, Vitadello T, et al. Value of PET ECG gating in a cross-validation study of cardiac function assessment by PET/MR imaging. J Nucl Cardiol 2022;30:1050–60.
20. Ruan W, Liu F, Sun X, et al. Evaluating two respiratory correction methods for abdominal PET/MRI imaging. EJNMMI Phys 2022;9:5.
21. Lassen ML, Rasul S, Beitzke D, et al. Assessment of attenuation correction for myocardial PET imaging using combined PET/MRI. J Nucl Cardiol 2019;26: 1107–18.
22. Edelson JB, Burstein DS, Paridon S, et al. Exercise stress testing: a valuable tool to predict

risk and prognosis. Prog Pediatr Cardiol 2019;54: 101130.

23. Maddahi J, Lazewatsky J, Udelson JE, et al. Phase-III clinical trial of fluorine-18 flurpiridaz positron emission tomography for evaluation of coronary artery disease. J Am Coll Cardiol 2020;76:391–401.

24. Maaniitty T, Knuuti J, Saraste A. 15O-Water PET MPI: current status and future perspectives. Semin Nucl Med 2020;50:238–47.

25. Celiker-Guler E, Ruddy TD, Wells RG. Acquisition, processing, and interpretation of PET (18)F-FDG viability and inflammation studies. Curr Cardiol Rep 2021;23:124.

26. Gowd BM, Heller GV, Parker MW. Stress-only SPECT myocardial perfusion imaging: a review. J Nucl Cardiol 2014;21:1200–12.

27. Knuuti J, Wijns W, Saraste A, et al. 2019 ESC Guidelines for the diagnosis and management of chronic coronary syndromes. Eur Heart J 2020;41:407–77.

28. Shaw LJ, Hage FG, Berman DS, et al. Prognosis in the era of comparative effectiveness research: where is nuclear cardiology now and where should it be? J Nucl Cardiol 2012;19:1026–43.

29. Nazir MS, Gould SM, Milidonis X, et al. Simultaneous (13)N-Ammonia and gadolinium first-pass myocardial perfusion with quantitative hybrid PET-MR imaging: a phantom and clinical feasibility study. Eur J Hybrid Imaging 2019;3:15.

30. Pezel T, Hovasse T, Sanguineti F, et al. Long-term prognostic value of stress CMR in patients with heart failure and preserved ejection fraction. JACC Cardiovasc Imaging 2021;14:2319–33.

31. Di Bella G, Pingitore A, Piaggi P, et al. Usefulness of late gadolinium enhancement MRI combined with stress imaging in predictive significant coronary stenosis in new-diagnosed left ventricular dysfunction. Int J Cardiol 2016;224:337–42.

32. Panza JA, Ellis AM, Al-Khalidi HR, et al. Myocardial viability and long-term outcomes in ischemic cardiomyopathy. N Engl J Med 2019;381:739–48.

33. Rahimtoola SH. A perspective on the three large multicenter randomized clinical trials of coronary bypass surgery for chronic stable angina. Circulation 1985;72:V123–35.

34. Tillisch J, Brunken R, Marshall R, et al. Reversibility of cardiac wall-motion abnormalities predicted by positron tomography. N Engl J Med 1986;314: 884–8.

35. Schinkel AF, Poldermans D, Elhendy A, et al. Assessment of myocardial viability in patients with heart failure. J Nucl Med 2007;48:1135–46.

36. Taegtmeyer H, Dilsizian V. Imaging myocardial metabolism and ischemic memory. Nat Clin Pract Cardiovasc Med 2008;5(Suppl 2):S42–8.

37. Allman KC, Shaw LJ, Hachamovitch R, et al. Myocardial viability testing and impact of revascularization on prognosis in patients with coronary artery disease and left ventricular dysfunction: a meta-analysis. J Am Coll Cardiol 2002;39:1151–8.

38. Kim RJ, Wu E, Rafael A, et al. The use of contrast-enhanced magnetic resonance imaging to identify reversible myocardial dysfunction. N Engl J Med 2000;343:1445–53.

39. Krone RJ, Friedman E, Thanavaro S, et al. Long-term prognosis after first Q-wave (transmural) or non-Q-wave (nontransmural) myocardial infarction: analysis of 593 patients. Am J Cardiol 1983;52:234–9.

40. Klein C, Nekolla SG, Bengel FM, et al. Assessment of myocardial viability with contrast-enhanced magnetic resonance imaging: comparison with positron emission tomography. Circulation 2002;105:162–7.

41. Priamo J, Adamopoulos D, Rager O, et al. Downstream indication to revascularization following hybrid cardiac PET/MRI: preliminary results. Nucl Med Commun 2017;38:515–22.

42. Rischpler C, Langwieser N, Souvatzoglou M, et al. PET/MRI early after myocardial infarction: evaluation of viability with late gadolinium enhancement transmurality vs. 18F-FDG uptake. Eur Heart J Cardiovasc Imaging 2015;16:661–9.

43. Nensa F, Poeppel TD, Beiderwellen K, et al. Hybrid PET/MR imaging of the heart: feasibility and initial results. Radiology 2013;268:366–73.

44. Beitzke D, Rasul S, Lassen ML, et al. Assessment of myocardial viability in ischemic heart disease by PET/MRI: comparison of left ventricular perfusion, hibernation, and scar burden. Acad Radiol 2020;27: 188–97.

45. Barrio P, Lopez-Melgar B, Fidalgo A, et al. Additional value of hybrid PET/MR imaging versus MR or PET performed separately to assess cardiovascular disease. Rev Esp Cardiol 2021;74:303–11.

46. Aletras AH, Tilak GS, Natanzon A, et al. Retrospective determination of the area at risk for reperfused acute myocardial infarction with T2-weighted cardiac magnetic resonance imaging: histopathological and displacement encoding with stimulated echoes (DENSE) functional validations. Circulation 2006; 113:1865–70.

47. Tilak GS, Hsu LY, Hoyt RF Jr, et al. In vivo T2-weighted magnetic resonance imaging can accurately determine the ischemic area at risk for 2-day-old nonreperfused myocardial infarction. Invest Radiol 2008;43:7–15.

48. Tsujioka H, Imanishi T, Ikejima H, et al. Impact of heterogeneity of human peripheral blood monocyte subsets on myocardial salvage in patients with primary acute myocardial infarction. J Am Coll Cardiol 2009;54:130–8.

49. O'Regan DP, Ariff B, Neuwirth C, et al. Assessment of severe reperfusion injury with T2* cardiac MRI in patients with acute myocardial infarction. Heart 2010;96:1885–91.

50. Slart R, Glaudemans A, Gheysens O, et al. Procedural recommendations of cardiac PET/CT imaging: standardization in inflammatory-, infective-, infiltrative-, and innervation- (4Is) related cardiovascular diseases: a joint collaboration of the EACVI and the EANM: summary. Eur Heart J Cardiovasc Imaging 2020;21:1320–30.

51. Caforio AL, Pankuweit S, Arbustini E, et al. Current state of knowledge on aetiology, diagnosis, management, and therapy of myocarditis: a position statement of the European Society of Cardiology Working Group on Myocardial and Pericardial Diseases. Eur Heart J 2013;34:2636–48, 2648a-2648d.

52. Friedrich MG, Sechtem U, Schulz-Menger J, et al. Cardiovascular magnetic resonance in myocarditis: a JACC white paper. J Am Coll Cardiol 2009;53:1475–87.

53. Ferreira VM, Schulz-Menger J, Holmvang G, et al. Cardiovascular magnetic resonance in nonischemic myocardial inflammation: expert recommendations. J Am Coll Cardiol 2018;72:3158–76.

54. Friedrich MG, Marcotte F. Cardiac magnetic resonance assessment of myocarditis. Circ Cardiovasc Imaging 2013;6:833–9.

55. Nensa F, Kloth J, Tezgah E, et al. Feasibility of FDG-PET in myocarditis: comparison to CMR using integrated PET/MRI. J Nucl Cardiol 2018;25:785–94.

56. Aggarwal NR, Snipelisky D, Young PM, et al. Advances in imaging for diagnosis and management of cardiac sarcoidosis. Eur Heart J Cardiovasc Imaging 2015;16:949–58.

57. Ahmadian A, Brogan A, Berman J, et al. Quantitative interpretation of FDG PET/CT with myocardial perfusion imaging increases diagnostic information in the evaluation of cardiac sarcoidosis. J Nucl Cardiol 2014;21:925–39.

58. Cabrera R, Ananthasubramaniam K. Diagnosis, therapeutic response assessment, and detection of disease recurrence in cardiac sarcoidosis: Integral role of cardiac PET. J Nucl Cardiol 2016;23:850–3.

59. Yaddanapudi K, Brunken R, Tan CD, et al. PET-MR imaging in evaluation of cardiac and paracardiac masses with histopathologic correlation. JACC Cardiovasc Imaging 2016;9:82–5.

60. Nensa F, Tezgah E, Poeppel TD, et al. Integrated 18F-FDG PET/MR imaging in the assessment of cardiac masses: a pilot study. J Nucl Med 2015;56:255–60.

61. Andrews JPM, Trivieri MG, Everett R, et al. 18F-fluoride PET/MR in cardiac amyloid: a comparison study with aortic stenosis and age- and sex-matched controls. J Nucl Cardiol 2022;29:741–9.

62. Park MA, Padera RF, Belanger A, et al. 18F-florbetapir binds specifically to myocardial light chain and transthyretin amyloid deposits: autoradiography study. Circ Cardiovasc Imaging 2015;8.

63. Cuddy SAM, Bravo PE, Falk RH, et al. Improved quantification of cardiac amyloid burden in systemic light chain amyloidosis: redefining early disease? JACC Cardiovasc Imaging 2020;13:1325–36.

64. ten Bokum AM, Hofland LJ, de Jong G, et al. Immunohistochemical localization of somatostatin receptor sst2A in sarcoid granulomas. Eur J Clin Invest 1999;29:630–6.

65. Hofman MS, Lau WF, Hicks RJ. Somatostatin receptor imaging with 68Ga DOTATATE PET/CT: clinical utility, normal patterns, pearls, and pitfalls in interpretation. Radiographics 2015;35:500–16.

66. Gormsen LC, Haraldsen A, Kramer S, et al. A dual tracer (68)Ga-DOTANOC PET/CT and (18)F-FDG PET/CT pilot study for detection of cardiac sarcoidosis. EJNMMI Res 2016;6:52.

67. Vachatimanont S, Kunawudhi A, Promteangtrong C, et al. Benefits of [(68)Ga]-DOTATATE PET-CT comparable to [(18)F]-FDG in patient with suspected cardiac sarcoidosis. J Nucl Cardiol 2022;29:381–3.

68. Corovic A, Wall C, Nus M, et al. Somatostatin receptor PET/MR imaging of inflammation in patients with large vessel vasculitis and atherosclerosis. J Am Coll Cardiol 2023;81:336–54.

69. Kwiecinski J, Tzolos E, Adamson PD, et al. Coronary (18)F-sodium fluoride uptake predicts outcomes in patients with coronary artery disease. J Am Coll Cardiol 2020;75:3061–74.

70. Krumm P, Greulich S, la Fougère C, et al. Hybrid-PET/MRT bei inflammatorischer Kardiomyopathie. Die Radiologie 2022;62:954–9.

Pediatric Imaging Using PET/MR Imaging

Chiara Giraudo, MD[a], Silvia Carraro, MD[b], Pietro Zucchetta, MD[a], Diego Cecchin, MD[a],*

KEYWORDS

• PET/MRI • Pediatric • Children • Oncology • Neurology • Imaging • [18F]FDG

INTRODUCTION

When comparing PET/MR imaging with PET/CT in adults, the literature supports the following: (a) higher contrast resolution in soft tissues (in particular in brain, liver, muscles, heart, and pelvic region) allowing a complete staging for head neck cancer (HNC),[1,2] better assessment of brain tumors[3] and tumors of the pelvic[4] region (not possible with PET/CT alone); (b) a real multiparametric approach[5,6] that could be exploited both in MR imaging (multiple sequences such as diffusion-weighted imaging (DWI), PWI, tractography, anatomic sequences) and PET (multiple tracers); (c) a lower exposure to ionizing radiation as compared with PET/CT; (d) real simultaneous acquisition of both modalities, which implies the identical positioning of the patient during image acquisition and the possibility to correct for movement using MR imaging data[7,8]; (e) partial volume correction of PET using MR imaging data[9]; (f) the possibility to use a contrast medium (CE) that does not interfere with attenuation, allowing for quantification.[10]

Although there are fewer comparison studies between PET/MR imaging and PET/CT in the pediatric population, it has been demonstrated that a significant (up to ~70–80%)[11,12] reduction of injected activity[13,14] and overall dose is achievable using PET/MR imaging (being based on modern digital detectors and avoiding the CT component) as compared with PET/CT (especially non-digital), with the same image quality. As in the adult population, PET/MR imaging has proven useful to achieve better contrast resolution in soft tissue pathologies

such as sarcomas, lymphomas, neurofibromatosis, histiocytosis, epilepsy, and brain tumors. Importantly, the simultaneous acquisition of a standard-of-care radiological examination (3T MR imaging) and state-of-the-art PET reduces sedation time (and number of sedations) in children.[15]

On the other hand, in adults and children, several clinical conditions have been identified where PET/CT could be superior as compared with PET/MR imaging such as the detection of small lung nodules[16,17] or sclerotic bone lesions.[18] Furthermore, PET/MR imaging has a less favorable profile in terms of cost, comfort/claustrophobia of the patient (mainly related to longer scan time and smaller gantry), increased metallic interference (not only because of incompatibility but also possible ferromagnetic artifacts), [11C] methionine ([11C]MET) complicated attenuation correction,[19,20] and respiratory motion correction (due to longer acquisition times). Furthermore, PET/MR imaging protocols are not yet fully standardized and there are relatively few physicians/technologists specifically trained in pediatric nuclear medicine in advanced hybrid imaging.

Specifically, as it concerns PET/MR imaging limitations, in a pediatric population, the use of attenuation correction algorithms is a major issue, as can be seen in atlas-based attenuation correction, where adult-derived factors could be inaccurate[11] being based on adult atlases. For example, in a young child, the attenuation correction of an incomplete myelination of the brain could be very challenging.

Regarding PET/MR imaging semi-quantification, it has been shown that similar to the adult

---

[a] Complex Unit of Nuclear Medicine, Department of Medicine (DIMED), University Hospital of Padova, Via Nicolo' Giustiniani 2, 35128, Padova, Italy; [b] Unit of Pediatric Allergy and Respiratory Medicine, Women's and Children's Health Department, University Hospital of Padova, Via Nicolo' Giustiniani 2, 35128, Padova, Italy
* Corresponding author.
E-mail address: diego.cecchin@unipd.it

Magn Reson Imaging Clin N Am 31 (2023) 625–636
https://doi.org/10.1016/j.mric.2023.06.001
1064-9689/23/© 2023 Elsevier Inc. All rights reserved.

population, there is a good correlation between parameters (SUVmean and SUVmax) obtained by PET/CT and PET/MR imaging, although the standardized uptake value (SUV) values are numerically different, largely depending[21] on the specific organ explored and the method used for atetnuation corrected (AC).

In the following paragraphs, the authors try to summarize the main clinical applications of PET/MR imaging in neuroimaging, oncology, and inflammatory and infectious diseases in the pediatric population.

NEUROIMAGING

One of the first applications of PET/MR imaging was for evaluation of the central nervous system (CNS). PET/MR imaging allows the simultaneous use of structural MR imaging sequences (such as isotropic T1 Flair and T2), advanced MR imaging sequences (such as perfusion-weighted imaging [PWI], DWI, and fMR imaging) and PET tracers for tumor evaluation (using [18F]Fluorodeoxyglucose ([18F]FDG), amino acid analogs, [18F]fluorothymidine [FLT]), epilepsy ([18F]FDG, amino acids, synaptic density tracers, neurotransmitters, and opioids) and mainly in adults, neurodegeneration ([18F]FDG and amyloid tracers). In the following two paragraphs, the authors summarize the main achievement of PET/MR imaging in pediatric epilepsy and pediatric neuro-oncology.

Pediatric Epilepsy and PET/MR Imaging

Several conditions contribute to pediatric epilepsy including focal cortical dysplasia (FCD), mesial temporal sclerosis (MTS), tumors (especially with a low-grade histology), perinatal CNS injuries, tuberous sclerosis complex (TSC), and epilepsy syndromes[22] such as Sturge–Weber and Rasmussen. The main indication for imaging in these settings is the presurgical localization of the epileptogenic foci usually accomplished coupling clinical data, MR imaging, and electroencephalography (EEG) (ictal and interictal).

However, despite many technical advancements (including fMR imaging to map motor and language functions), MR imaging still fails to reveal any structural abnormality (Fig. 1) in about 20% of cases.[23]

The PET hypometabolism (mainly due to postictal disconnections or loss of neurons and synaptic density) seen in interictal phase, using [18F]FDG, could help[24] to establish the laterality of the lesion but lacks anatomic precision. Several studies[25] have therefore, in the past, demonstrated that the co-registration of PET and MR imaging[26,27] could improve both sensitivity and the localization

of the epileptogenic focus. Furthermore, the investigators demonstrated that in about 40% of cases, the area of hypometabolism on PET helped finding subtle lesions not reported on MR imaging.

Therefore, when MR imaging reveals normal findings[28] or in the case of multiple structural abnormalities (lesions in the contralateral hemisphere could influence surgical outcome) with respect to PET/CT and fused MR, a "real," co-acquired PET/MR imaging could be more accurate (in contrast to PET/CT and fused MR imaging), revealing foci of epilepsy[29] without significant artifacts due to MR imaging-derived attenuation correction.[30]

- *Focal cortical dysplasia*: About 20% of malformations of cortical development (FCD) type 2 and from 30% to 70% of FCD type 1 could present with a negative or inconclusive MR imaging. In the setting of a doubtful or negative MR imaging, Kim and colleagues[31] demonstrated positive PET findings in 86% of cases demonstrating a role for combined PET/MR imaging.
- *Mesial temporal sclerosis*: The PET hypometabolism detected in mesial temporal lobe epilepsy (MTLE) is mainly due to MTS. PET seems more sensitive in temporal lobe than extratemporal lobe epilepsy for detection of the seizure focus showing a metabolism that exceeds the temporal lobe and involving mainly the frontal regions, thalamus, and basal ganglia. The hypometabolism in these areas usually ameliorates after surgical resection. When MR imaging findings are subtle or inconsistent with symptoms or EEG, PET has shown hypometabolism in 80% of unilateral MTLE[32] with frequent involvement of the thalamus. Furthermore, extra-temporal or bitemporal hypometabolism correlates with worse postsurgical results.[33] Unilateral temporal PET findings correlate with excellent[34] postsurgical outcomes (96% Engel class I or II), especially if the area to be resected is tailored to the extent of the hypometabolism.[35]
- *Tumors*: Attempts have been made to use [18F]FDG in the differential diagnosis between FCD and dysembrioblastic neuroepithelial tumor (DNET) or gangliogliomas suggesting a role for amino acids in this setting.[36] However, [18F]FDG could prove useful in this scenario identifying FCDs located outside the tumor burden. The incomplete seizure control was associated with the presence of FCDs in patients with gangliogliomas.[37]
- *Epilepsy syndromes*: Although a complete discussion on pediatric epilepsy syndromes is complicated and goes beyond the scope

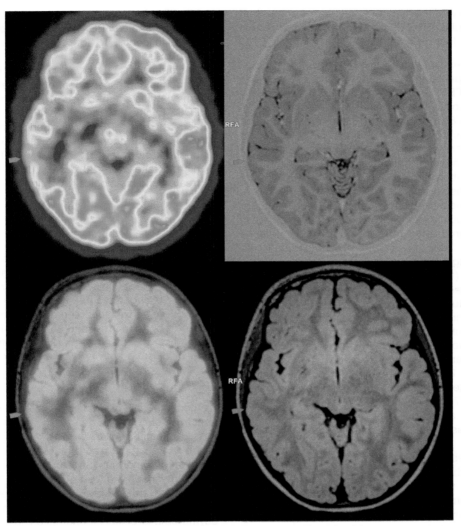

Fig. 1. PET/MR imaging in epilepsy: [18F]FDG (*upper left*) PET showing (*red arrow*) clear right temporal hypometabolism not corresponding to anatomic defects in inversion recovery (*upper right*) or Flair (*lower right*) sequences. Fused Flair and PET showing the area of abnormality (*lower left*).

of this article, it has been shown that [18F] FDG PET/MR imaging is useful for excluding bihemispheric involvement in syndromes such as in Rasmussen encephalitis[38] or hemimegalencephaly. It is also useful for predicting epilepsy by showing areas of hypermetabolism in patients affected by Sturge–Weber syndrome[39] correlating with hyperperfusion at single photon Emissio Tomography (SPET) and accelerated myelination at MR imaging. In TSC syndrome, the outcome of surgery is highly dependent on the resection of the epileptogenic tuber[40] that is detected with a combination of DWI and [18F]FDG using PET/MR imaging.[41]

Pediatric Neuro-Oncology and PET/MR Imaging

Approximately 20% of all pediatric tumors are malignancies of the CNS[42] with more than 80%[43] represented by astrocytomas (~80% of low grade including pilocytic astrocytomas), medulloblastomas (~15% of all CNS tumors), and ependymomas. Usually, CT and MR imaging plays a major role in the initial workup. Low-grade masses are hypointense on MR imaging with minimal mass effect and variable post-contrast enhancement. Conventional MR imaging, however, provides little information regarding the true biological behavior of the tumor.

A review of the most relevant studies shows that the combination of PET and MR imaging can prove useful in four main settings:

1. *Differentiation of tumors versus non-tumors:* Two pediatric PET studies using, respectively, [18F]FET[44] in 26 and [11C]MET[45] in 27 newly diagnosed CNS masses showed similar (77% and 78%) accuracy in differentiating tumoral versus non-tumoral lesions. The investigators also showed that (1)H-MR imaging spectroscopy acquired with a separate MR imaging examination could complement PET data, increasing accuracy in differentiating lesions. We speculate that a co-acquired PET/MR imaging could perform even better in this setting. In fact, in a very large series of pediatric patients (N = 169), researchers[46] demonstrated that adding [18F]FET to MR imaging increased specificity (1.0 vs 0.48) and accuracy (0.91 vs 0.81).

2. *Differential diagnosis of low-grade tumors*: Non-tumoral lesions, a number of low-grade and intermediate-grade tumors can show normal or even reduced uptake of [18F]FDG; therefore, labeled amino acids are usually recommended to study these lesions. Nevertheless, DNETs demonstrated no to minimal uptake of [11C]MET PET in a small series of 5 and 27 children.[47,48] This was in contrast to gliomas and gangliogiomas that present with an increased [11C]MET uptake and high (and variable) uptake in a [18F]FET study.[49] Both studies also suggest a role for fused MR imaging (thus for PET/MR imaging) in functional brain mapping to characterize and provide anatomic definition using CE.

3. *Assessment of tumoral grade:* A study[50] in 38 children showed that [18F]FDG PET correlates with malignancy grade and that digitally performed PET/MR imaging co-registration increased characterization in 90% of cases, although pilocytic astrocytoma, choroid plexus, and occasionally gangliogliomas can present with hypermetabolism. Tumoral grade assessment using amino acid PET ([11C]MET and [18F]FET) is usually accomplished by means of a kinetic or semiquantitative analysis due to the frequent increased uptake in low-grade tumors.[51]

   [18F]DOPA seems to correlate (with a certain overlap) with tumoral grade, and[52] PET/MR imaging fusion was relevant in 9 of 13 patients (69%) prompting treatment change in 5 patients.

4. *Targeting a biopsy:* In a large pediatric study[53] where MR imaging was unable to assist in selecting accurately the site for biopsy, all PET-guided targets (33 patients) lead to tumor identification on histologic examination. Therefore, a combined PET/MR imaging seems very useful in identifying hot spots in diffuse pediatric gliomas.

5. *Posttreatment evaluation:* For posttreatment response and assessment of residual disease, amino acids seem to perform better than [18F]FDG. In 48 children,[44] [18F]FET showed an accuracy of 79% (82% considering kinetic analysis) in identifying recurrent disease. In another pediatric study using [11C]MET,[54] PET revealed high uptake in 14/20 cases (11/14 surgically treated and histologically confirmed).

ONCOLOGICAL IMAGING
Musculoskeletal Tumors

Various pediatric oncological diseases can primarily or secondarily affect the skeletal system. These are successfully investigated by PET/MR imaging, taking advantage of the whole-body assessment as well as of the accurate characterization of bone marrow and soft tissue infiltration enabled by MR imaging, in addition to the evaluation of disease activity by the PET component (Table 1).

Langerhans cell histiocytosis

Langerhans cell histiocytosis (LCH) includes a spectrum of rare disorders, with unknown origin, mostly affecting children up to 14 years of age and being characterized by infiltration and accumulation of abnormal Langerhans cells (ie, histiocytes) in various organs and tissues.[55] Thus, the symptoms and overall clinical presentation depend on the affected areas and vary from an asymptomatic solitary bone lesion to multiorgan disease, with skeletal involvement representing the most frequent expression of the disease.[55] Even if the diagnosis relies on tissue sampling of the most easily accessible lesion, diagnostic imaging plays a significant role.[55] For instance, for bone lesions radiography often represents the first approach despite its low sensitivity for lytic lesions, particularly in pelvic bones. PET/CT and PET/MR imaging can be used to better characterize disease extension, allowing for a whole-body assessment and providing information about disease activity and response to treatment.[56] Recently, Sher and colleagues compared these two techniques in 10 children with LCH and seven with Rosai–Dorfman disease (ie, aka sinus histiocytosis with severe lymphadenopathy) demonstrating comparable diagnostic performance, image quality, and quantitative assessment.[57] In particular, PET/MR imaging identified 74 out 77 lesions in various organs and tissues (eg, bone, lymph nodes, spleen, skin)

Table 1
Typical MR imaging parameters used in pediatric PET/MR imaging oncologic imaging

T2 Tirm, transaxial

Pat Mode	Acc Factor PE	TR (ms)	TE (ms)	Averages	TI (ms)	Flip Angle	Slice Thickness (mm)
Grappa	2	6320	51	2	220	120°	4

T2 Haste, transaxial

Pat Mode	Acc Factor PE	TR (ms)	TE (ms)	Averages	Phase Resol	Flip angle	Slice Thickness (mm)
Grappa	2	1600	95	1	81%	160°	5

EP2D DWI weighted imaging (b50, b800), transaxial

Pat Mode	Acc Factor PE	TR (ms)	TE (ms)	Averages	Phase Resol	FoV Phase	Slice Thickness (mm)
Grappa	2	4900	53	1	100%	80%	5

T2 TSE STIR, coronal

Pat Mode	Acc Factor PE	TR (ms)	TE (ms)	Averages	TI (ms).	FoV Phase	Slice Thickness (mm)
Grappa	3	7390	53	2	220	100%	5

Abbreviations: Acc, acceleration; PE, phase encode; Resol, resolution; TI, inversion time; TIRM, turbo inversion recovery magnitude; TR, repetition time; TSE, turbo spin echo.

with a detection rate of 96%.[57] Wang and colleagues successfully used PET/MR imaging to assess 52 children with LCH identifying systemic involvement in 21 cases.[58]

PET/MR imaging also allows for the simultaneous collection of functional information by DWI. This was demonstrated by Baratto and colleagues in a population of 23 children and young adults with 65 lesions at baseline, where DWI was shown to be complementary to PET imaging at baseline and after chemotherapy with high agreement (100% sensitivity of DWI for all investigated regions excluding spine and chest and 100% specificity for all areas).[59] Further studies are needed to investigate if PET/MR imaging with or without DWI can predict the response to treatment.

Sarcomas

Sarcomas include a heterogeneous group of tumors which account for 10% of all solid pediatric cancers. Osteosarcoma, Ewing sarcoma, and rhabdomyosarcoma are the most common malignant musculoskeletal tumors.[60]

Despite the potential diagnostic value of this technique, only a few studies investigated the role of PET/MR imaging for children (Fig. 2) with sarcomas by a fully integrated device. Pfluger and colleagues obtained very good results using postprocessing fusion of the data set acquired via two separate scanners (ie, PET/CT and MR imaging) in a cohort of 132 oncological patients, 36 of which had sarcomas.[61]

Aghighi and colleagues fused PET imaging with separately acquired MR imaging images in a study on 33 children and young adults with cancer including also six patients with Ewing and osteosarcoma (ie, three patients each).[62] They demonstrated the utility of a fast protocol.

Chodyla and colleagues examined 11 children with Ewing sarcoma before, during and after treatment showing that PET/MR imaging is a valuable imaging tool for this type of tumor.[63]

Given the tendency of sarcomas to metastasize to the lungs, it cannot be overlooked that PET/MR imaging has a lower diagnostic performance than CT for pulmonary assessment. Thus, despite the recent technological improvements and the recent recommendations for lung MR imaging,[64,65] chest CT is still mandatory for the global assessment in children examined by PET/MR imaging.

Several quantitative studies have shown promising results taking advantage of the simultaneous collection of functional and metabolic information.[66–68] For instance, histogram analysis demonstrated that SUVs and ADCs are dependent biomarkers in pediatric [18F]FDG-avid sarcomas and radiomics variables extracted from ADC maps seem to act as biomarkers of pediatric soft tissue sarcoma grade and histotype.[66,67]

Neuroblastoma

Neuroblastoma is the most common extracranial pediatric solid tumor accounting for around 15% of all cancer-related deaths in children and 90%

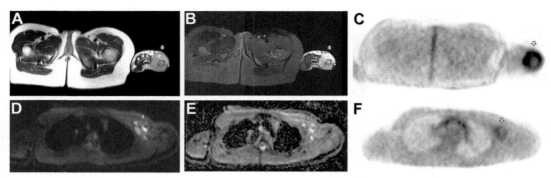

Fig. 2. PET/MR imaging in rhabdomyosarcoma. A 11-year-old girl affected by alveolar rhabdomyosarcoma of the left hand (*yellow arrows* on the axial turbo inversion recovery, Half Fourier single-shot turbo spin-echo, and PET images, respectively, in *A*, *B*, and *C*). There is a large skip lesion in the soft tissue of the chest wall (*orange arrows* on axial diffusion weighted imaging, apparent diffusion coefficient map, and PET respectively in *D*, *E*, and *F*).

of cases are diagnosed before the age of 5 years.[69,70] Although most of the lesions affect the abdomen (65%) and the medulla of the adrenal gland in particular, this type of tumor may occur in different areas such as chest, pelvis, or neck.[70] Around half of patients have a localized disease while 35% have nodal involvement; other common metastatic sites include bone and bone marrow and liver.[70]

Imaging plays a pivotal role with ultrasound being often the first-line modality and computed tomography and magnetic resonance being considered the main diagnostic tools with high accuracy rates. It has been recently shown that the MR imaging outperforms CT in the pretreatment evaluation for metastatic assessment.[71] Regarding nuclear medicine imaging, [123I]meta-iodobenzylguanidine ([123I]MIBG) scintigraphy, labeling chromaffin tissues, is routinely used to assess bone marrow metastases, but PET/CT with different tracers (eg, [68 Ga]DOTA peptides, [18F]dihydroxy-phenylalanine (DOPA), and [18F] meta-fluorobenzyl guanidine) has also been proposed.[72,73] It has been shown that [18F]FDG uptake in neuroblastoma can vary and that tumor uptake represents a negative prognostic factor.[74] Thus, it has been proposed to use [18F]FDG PET in association with [123I]MIBG scintigraphy in high-risk neuroblastomas.[75] In a study comparing PET/MR imaging and PET/CT in children affected by various types of tumors, using DWI and short time inversion recovery (STIR) in the PET/MR imaging protocol, a precise diagnosis of bone marrow infiltration was achieved in disseminated neuroblastoma, demonstrating the utility of this technique for this cancer.[76] A recent abstract exploring the diagnostic performance of PET/MR imaging in 72 children with neuroblastoma suggested that it is superior to clinical assessment for staging especially in detecting the invasion

and metastasis.[77] Further longitudinal studies assessing the role of PET/MR imaging, also with different tracer, and taking into account a systematic application of DWI should be performed to better define all the potential applications of this technique in staging and after treatment assessment.

Lymphoma

Lymphomas represent up to 10% of cancers diagnosed in children and adolescents and are subdivided in two main types: Hodgkin and non-Hodgkin lymphoma (HL and NHL).[78] NHL includes a heterogeneous group of lymphoid malignancies (eg, Burkitt lymphoma, diffuse large B-cell lymphoma) nowadays defined according to the 2022 WHO classification.[79] NHL is the fourth most common malignancy among children and the vast majority of childhood NHL is of high-grade and B-cell origin.[80]

HL is a unique monoclonal lymphoid malignancy with a first large peak of incidence in adolescents and young adults (15–24 year old)[81] with a 5-year overall survival rate above 90%.[82]

In terms of imaging, all main radiological techniques can be used but especially whole-body examinations also with hybrid devices allow an accurate staging and disease monitoring during and after treatment.[83] In fact, for instance, functional imaging with [18F]FDG PET has become the standard of care in the initial evaluation and management of HL because this tumor is very [18F]FDG–avid.[84] PET/MR imaging assessment is recommended for both adults and children[76,85–87] providing low radiation exposure and does not require contrast injection. There is some controversy about the benefits of DWI for evaluation of these tumors. Kirchner and colleagues recently suggested that DWI does not lead to any noticeable improvement to PET/MR imaging protocols which is in contrast with previous literature especially on adults. The inconsistency might be due to the different histotypes of their population because DWI is especially useful in patients with low [18F]FDG–avid tumors such as mucosa-associated lymphoid tissue (MALT)[85] or for extranodal involvement.[88] If this is true, optimization of the imaging protocol (ie, dropping whole-body DWI) can shorten the acquisition duration, improving tolerability and reducing the need for sedation.[89]

PET/MR imaging also has the advantage of an accurate assessment of bone marrow which can be especially useful in children with infiltration due to lymphoma[75,76] or primary bone lymphomas.[87] Primary NHL of the bone was initially described in 1928 by Oberling[90,91] and now it is a well-established condition listed in the WHO classification of tumors of soft tissue and bone.[92] It is defined as a malignant cancer causing at least one mass within the bone, without involvement of supraregional nodes or other extra nodal areas. Primary bone lymphomas account for 2% to 9% of NHL in children being diffuse large B-cell the most common type.[90] In the study of 10 patients with NHL, PET/MR imaging demonstrated skeletal involvement due to osseous diffuse large B-cell lymphoma in two children.[87]

PET/MR imaging has achieved excellent results for evaluation of therapy response (**Fig. 3**), particularly in early response assessment in lymphomas.[93]

PET/MR imaging also allows for accurate detection and characterization of ischemic skeletal lesions occurring in children with HL under treatment.[94]

Metastases

In the global assessment of cancer burden PET/MR imaging enables an accurate detection of metastatic spread. Challenges related to the lack of detection of metastases in the lung on MR imaging cannot be ignored. Despite the technical improvements in MR imaging pulmonary imaging, as shown by Schaefer and colleagues, lung lesions were only partly visible in two patients with sarcoma examined by PET/MR imaging.[76] For this reason, as previously stated for sarcomas, a chest CT is usually recommended in addition to the PET/MR imaging scan for tumors potentially associated with lung metastases.

Miscellaneous

In addition to the types of tumors previously addressed, various other types of cancer (**Fig. 4**) have been successfully investigated by PET/MR imaging in children.[76] For instance, the diagnosis of a rare case of pediatric solid pseudopapillary pancreatic tumor was achieved combining morphologic characteristics, features on DWI and metabolic activity.[95] Preliminary results summarized in a recent abstract on 77 patients demonstrated the potential role of PET/MR imaging for staging of nephroblastoma.[77] The association of high soft tissue contrast on MR imaging and metabolic activity on PET has been shown to be especially suitable for patients with neurofibromatosis in a study on 28 patients including 15 subjects less than 18 year old, and the investigators also identified SUVmax $\geq$ 2.78 as a significant cutoff value to differentiate between still benign peripheral neurofibromatosis and malignant peripheral nerve sheath tumor.[96]

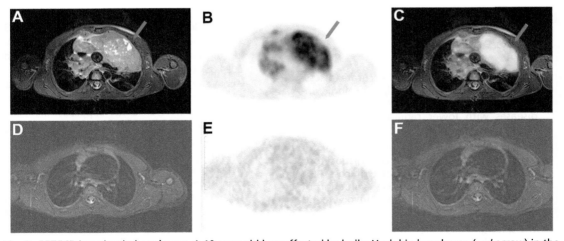

Fig. 3. PET/MR imaging in lymphoma. A 10-year-old boy affected by bulky Hodgkin lymphoma (*red arrow*) in the chest (axial turbo inversion recovery in *A*) with pathologic [18F] FDG uptake (axial PET image in *B*; fused image in *C*). The PET/MR performed after chemotherapy demonstrated a complete metabolic response with significant reduction of the mass (axial TIRM image in *D*, PET image in *E*, and fused image in *F*).

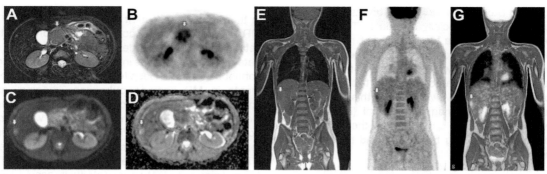

Fig. 4. PET/MR imaging in pancreatoblastoma. A 9-year-old girl affected by histologically proven metastatic pancreatoblastoma. The large primary tumor in the head of the pancreas (*yellow arrow* on the axial T2-weigthed fat-sat axial image in *A*) showed pathologic [18F]FDG uptake (*yellow arrow* on the axial positron emission tomography image in *B*). Axial diffusion-weighted imaging (*C*) and apparent diffusion coefficient map (*D*), coronal T1-weighted (*E*), coronal PET (*F*), and coronal fused (*G*) images show the hepatic metastasis (*white arrows*).

INFLAMMATORY AND INFECTIOUS DISEASES

In addition to the numerous oncological applications mentioned above, PET/MR imaging can also be used for diagnosis and monitoring of treatment response of inflammatory or infectious diseases. Promising PET/CT results, useful for detecting a source in children with fever of unknown origin could also be seen using PET/MR imaging.[97] PET/MR imaging could also play a role in pediatric inflammatory bowel disease, as recently shown in adults.[98] Promising results have also been published for PET/MR imaging in pediatric fungal infections.[99]

A three-center cross-sectional study showed that in 17 children with Takayasu arteritis, PET/MR imaging adds crucial information regarding vessel inflammation.[100]

CLINICS CARE POINTS

- PET/MR imaging allows an accurate assessment of various oncological, neurologic, inflammatory, and infectious pediatric diseases with lower radiation exposure as compared with PET/CT.
- In children affected by musculoskeletal tumors such as Langerhans cell histiocytosis and sarcomas, [18F]Fluorodeoxyglucose PET/MR imaging enables a precise evaluation of bone infiltration, soft tissue involvement, and metastatic spread.
- The simultaneous collection of metabolic and functional information obtained by PET/MR imaging allows complex quantitative analyses and the potential identification of imaging biomarkers.

- The simultaneous acquisition of PET/MR imaging images could be of great value for assessment of pediatric resistant epilepsy and pediatric neuro-oncology.
- The simultaneous acquisition of a standard-of-care radiological examination (3T MR imaging) and state-of-the-art PET results in decreasing the number and duration of sedations in children.
- PET/MR demonstrated lower sensitivity as compared with CT in detecting lung nodules.

DISCLOSURE

The authors have nothing to disclose.

REFERENCES

1. Crimì F, Borsetto D, Stramare R, et al. [18F]FDG PET/MRI versus contrast-enhanced MRI in detecting regional HNSCC metastases. Ann Nucl Med 2021;35:260–9.
2. Kubiessa K, Purz S, Gawlitza M, et al. Initial clinical results of simultaneous 18F-FDG PET/MRI in comparison to 18F-FDG PET/CT in patients with head and neck cancer. Eur J Nucl Med Mol Imaging 2014;41:639–48.
3. Neuner I, Kaffanke JB, Langen K-J, et al. Multimodal imaging utilising integrated MR-PET for human brain tumour assessment. Eur Radiol 2012;22:2568–80.
4. Wetter A, Grueneisen J, Umutlu L. PET/MR imaging of pelvic malignancies. Eur J Radiol 2017;94:A44–51.
5. Cecchin D, Palombit A, Castellaro M, et al. Brain PET and functional MRI: why simultaneously using hybrid PET/MR systems? Q J Nucl Med Mol Imaging 2017;61:345–59.

6. Lombardi G, Spimpolo A, Berti S, et al. PET/MR in recurrent glioblastoma patients treated with regorafenib: [18F]FET and DWI-ADC for response assessment and survival prediction. Br J Radiol 2022;95:20211018.

7. Chun SY, Reese TG, Ouyang J, et al. MRI-based nonrigid motion correction in simultaneous PET/MRI. J Nucl Med 2012;53:1284–91.

8. Catana C. Motion correction options in PET/MRI. Semin Nucl Med 2015;45:212–23.

9. Cecchin D, Barthel H, Poggiali D, et al. A new integrated dual time-point amyloid PET/MRI data analysis method. Eur J Nucl Med Mol Imaging 2017;44:2060–72.

10. Lois C, Bezrukov I, Schmidt H, et al. Effect of MR contrast agents on quantitative accuracy of PET in combined whole-body PET/MR imaging. Eur J Nucl Med Mol Imaging 2012;39:1756–66.

11. Kwatra NS, Lim R, Gee MS, et al. PET/MR Imaging:: Current Updates on Pediatric Applications. Magn Reson Imaging Clin N Am 2019;27:387–407.

12. Martin O, Schaarschmidt BM, Kirchner J, et al. PET/MRI Versus PET/CT for Whole-Body Staging: Results from a Single-Center Observational Study on 1,003 Sequential Examinations. J Nucl Med 2020;61:1131–6.

13. Zucchetta P, Branchini M, Zorz A, et al. Quantitative analysis of image metrics for reduced and standard dose pediatric 18F-FDG PET/MRI examinations. Br J Radiol 2019;92:20180438.

14. Branchini M, Zorz A, Zucchetta P, et al. Impact of acquisition count statistics reduction and SUV discretization on PET radiomic features in pediatric 18F-FDG-PET/MRI examinations. Phys Med 2019;59:117–26.

15. States LJ, Reid JR. Whole-Body PET/MRI Applications in Pediatric Oncology. AJR Am J Roentgenol 2020;215:713–25.

16. Rauscher I, Eiber M, Fürst S, et al. PET/MR imaging in the detection and characterization of pulmonary lesions: technical and diagnostic evaluation in comparison to PET/CT. J Nucl Med 2014;55:724–9.

17. Sawicki LM, Grueneisen J, Buchbender C, et al. Evaluation of the Outcome of Lung Nodules Missed on 18F-FDG PET/MRI Compared with 18F-FDG PET/CT in Patients with Known Malignancies. J Nucl Med 2016;57:15–20.

18. Samarin A, Burger C, Wollenweber SD, et al. PET/MR imaging of bone lesions–implications for PET quantification from imperfect attenuation correction. Eur J Nucl Med Mol Imaging 2012;39:1154–60.

19. Werner P, Rullmann M, Bresch A, et al. Impact of attenuation correction on clinical [(18)F]FDG brain PET in combined PET/MRI. EJNMMI Res 2016;6:47.

20. Olin A, Ladefoged CN, Langer NH, et al. Reproducibility of MR-Based Attenuation Maps in PET/MRI and the Impact on PET Quantification in Lung Cancer. J Nucl Med 2018;59:999–1004.

21. Lyons K, Seghers V, Sorensen JIL, et al. Comparison of Standardized Uptake Values in Normal Structures Between PET/CT and PET/MRI in a Tertiary Pediatric Hospital: A Prospective Study. AJR Am J Roentgenol 2015;205:1094–101.

22. Wirrell EC, Nabbout R, Scheffer IE, et al. Methodology for classification and definition of epilepsy syndromes with list of syndromes: Report of the ILAE Task Force on Nosology and Definitions. Epilepsia 2022;63:1333–48.

23. Lehéricy S, Semah F, Hasboun D, et al. Temporal lobe epilepsy with varying severity: MRI study of 222 patients. Neuroradiology 1997;39:788–96.

24. Salamon N, Kung J, Shaw SJ, et al. FDG-PET/MRI coregistration improves detection of cortical dysplasia in patients with epilepsy. Neurology 2008;71:1594–601.

25. Lee KK, Salamon N. [18F] fluorodeoxyglucose-positron-emission tomography and MR imaging coregistration for presurgical evaluation of medically refractory epilepsy. AJNR Am J Neuroradiol 2009;30:1811–6.

26. Murphy MA, O'Brien TJ, Morris K, et al. Multimodality image-guided surgery for the treatment of medically refractory epilepsy. J Neurosurg 2004;100:452–62.

27. Rubí S, Setoain X, Donaire A, et al. Validation of FDG-PET/MRI coregistration in nonlesional refractory childhood epilepsy. Epilepsia 2011;52:2216–24.

28. LoPinto-Khoury C, Sperling MR, Skidmore C, et al. Surgical outcome in PET-positive, MRI-negative patients with temporal lobe epilepsy. Epilepsia 2012;53:342–8.

29. Shin HW, Jewells V, Sheikh A, et al. Initial experience in hybrid PET-MRI for evaluation of refractory focal onset epilepsy. Seizure 2015;31:1–4.

30. Paldino MJ, Yang E, Jones JY, et al. Comparison of the diagnostic accuracy of PET/MRI to PET/CT-acquired FDG brain exams for seizure focus detection: a prospective study. Pediatr Radiol 2017;47:1500–7.

31. Kim SK, Na DG, Byun HS, et al. Focal cortical dysplasia: comparison of MRI and FDG-PET. J Comput Assist Tomogr 2000;24:296–302.

32. Henry TR, Mazziotta JC, Engel J. Interictal metabolic anatomy of mesial temporal lobe epilepsy. Arch Neurol 1993;50:582–9.

33. Choi JY, Kim SJ, Hong SB, et al. Extratemporal hypometabolism on FDG PET in temporal lobe epilepsy as a predictor of seizure outcome after temporal lobectomy. Eur J Nucl Med Mol Imaging 2003;30:581–7.

34. Gok B, Jallo G, Hayeri R, et al. The evaluation of FDG-PET imaging for epileptogenic focus

localization in patients with MRI positive and MRI negative temporal lobe epilepsy. Neuroradiology 2013;55:541–50.

35. Vinton AB, Carne R, Hicks RJ, et al. The extent of resection of FDG-PET hypometabolism relates to outcome of temporal lobectomy. Brain 2007;130:548–60.

36. Phi JH, Paeng JC, Lee HS, et al. Evaluation of focal cortical dysplasia and mixed neuronal and glial tumors in pediatric epilepsy patients using 18F-FDG and 11C-methionine pet. J Nucl Med 2010;51:728–34.

37. Im S-H, Chung CK, Cho B-K, et al. Supratentorial ganglioglioma and epilepsy: postoperative seizure outcome. J Neuro Oncol 2002;57:59–66.

38. Fiorella DJ, Provenzale JM, Coleman RE, et al. (18)F-fluorodeoxyglucose positron emission tomography and MR imaging findings in Rasmussen encephalitis. AJNR Am J Neuroradiol 2001;22:1291–9.

39. Chugani HT. Hypermetabolism on Pediatric PET Scans of Brain Glucose Metabolism: What Does It Signify? J Nucl Med 2021;62:1301–6.

40. Koh S, Jayakar P, Dunoyer C, et al. Epilepsy surgery in children with tuberous sclerosis complex: presurgical evaluation and outcome. Epilepsia 2000;41:1206–13.

41. Chandra PS, Salamon N, Huang J, et al. FDG-PET/MRI coregistration and diffusion-tensor imaging distinguish epileptogenic tubers and cortex in patients with tuberous sclerosis complex: a preliminary report. Epilepsia 2006;47:1543–9.

42. Jadvar H, Connolly LP, Fahey FH, et al. PET and PET/CT in pediatric oncology. Semin Nucl Med 2007;37:316–31.

43. Panigrahy A, Blüml S. Neuroimaging of pediatric brain tumors: from basic to advanced magnetic resonance imaging (MRI). J Child Neurol 2009;24:1343–65.

44. Dunkl V, Cleff C, Stoffels G, et al. The usefulness of dynamic O-(2-18F-fluoroethyl)-L-tyrosine PET in the clinical evaluation of brain tumors in children and adolescents. J Nucl Med 2015;56:88–92.

45. Morana G, Piccardo A, Puntoni M, et al. Diagnostic and prognostic value of 18F-DOPA PET and 1H-MR spectroscopy in pediatric supratentorial infiltrative gliomas: a comparative study. Neuro Oncol 2015;17:1637–47.

46. Marner L, Lundemann M, Sehested A, et al. Diagnostic accuracy and clinical impact of [18F]FET PET in childhood CNS tumors. Neuro Oncol 2021;23:2107–16.

47. Kaplan AM, Lawson MA, Spataro J, et al. Positron emission tomography using [18F] fluorodeoxyglucose and [11C] l-methionine to metabolically characterize dysembryoplastic neuroepithelial tumors. J Child Neurol 1999;14:673–7.

48. Rosenberg DS, Demarquay G, Jouvet A, et al. [11C]-Methionine PET: dysembryoplastic neuroepithelial tumours compared with other epileptogenic brain neoplasms. J Neurol Neurosurg Psychiatry 2005;76:1686–92.

49. Kasper BS, Struffert T, Kasper EM, et al. 18Fluoroethyl-L-tyrosine-PET in long-term epilepsy associated glioneuronal tumors. Epilepsia 2011;52:35–44.

50. Borgwardt L, Højgaard L, Carstensen H, et al. Increased fluorine-18 2-fluoro-2-deoxy-D-glucose (FDG) uptake in childhood CNS tumors is correlated with malignancy grade: a study with FDG positron emission tomography/magnetic resonance imaging coregistration and image fusion. J Clin Oncol 2005;23:3030–7.

51. Utriainen M, Metsähonkala L, Salmi TT, et al. Metabolic characterization of childhood brain tumors: comparison of 18F-fluorodeoxyglucose and 11C-methionine positron emission tomography. Cancer 2002;95:1376–86.

52. Morana G, Piccardo A, Milanaccio C, et al. Value of 18F-3,4-dihydroxyphenylalanine PET/MR image fusion in pediatric supratentorial infiltrative astrocytomas: a prospective pilot study. J Nucl Med 2014;55:718–23.

53. Pirotte BJM, Lubansu A, Massager N, et al. Clinical impact of integrating positron emission tomography during surgery in 85 children with brain tumors. J Neurosurg Pediatr 2010;5:486–99.

54. Pirotte B, Levivier M, Morelli D, et al. Positron emission tomography for the early postsurgical evaluation of pediatric brain tumors. Childs Nerv Syst 2005;21:294–300.

55. Khung S, Budzik J-F, Amzallag-Bellenger E, et al. Skeletal involvement in Langerhans cell histiocytosis. Insights Imaging 2013;4:569–79.

56. Kaste SC, Rodriguez-Galindo C, McCarville ME, et al. PET-CT in pediatric Langerhans cell histiocytosis. Pediatr Radiol 2007;37:615–22.

57. Sher AC, Orth R, McClain K, et al. PET/MR in the Assessment of Pediatric Histiocytoses: A comparison to PET/CT. Clin Nucl Med 2017;42:582–8.

58. Wang F, Xu Y. The diagnostic value of 18F-FDG PET/MR in Langerhans histiocytosis in children. J Nucl Med 2013;63.

59. Baratto L, Nyalakonda R, Theruvath A, et al. Comparing 18F-FDG PET/MRI and Diffusion-Weighted MRI for staging a restaging of Langerhans Cell Histiocytosis in children. J Nucl Med 2022;63.

60. Carola AS, Peter SR, Andrew LF, et al. Common musculoskeletal tumors of childhood and adolescence. Mayo Clin Proc 2012;87(5):475–87.

61. Pfluger T, Melzer HI, Mueller WP, et al. Diagnostic value of combined 18F-FDG PET/MRI for staging and restaging in paediatric oncology. Eur J Nucl Med Mol Imaging 2012;39:1745–55.

62. Aghighi M, Pisani LJ, Sun Z, et al. Speeding up PET/MR for cancer staging of children and young adults. Eur Radiol 2016;26:4239–48.

63. Chodyla M, Barbato F, Dirksen U, et al. Utility of Integrated PET/MRI for the Primary Diagnostic Work-Up of Patients with Ewing Sarcoma: Preliminary Results. Diagnostics 2022;12.

64. Gräfe D, Anders R, Prenzel F, et al. Pediatric MR lung imaging with 3D ultrashort-TE in free breathing: Are we past the conventional T2 sequence? Pediatr Pulmonol 2021;56:3899–907.

65. Hatabu H, Ohno Y, Gefter WB, et al. Expanding Applications of Pulmonary MRI in the Clinical Evaluation of Lung Disorders: Fleischner Society Position Paper. Radiology 2020;297:286–301.

66. Orsatti G, Zucchetta P, Varotto A, et al. Volumetric histograms-based analysis of apparent diffusion coefficients and standard uptake values for the assessment of pediatric sarcoma at staging: preliminary results of a PET/MRI study. Radiol Med 2021;126:878–85.

67. Giraudo C, Fichera G, Stramare R, et al. Radiomic features as biomarkers of soft tissue paediatric sarcomas: preliminary results of a PET/MR study. Radiol Oncol 2022;56:138–41.

68. Maennlin S, Chaika M, Gassenmaier S, et al. Evaluation of functional and metabolic tumor volume using voxel-wise analysis in childhood rhabdomyosarcoma. Pediatr Radiol 2022;53(3):438–49.

69. Littooij AS, de Keizer B. Imaging in neuroblastoma. Pediatr Radiol 2022;53(4):783–7.

70. Colon NC, Chung DH. Neuroblastoma. Adv Pediatr 2011;58:297–311.

71. Sarioglu FC, Salman M, Guleryuz H, et al. Radiological staging in neuroblastoma: computed tomography or magnetic resonance imaging? Polish J Radiol 2019;84:e46–53.

72. Samim A, Tytgat GAM, Bleeker G, et al. Nuclear Medicine Imaging in Neuroblastoma: Current Status and New Developments. J Pers Med 2021;11.

73. Piccardo A, Morana G, Puntoni M, et al. Diagnosis, Treatment Response, and Prognosis: The Role of 18F-DOPA PET/CT in Children Affected by Neuroblastoma in Comparison with 123I-mIBG Scan: The First Prospective Study. J Nucl Med 2020;61:367–74.

74. Papathanasiou ND, Gaze MN, Sullivan K, et al. 18F-FDG PET/CT and 123I-metaiodobenzylguanidine imaging in high-risk neuroblastoma: diagnostic comparison and survival analysis. J Nucl Med 2011;52:519–25.

75. Hirsch FW, Sattler B, Sorge I, et al. PET/MR in children. Initial clinical experience in paediatric oncology using an integrated PET/MR scanner. Pediatr Radiol 2013;43:860–75.

76. Schäfer JF, Gatidis S, Schmidt H, et al. Simultaneous whole-body PET/MR imaging in comparison to PET/CT in pediatric oncology: initial results. Radiology 2014;273:220–31.

77. Liang J, Xu Y, Wang F, et al. The value of 18F-FDG PET/MR whole body imaging in staging of pediatric neuroblastoma. J Nucl Med 2020;61.

78. Chun GYC, Sample J, Hubbard AK, et al. Trends in pediatric lymphoma incidence by global region, age and sex from 1988-2012. Cancer Epidemiol 2021;73:101965.

79. Alaggio R, Amador C, Anagnostopoulos I, et al. The 5th edition of the World Health Organization Classification of Haematolymphoid Tumours: Lymphoid Neoplasms. Leukemia 2022;36:1720–48.

80. Minard-Colin V, Brugières L, Reiter A, et al. Non-Hodgkin Lymphoma in Children and Adolescents: Progress Through Effective Collaboration, Current Knowledge, and Challenges Ahead. J Clin Oncol 2015;33:2963–74.

81. Nagpal P, Akl MR, Ayoub NM, et al. Pediatric Hodgkin lymphoma: biomarkers, drugs, and clinical trials for translational science and medicine. Oncotarget 2016;7:67551–73.

82. Garaventa A, Parodi S, Guerrini G, et al. Outcome of Children and Adolescents with Recurrent Classical Hodgkin Lymphoma: The Italian Experience. Cancers 2022;14.

83. Rosolen A, Perkins SL, Pinkerton CR, et al. Revised International Pediatric Non-Hodgkin Lymphoma Staging System. J Clin Oncol 2015;33:2112–8.

84. McCarten KM, Nadel HR, Shulkin BL, et al. Imaging for diagnosis, staging and response assessment of Hodgkin lymphoma and non-Hodgkin lymphoma. Pediatr Radiol 2019;49:1545–64.

85. Giraudo C, Raderer M, Karanikas G, et al. 18F-Fluorodeoxyglucose Positron Emission Tomography/Magnetic Resonance in Lymphoma: Comparison With 18F-Fluorodeoxyglucose Positron Emission Tomography/Computed Tomography and With the Addition of Magnetic Resonance Diffusion-Weighted Imaging. Invest Radiol 2016;51:163–9.

86. Giraudo C, Karanikas G, Weber M, et al. Correlation between glycolytic activity on [18F]-FDG-PET and cell density on diffusion-weighted MRI in lymphoma at staging. J Magn Reson Imaging 2018;47:1217–26.

87. Kurch L, Kluge R, Sabri O, et al. Whole-body [18F]-FDG-PET/MRI for staging of pediatric non-Hodgkin lymphoma: first results from a single-center evaluation. EJNMMI Res 2021;11:62.

88. Giraudo C, Simeone R, Fosio M, et al. Diagnostic Value of PET/MR with DWI for Burkitt Lymphoma. Diagnostics 2021;11.

89. Georgi TW, Stoevesandt D, Kurch L, et al. Optimized Whole-Body PET MRI Sequence Workflow in Pediatric Hodgkin Lymphoma Patients. J Nucl Med 2023;64:96–101.

90. Chisholm KM, Ohgami RS, Tan B, et al. Primary lymphoma of bone in the pediatric and young adult population. Hum Pathol 2017;60:1–10.

91. Oberling C. Les reticulosarcomes et les reticuloendotheliosarcomes de la moelle osseuse (sarcomes d'Ewing) Bull Assoc Fr Etude Cancer, (Paris), 17, 1928, 259–296.

92. Fletcher C, Bridge J, Hogendoorn P and Mertens F. WHO classification of tumours of soft tissue and bone, 5, 2013.

93. Daldrup-Link HE, Theruvath AJ, Baratto L, et al. One-stop local and whole-body staging of children with cancer. Pediatr Radiol 2022;52:391–400.

94. Giraudo C, Carraro E, Cavallaro E, et al. [18F]FDG PET-MR in the Evaluation and Follow-Up of Incidental Bone Ischemic Lesions in a Mono-Center Cohort of Pediatric Patients Affected by Hodgkin's Lymphoma. Diagnostics 2023;13.

95. Cavaliere A, Giraudo C, Zuliani M, et al. 18F-FDG PET/MR in an Atypical Pediatric Solid Pseudopapillary Pancreatic Tumor. Clin Nucl Med 2019;44:e522–3.

96. Reinert CP, Schuhmann MU, Bender B, et al. Comprehensive anatomical and functional imaging in patients with type I neurofibromatosis using simultaneous FDG-PET/MRI. Eur J Nucl Med Mol Imaging 2019;46:776–87.

97. Pijl JP, Kwee TC, Legger GE, et al. Role of FDG-PET/CT in children with fever of unknown origin. Eur J Nucl Med Mol Imaging 2020;47:1596–604.

98. Pellino G, Nicolai E, Catalano OA, et al. PET/MR Versus PET/CT Imaging: Impact on the Clinical Management of Small-Bowel Crohn's Disease. J Crohns Colitis 2016;10:277–85.

99. Varotto A, Orsatti G, Crimì F, et al. Radiological Assessment of Paediatric Fungal Infections: A Pictorial Review With Focus on PET/MRI. In Vivo 2019;33:1727–35.

100. Clemente G, de Souza AW, Leão Filho H, et al. Does [18F]F-FDG-PET/MRI add metabolic information to magnetic resonance image in childhood-onset Takayasu's arteritis patients? A multicenter case series. Adv Rheumatol (London, England) 2022;62:28.

Metabolic Imaging for Radiation Therapy Treatment Planning
The Role of Hybrid PET/MR Imaging

Letizia Deantonio, MD[a,b], Francesco Castronovo, MD[a],
Gaetano Paone, MD[b,c], Giorgio Treglia, MD[b,c,d], Thomas Zilli, MD[a,b,e],*

KEYWORDS

- PET/MR imaging • Metabolic imaging • Radiotherapy • Treatment planning • Tumor delineation
- Tumor response • Contouring

KEY POINTS

- Modern radiotherapy requires diagnostic images that can offer excellent spatial resolution and high soft tissue contrast.
- Tumor staging, target volume delineation, and treatment response assessment mainly rely on MR imaging and PET/CT using different radiotracers.
- Combination of PET and MR imaging in one imaging session may improve image definition and reduce tumor and organs displacements caused by different scanning times and patient's setup.
- Tumor volume delineation, dose painting, treatment planning using an MR imaging-only workflow and treatment response assessment are the main fields of application of hybrid PET/MR imaging in radiotherapy planning.
- Current clinical evidence stems from single-center studies with a small sample size.

INTRODUCTION

Radiotherapy (RT) is a mainstay of oncological treatments, and more than half of patients require RT in both curative and palliative settings during their disease management. RT provides excellent local tumor control along with appropriate cosmesis and function preservation. The improvement of local control and the reduction of late side effects are based on both advances for treatment delivery with intensity-modulated radiation therapy (IMRT) techniques, which achieves highly conformal and accurate radiation dose distribution to complex targets while sparing nearby critical tissues, and on on-board image guidance technologies during daily treatment delivery.[1]

These advances require diagnostic images that can offer excellent spatial resolution and high soft tissue contrast between tissues, bone, and fat, as well as functional information on tumor behavior and aggressiveness to optimize target volume delineation and therapeutic adaptations.

RT was revolutionized in the 1990s by computed tomography (CT), which made possible to visualize the tumor as a target and the nearby organs as organs at risk. Since then, CT has become the standard imaging for RT planning. However, CT results in extradose exposure and has a lack of contrast in

[a] Radiation Oncology Clinic, Oncology Institute of Southern Switzerland, Ente Ospedaliero Cantonale, Bellinzona 6500, Switzerland; [b] Faculty of Biomedical Sciences, Università della Svizzera italiana, Lugano 6900, Switzerland; [c] Clinic for Nuclear Medicine and Molecular Imaging, Imaging Institute of Southern Switzerland, Ente Ospedaliero Cantonale, Bellinzona 6500, Switzerland; [d] Faculty of Biology and Medicine, University of Lausanne, Lausanne 1015, Switzerland; [e] Faculty of Medicine, University of Geneva, Geneva 1211, Switzerland
* Corresponding author. Via Gallino 12, Bellinzona 6500, Switzerland.
E-mail address: thomas.zilli@eoc.ch

Magn Reson Imaging Clin N Am 31 (2023) 637–654
https://doi.org/10.1016/j.mric.2023.06.005
1064-9689/23/© 2023 Elsevier Inc. All rights reserved.

soft tissue and artifacts when metal is present.[2] In this regard, MR imaging with its excellent spatial resolution (1 mm), high soft tissue contrast, and functional measurements performed by diffusion-weighted imaging (DWI) sequences, has recently become the gold standard for tumor staging and response assessment in several cancer types (eg, prostate, rectal, and head and neck).[3] As a complement to these imaging modalities, PET can visualize biological processes with different radiotracers and is commonly coupled with CT to compensate low spatial resolution. Both PET/CT and MR imaging are widely used in RT workflow for volume delineation; however, their integration into the CT scan used for treatment planning has required multistep coregistration and adjustment of both images, which can generate image registration distortions and uncertainties in target contouring.[4] These aspects made the use of hybrid PET/MR imaging machines appealing.

In clinical practice, hybrid PET/MR imaging allows simultaneous acquisition of both examinations since digital PET detectors are insensitive to the magnetic field.[3]

In 2010, the first PET/MR imaging tomograph for clinical applications was installed. Since then, hybrid imaging has been considered superior to PET/CT for diagnostic purposes such as detection and characterization of breast cancer bone metastases, colorectal cancer liver metastases, and pelvic recurrences of various cancers.[3] However, the adoption of PET/MR imaging has been slower than PET/CT due to equipment costs and logistics.[4]

The possibility to acquire both modalities simultaneously is attractive for RT planning because hybrid PET/MR imaging minimizes intermodality registration errors on CT simulation scan and reduces the number of examinations.[5] In addition, several studies have been published since the first application of gallium-68-labeled somatostatin-receptor ligand 1,4,7,10-tetraazacyclododecane 1,4,7,10-tetraacetic acid (DOTA)-D-Phe1-Tyr3-octreotide (TOC) ([68Ga]DOTATOC) PET/MR imaging for RT in Tubingen in 2011, reporting a case of a patient with a meningioma treated with IMRT and showing better visualization and target volume delineation with a simultaneous acquisition of PET/MR imaging than with PET/CT and MR imaging separately.[5]

The role of hybrid PET/MR imaging in RT workflow is not clearly established, and its applications are mostly reported from single-center institutional experiences (Table 1). Therefore, the aim of the present review is to present the clinical evidence of hybrid PET/MR imaging for RT workflow, focusing on 4 main topics.

- Definition/delineation of target volumes for radiation treatment planning;
- Understanding the complexity of tumor, exploring the concept of the biological tumor volume (BTV) and dose painting;
- Tumor response assessment and predictive value to achieve a complete remission; and
- Integration as a MR imaging-only workflow generating synthetic CT for dose distribution calculation.

Target Volume Delineation

Target identification and volume delineation are crucial parts of the RT workflow. PET/CT using different radiotracers for treatment planning can modify the gross tumor volume (GTV) boundaries and tumor staging, resulting in the identification of new pathological lymph nodes and, in some cases, distant metastases.[6,7] In this regard, the better soft tissue contrast of MR imaging, combined with the metabolic information from PET, may improve the delineation of GTV. These modifications could have clinical implications for disease control and risk of sequelae for organs at risk. Several reports have explored this hypothesis by studying integrated PET/MR imaging for different tumor sites. Wang and colleagues[8] compared GTV-PET/MR imaging using fluorine-18 fluorodeoxyglucose ([18F]FDG) to GTV-CT used as a reference in a cohort of patients with oropharyngeal cancer. GTV defined using PET/MRIs were similar to GTV based on CT imaging, with minimal overall discrepancies in spatial overlap. The authors did not report a benefit from [18F]FDG PET/MR imaging because these differences did not seem to negatively affect the dose coverage distribution; however, improved confidence in target delineation with hybrid imaging could result in reduced clinical target volume (CTV) margins and improved separation of organs at risk. Similarly, in a recent study by Samolyk-Kogaczewska and colleagues,[9] a series of patients with tongue cancer underwent hybrid PET/MR imaging with [18F]FDG and the derived target volumes were compared with those from CT serving as reference image. Tumor and lymph node volumes detected by MR imaging were larger than those detected by CT due to the better soft tissue contrast of MR imaging, whereas most GTV-PET volumes, defined with visual and fixed-threshold methods, were smaller than GTV-CT due to low spatial resolution. The study raised another issue that is still a matter of debate: the difficulty to identify the ideal method for PET delineation. Currently, the most applied are visual methods more prone to interobserver variation, while threshold methods generate

Table 1
Summary of most relevant clinical studies with hybrid PET/MR imaging

Authors	Country and Publication year	Type of Study	Topic	Tumor	PET/MR Imaging Tomograph	No. of pts	Aim	Main Results
Terzidis et al,[17] 2023	Denmark 2023	Prospective	Target volume delineation	HNSCC	Siemens Biograph mMR	25	To evaluate mismatch and potential clinical impact between the volumes defined from imaging and pathology	The mean mismatch between GTVpatho and GTVonco was 27.9%. An isotropic 5 mm expansion to GTVonco sufficient to cover the GTVpatho
Scharl et al,[14] 2020	Germany 2022	Prospective	Target volume delineation	Cervical cancer	Siemens Biograph mMR	19	To access dose prescription and target volume variation with PET	PET imaging altered RT procedure in 68% of pts; dose prescription and target volume in 70% of pts
Zhang et al,[18] 2020	China 2022	Retrospective	Target volume delineation	Prostate cancer	United imaging PET/MR imaging	69	To evaluate clinical value of PSMA-PET/MR imaging in the GTV delineation of RT compared with histopathology (longest tumor length, L_{path})	DSC MR imaging >0.70 between GTV-MR imaging and GTV-PET $L_{PET/MRI}$ was most correlated with L_{path} in PSMA PET ($P < .001$)
Cao et al,[10] 2021	China 2021	Retrospective	Target volume delineation	HNSCC	GE SIGNA PET/MR imaging	331	To define the locoregional extension patterns by PET/MR imaging and CTV improvement	PET/MR imaging improves CTV delineation based on the locoregional extension patterns

(continued on next page)

Table 1
(continued)

Authors	Country and Publication year	Type of Study	Topic	Tumor	PET/MR Imaging Tomograph	No. of pts	Aim	Main Results
Zhang et al,[12] 2021	China 2021	Prospective	Target volume delineation	Colon cancer liver metastases	Unspecified	24	To compare GTV-PET/MR imaging with GTV-MR imaging during RT	83.33% of GTV-PET/MR imaging and 63.33% of GTV-PET were larger than the reference GTV-MR imaging DSC = 0.51 between GTV-MR imaging and GTV-PET DSC = 0.72 between GTV-MR imaging and GTVPET/MR imaging GTV-PET/MR imaging and GTV-PET were larger than GTV-MR imaging
Graef et al,[11] 2021	Germany 2021	Retrospective	Target volume delineation	Optic nerve sheath meningiomas (ONSM)	Siemens Biograph mMR	8	Feasibility of [68Ga] DOTATOC-PET/MR imaging for diagnostic and PTV contouring for SRS	PET/MR imaging improved margins in 7 out of 10 lesions
Scobioala et al,[15] 2021	Germany 2021	Prospective	Target volume delineation	Prostate cancer	Siemens Biograph mMR	35	Accuracy of PSMA-PET/CT, PSMA-PET/MR imaging, and mpMRI for the delineating of dominant IPL	No IPL delineation improvement by PSMA PET/CT and mpMRI compared with PET/CT alone

Study	Country Year	Design	Application	Cancer	Scanner	N	Objective	Findings
Acker et al,[40] 2019	Germany 2019	Retrospective	Target volume delineation	Meningioma	Siemens Biograph mMR	10	Impact of [68Ga]DOTATOC PET/MR imaging on treatment planning for image-guided SRS by CyberKnife	Smaller PTV of less-experienced physician than experienced ones, (P = .003). Best spatial congruency between experienced physicians
Samolyk-Kogaczewska et al,[9] 2019	Poland 2019	Retrospective	Target volume delineation	HNSCC	Siemens Biograph mMR	10	To evaluate the usefulness and accuracy of PET/MR imaging in GTV delineation	80% GTV-MR imaging and 40% of GTV-PET$_{vis}$ were larger than the reference GTV-CT. [18F]FDG-PET with MR imaging decreases the risk of marginal miss
Wang et al,[8] 2017	USA 2017	Prospective	Target volume delineation	HNSCC	Siemens Biograph mMR	11	To assess differences in GTV delineation/dose coverage hybrid PET/MR imaging vs CT	PET/MR imaging vs CT: mean DSC = 0.63 for T mean DSC = 0.69 for N Discrepancy between GTV-CT and GTV-PET/MR imaging, did not affect treatment plans

(continued on next page)

Table 1
(continued)

Authors	Country and Publication year	Type of Study	Topic	Tumor	PET/MR Imaging Tomograph	No. of pts	Aim	Main Results
Ma et al,[20] 2017	China 2017	Prospective	Target volume delineation	HNSCC	Fused PET/MR imaging Philips Fusion Viewer software on the Extended Brilliance Workspace	18	To evaluate the feasibility of contouring GTV by PET/MR imaging and to define an adaptive threshold level (aTL) for delineating the BTV	Delineating GTV on hybrid PET/MRIs is feasible, and aTL, for delineating BTV, was correlated inversely with SUVmax
Zhang et al,[13] 2014	China 2014	Retrospective	Target volume delineation	Cervical cancer	Philips Ingenuity TF PET/MR imaging	27	To compare different PET-GTV delineation methods with MR-GTV to assess the tumor volume and overlap	PET_{vis}-GTV, $PET_{2.5}$-GTV, and PET_{40}-GTV: not suitable for target delineation. The PET_{DSC}-GTV may increase the accuracy in target volume delineation
Witek et al,[22] 2022	USA 2022	Prospective	Dose painting/personalized RT	HNSCC	GE SIGNA PET/MR imaging	24	To examine tumor response with PET/MR imaging during CRT as a predictor of outcome in p16+ pts	Intermediate risk p16+ pts exhibit heterogeneity in their PET/MR imaging response to CRT
McDonald et al,[43] 2019	USA 2019	Retrospective	Dose painting/personalized RT	Prostate cancer	GE SIGNA PET/MR imaging	12	To report the treatment planning feasibility of dose escalation to [18F] fluciclovine PET/MR imaging suspicious lymph nodes	PET/MR imaging directed dose escalation of suspicious pelvic lymph nodes is feasible in the setting of definitive RT

Study	Country/Year	Design	Application	Cancer	Scanner	N	Aim	Results
Rasmussen et al,[21] 2017	Denmark 2016	Prospective	Dose painting/personalized RT	HNSCC	Siemens Biograph mMR	21	Correlation and reproducibility of multiparametric imaging ($[^{18}F]$ FDG PET and DWI) in VOI contouring	No correlation between FDG PET and DWI. The median tumor overlaps between VOI_{DWI} and VOI_{PET} was 82% (VOI_{DWI} in VOI_{PET}) and 62% (VOI_{PET} in VOI_{DWI}) on scan 1 and scan 2. The VOIs from DWI and FDG PET were both within the target volume for RT planning
Vojtíšek et al,[41] 2021	Czech Republic 2021	Prospective	Tumor response assessment/predictive value	Cervical cancer	Siemens Biograph mMR	66	To find metabolic, morphological characteristics of the tumor predicting non-CMR by the midtreatment PET/MR imaging	Mid-MTV-sum best for prediction of non-CMR (AUC 0.74)
Evangelista et al,[35] 2021	Italy 2021	Retrospective	Tumor response assessment	Prostate cancer	Siemens Biograph mMR	70	To examine PCa detection rate of $[^{18}F]$ fluorocholine PET/MR imaging and to assess the impact of PET/MR imaging findings using PSA response as a biomarker	The overall PCa detection rates for MR imaging, PET, and PET/MR imaging were 65.7%, 37.1%, and 74.3%. PET/MR imaging has a higher detection rate than MR imaging or PET for PCa pts with OMD and PSA levels >0.5 ng/mL

(continued on next page)

Table 1
(*continued*)

Authors	Country and Publication year	Type of Study	Topic	Tumor	PET/MR Imaging Tomograph	No. of pts	Aim	Main Results
Fraioli et al,[30] 2020	UK 2020	Prospective	Tumor response assessment	Glioma	Siemens Biograph mMR	40	To assess benefit of a hybrid [18F] FDOPA PET/MR imaging vs cross-sectional MR imaging for the evaluation of active disease in posttreatment patients and to recognize different tumor features	Significant differences in volume for low-grade/high-grade glioma between [18F] FDOPA PET and MR imaging, both bigger at [18F]FDOPA PET. Overlap percentage significantly higher for low-grade than high-grade. The overlap areas between the tumors were 60% for high-grade and 80% for low-grade
Ivanidze et al,[44] 2019	USA 2019	Retrospective	Tumor response assessment	Meningiomas	Siemens Biograph mMR or GE SIGNA PET/MR imaging	20	To assess postsurgical/postradiation recurrence	Differentiation between meningioma and posttreatment change based on our approach of target lesion/superior sagittal sinus maximum SUVs ratio (16.6 vs 1.6, $P < .0001$)

Study	Country/Year	Design		Cancer	Scanner	N	Objective	Results
Mongula et al,[31] 2018	Netherlands 2018	Prospective	Tumor response assessment	Cervical cancer	Siemens Biograph mMR	10	To evaluate residual disease/metastasis	PET/MR imaging increased in diagnostic confidence in 80%–90% of all pts. Change of opinion was observed in 70% and change of policy in 50%. Good diagnostic accuracy for PET-MR imaging (AUC 0.83)
Becker et al,[32] 2018	Switzerland 2017	Prospective	Tumor response assessment	HNSCC	Philips Ingenuity TF PET/MR imaging	74	To determine the diagnostic performance of [18F]FDG PET/MR imaging after CRT	Sensitivity, specificity, and positive and negative predictive value of PET/DWI-MR imaging were 97.4%, 91.7%, 92.5% and 97.1% per pts, and 93.0%, 93.5%, 90.9%, and 95.1% per lesion, respectively. Agreement between imaging-based and pathological T-stage was excellent (P < .001)

(continued on next page)

Table 1
(continued)

Authors	Country and Publication year	Type of Study	Topic	Tumor	PET/MR Imaging Tomograph	No. of pts	Aim	Main Results
Hojjati et al,[29] 2018	USA 2017	Retrospective	Tumor response assessment	Glioblastoma	Philips Ingenuity TF PET/MR imaging	24	To compare the utility of quantitative PET/MR imaging and PET/CT in differentiating radiation necrosis (RN) from tumor recurrence (TR) in pts with treated glioblastoma	The joint model using PET/MR imaging and CBV mode (pMRI) resulted in AUC of 1.0. Quantitative PET/MR imaging parameters in combination with DSC pMRI provide the best diagnostic utility in distinguishing RN from TR in treated GBMs
Capelli et al,[27] 2022	Italy 2022	Retrospective	Predictive value to response	Rectal cancer	Siemens Biograph mMR	50	To assess the ability of [18F]FDG PET/MR imaging to predict response to nCRT among pts undergoing surgery	28% achieved CR. Second-order textural features (9 in ADC, 6 in PET, 4 in T2W) ROC 0.86 with 100% sensitivity, 64% specificity, 74% accuracy

Freihat et al,[25] 2021	Hungary 2021	Retrospective	Predictive value to response	HNSCC	Siemens Biograph mMR	33	To determine the feasibility of pretreatment primary tumor [^{18}F]FDG PET and DWI-MR imaging parameters in predicting HPV status and the second aim was to assess the feasibility of those imaging parameters to predict response to therapy	Pretreatment ADC of the primary tumor can predict HPV status and treatment response. Metabolic PET parameters (TLG, and MTV) were able to predict primary tumor response to therapy
F. Crimi et al,[24] 2020	Italy 2020	Prospective	Predictive value to response	Rectal cancer	Siemens Biograph mMR	36	To predict pathological stage of [^{18}F]FDG PET/MR imaging after preoperative CTRT in locally advanced rectal cancer	Higher accuracy of PET/MR imaging (92%) than MR imaging (86%) for predicting nodal disease ($P = .1$). Planned treatment strategy was changed in 11% (4/36) of pts

(continued on next page)

Table 1
(continued)

Authors	Country and Publication year	Type of Study	Topic	Tumor	PET/MR Imaging Tomograph	No. of pts	Aim	Main Results
Romeo et al,[42] 2018	Italy 2018	Retrospective	Predictive value to response	HNSCC	Siemens Biograph mMR	5	To assess the response to CHT and/or RT by extracting morphologic, metabolic and functional PET/MR imaging parameters	Useful tool to assess and predict the response to chemotherapy and/or RT
Ahangari et al,[39] 2021	Denmark 2021	Prospective	MR imaging-only planning	Cervical cancer	Siemens Biograph mMR	34	To investigate the feasibility of a PET/MR imaging only RT planning workflow	Good accuracy: dosimetric analysis of the synthetic CT-based dose planning showed a mean absolute error of 0.17 ± 0.12 Gy inside PTV

Abbreviations: CRT, Chemoradiotherapy; CTV, Clinical target volume; CMR, Complete metabolic response; DSC, Dice similarity coefficient; GTV, Gross tumor volume; HNSCC, Head and neck Squamous cell carcinoma; IPL, Intraprostatic lesions; mp, Multiparametric; NPC, Nasopharyngeal carcinoma; nCRT, Neoadjuvant chemoradiotherapy; OMD, Oligometastatic disease; ONSM, Optic nerve sheath meningiomas; pts, Patients; PTV, Planning target volume; RT, Radiotherapy; SRS, Stereotactic radiosurgery; sCT, Synthetic CT; VOI, Volume of interest.

different volumes depending on the fixed threshold chosen.[9]

More recently, Cao and colleagues[10] retrospectively analyzed a cohort of 331 patients with nasopharyngeal carcinoma and showed that the detection of the primary tumor extension with [18F]FDG PET/MR imaging translated in an improved risk stratification of CTVs.

The potential benefit of hybrid PET/MR imaging has also been hypothesized for radiosurgery, where the high-dose gradient combined with the steep fall dose emphasizes the need of an improved accuracy in target volume definition. This issue has been explored in stereotactic radiosurgery of optic nerve meningiomas. Hybrid [68Ga]DOTATOC PET/MR imaging was investigated for target volume delineation and resulted in a more accurate detection of tumor boundaries, useful to eliminate for the majority of lesions additional safety margins for radiation planning.[11] In another setting of stereotactic RT, the feasibility of GTV delineation with hybrid [18F]FDG PET/MR imaging was tested in liver metastases.[12] Interestingly, there was no significant interobserver difference in the contouring of target volumes using a PET/MR imaging, a PET, or a MR imaging technique. Moreover, PET/MR imaging-GTV and PET-GTV were larger than MR imaging-GTV, and PET/MR imaging-GTV differed significantly from MR imaging-GTV, probably because the PET component can easily detect microscopic tumor extension beyond morphological limits, making the hybrid PET/MR imaging technology worthy of consideration.[12]

In gynecological cancers, MR imaging has a central diagnostic role, and [18F]FDG PET is increasingly used in target volume definition. In this regard, hybrid [18F]FDG PET/MR imaging has been implemented in the diagnostic and planning workflow of cervical cancer. Zhang and colleagues explored, in a series of patients with cervical cancer who underwent hybrid [18F]FDG PET/MR imaging, different delineation methods of PET-GTV that were compared with the gold standard imaging of MR imaging-GTV. The PET-GTVs defined by the 30% SUVmax threshold were not different from MR imaging-GTVs; in contrast, other thresholds and visual methods seemed inadequate to define the target volume.[13] Furthermore, in an article by Scharl and colleagues[14] on cervical cancer, [18F]FDG PET findings mainly influenced lymph node staging, leading to altered target volume in nearly 70% of cases and variation in the dose prescription of the integrated simultaneous boost on PET-positive lymph nodes.

The recognized role of MR imaging and, more recently, prostate-specific membrane antigen (PSMA)-PET in the diagnosis and staging of prostate cancer is gaining relevance in target contouring. Scobioala and colleagues[15] evaluated the accuracy of delineation of dominant intraprostatic lesions with hybrid PET/MR imaging. The authors showed the significant diagnostic performance of PSMA-based imaging compared with multiparametric MR imaging. PSMA-PET also achieved superior contouring definition of prostate lesions compared with multiparametric-MR imaging (Fig. 1). No improvement in delineation of intraprostatic lesions was obtained with the combination of PSMA-PET/CT and multiparametric MR imaging compared with PSMA-PET/CT alone.

The gold standard reference for the correct definition of tumor volume should be the pathological extension on surgical specimens; however, since the publication of Daisne and colleagues[16] that stated no single imaging modality completely encompasses the tumor, few studies have included such a comparison. One of the most recent publications was performed by Terzidis and colleagues[17] on 13 head and neck squamous cell carcinoma scanned on an integrated [18F]FDG PET/MR imaging tomograph before surgery. Three GTVs were defined from MR imaging (GTV$_{MR\ imaging}$), PET (GTV$_{PET}$), and both anatomical images and clinical information (GTVonco) and compared with a pathological 3D tumor volume (GTVpato) derived from pathological tumor areas in all specimens. Even though the advances of imaging modalities, the GTVonco were found to be significantly larger than GTVpato, with a 28% mismatch. Of note, by adding the typical 5-mm margin around the GTVonco, the inclusion of all pathological volumes was ensured in most cases.[17] Similarly, Zhang and colleagues assessed the performance of [18F]PSMA-1007 or [68Ga]PSMA-11 PET/MR imaging in delineating GTV for prostate cancer and by comparing it with surgical specimens. The authors found that the longer tumor length based on GTV-PET/MR imaging had the highest consistency with the gold standard of pathology.[18] Both studies highlighted the potential benefit of combining PET and MR imaging.

Dose Painting and Personalized Radiotherapy

Intratumor heterogeneity must be considered when attempting to define tumor volume and dose prescription. Biologically different subvolumes can be studied using DWI sequences, quantified as the apparent diffusion coefficient (ADC), and radiotracer uptake, quantified as the standardized uptake value (SUV). These subvolumes can be identified and targeted before and during treatment with radiation dose painting.[19] Ma and

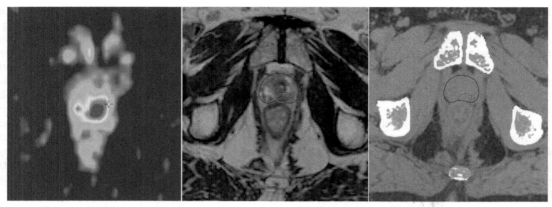

Fig. 1. A 57-year-old man with high-risk prostate cancer. From left to right: [^{18}F]PSMA-1007 PET uptake of the intraprostatic tumor; the dominant intraprostatic lesion (DIL) on T2-weighted MR imaging sequences; MRCAT (MR for calculating attenuation). The red line represents the DIL, the blue line the prostate CTV.

colleagues[20] explored this issue by hypothesizing that a hybrid PET/MR imaging is feasible and advantageous to define an adaptive threshold level to delineate the BTV. The authors used GTV-MR imaging as standard reference for selecting the adaptive BTV. All adaptive BTV generated within the GTV-PET, using different percentile thresholds, were easily delineated on hybrid images with significant correlation with GTV-MR imaging. However, Rasmussen and colleagues[21] in a similar setting of patients with head and neck cancer, assessed the correlation between DWI and [^{18}F] FDG PET uptake using an integrated PET/MR imaging scan to study tumor heterogeneity. The volumes of interest (VOI) generated from DWI and [^{18}F]FDG PET were both within the RT target volume; however, the correlation between DWI and [^{18}F]FDG uptake was weak, with a noncomplete volume overlap. This finding is of interest because both information should be considered complementary and relevant for treatment planning.

Image-based biomarkers can influence treatment approaches, and the use of PET/MR imaging would be of interest. In oropharyngeal cancer, staging and prognosis are strongly influenced by HPV status, and several studies are exploring the intensification and deintensification of the therapy. The combination of the ADC signal and [^{18}F]FDG uptake with HPV status was studied by Witek and colleagues[22] by examining hybrid [^{18}F]FDG PET/MR imaging performed at baseline and 10 days after initiation of RT in a series of 18 low-risk and intermediate-risk p16-positive oropharyngeal cancers. The authors found that pretreatment PET/MR imaging showed no differences between low-risk and intermediate-risk tumors, whereas intratreatment changes in radiographic parameters (ie, SUV and DWI) identified a cluster of intermediate-risk cancers amenable of treatment deintensification. In addition, hypoxia as a biomarker of radio-resistance is an interesting topic of study. In a prospective study of patients with high-grade prostate cancer candidates for curative RT, fluorine-18 misonidazole PET/MR imaging was used to detect hypoxia before and after the start of androgen deprivation therapy.[23] The authors showed a decrease in the baseline uptake after 3 months of neoadjuvant hormonal manipulation, suggesting a reoxygenation and a modulation of radio-resistance inside these intraprostatic lesions, thereby improving treatment outcome.

Response Assessment and Predictive Value

Another crucial issue is response assessment and noninvasive methods that can predict treatment response. Both morphologic and functional imagings are studied. This topic is a matter of debate in rectal cancer with the advent of the wait-and-see strategy, which requires methods that can identify complete responders. Crimi and colleagues[24] performed hybrid [^{18}F]FDG PET/MR imaging after neoadjuvant radio-chemotherapy and compared these results to pelvic MR imaging for predicting patients in complete pathological response and to a CT scan to identify the occurrence of metastases. The accuracy for ypT and ypN staging was slightly in favor of [^{18}F]FDG PET/MR imaging. Compared with CT, [^{18}F]FDG PET/MR imaging correctly diagnosed 4 of 5 metastases. In 11% of patients, [^{18}F]FDG PET/MR imaging changed the treatment strategy. The predictive value of baseline [^{18}F]FDG PET/MR imaging was also assessed in a population of patients with oropharyngeal cancer.[25] The authors showed that pretreatment ADC could predict HPV status and treatment response, whereas total lesion glycolysis (TLG) and metabolic tumor volume (MTV) were significantly different between patients with complete response and those without, potentially identifying patients amenable of treatment intensification.

Nowadays, among noninvasive approaches that can predict treatment response, radiomics, which is the analysis of radiologic images based on the extraction of quantitative features, is gaining interest and may represent an interesting modality.[26] Radiomics features derived from hybrid imaging combining PET and MR imaging undertaken simultaneously would be of interest. In this regard, Capelli and colleagues[27] analyzed features of [18F]FDG PET/MR imaging realized after a neoadjuvant treatment of rectal cancer. The [18F]FDG PET/MR imaging texture analysis (ie, ADC, PET and T2W images) seemed to be a valuable tool for identifying patients with rectal cancer in complete pathological response after neoadjuvant radio-chemotherapy (area under the curve value of 0.863).

Evaluating images after RT, the distinction between radionecrosis and disease progression in gliomas is a controversial issue.[28,29] The complementary use of radiolabeled amino acid PET/MR imaging can assess treatment response and residual tumor volume in gliomas, offering an improvement for the diagnosis of active residual disease compared with PET and MR imaging.[30] In gynecological cancer, combined evaluation of [18F]FDG PET/MR imaging changes after RT helped to discriminate between postradiation-induced fibrosis or edema and residual tumor. Mongula and colleagues[31] showed that [18F]FDG PET discriminated and corrected doubtful images on the MR imaging in the pelvic region. Thus, subsequent management changed in half of the patients. In a study by Becker and colleagues,[32] [18F]FDG PET and DWI sequences performed with a hybrid system yielded excellent results in detecting tumor recurrence and extension after radio-chemotherapy of head and neck squamous cell carcinoma compared with pathologic findings. In addition, a challenging scenario is the optimal imaging modality for detecting clinical recurrences in patients with prostate cancer with biochemical recurrence.[33–35] The potential value of combining high soft tissue contrast with MR imaging and metabolic information from PET has been studied by Evangelista and colleagues,[35] who showed that [18F]fluorocholine PET/MR imaging performed better than MR imaging and PET alone for patients with prostate cancer in detecting oligometastatic disease in patients with a PSA level greater than 0.5 ng/mL. Similarly, Achard and colleagues analyzed a cohort of patients in biochemical relapse after radical prostatectomy restaged with [18F]fluorocholine PET/MR imaging and compared the performance of hybrid imaging to pelvic multiparametric MR imaging. A PSA level of 1.5 ng/mL or greater was found to be a significant predictor of [18F]fluorocholine PET/MR imaging positivity. Compared with PET, mpMRI identified more local recurrences in the prostate bed.[34]

Dose Distribution Calculation

Dose distribution calculation is based on planning CT, and additional imaging modalities (eg, PET/CT and MR imaging) are used to improve tumor delineation. Each imaging modality needs specific set-up devices to perform the examination in treatment position to limit set-up variations. Compared with separate PET/CT and MR imaging, the integration of hybrid PET/MR imaging would reduce the number of RT steps needed for a treatment simulation. Paulus and colleagues[36] tested the integration in a hybrid PET/MR imaging of a prototype flat RT table, radiofrequency coil holders for head imaging, and radiofrequency body bridges. Implementation of this dedicated RT equipment in the clinical workflow was technically feasible. Although the "signal-to-noise" ratio of the images was reduced by about 20% to 30% compared with diagnostic MR imaging, the image quality was considered overall good. All the devices tested were PET compatible and did not produce visible artifacts or alter image quality. RT devices showed a satisfactory repositioning accuracy.

Another prototype by Brynolfsson and colleagues that was tested on a hybrid PET/MR imaging scanner adapted to image patients for RT treatment planning showed that the activity quantitation errors in PET imaging were within 5% when correcting for attenuation of the flat tabletop, coil holder, and flex coil. The "signal-to-noise" ratio of MR imaging images was reduced to 66% to 74% with dedicated RT components.[37] The complexity of integrating PET/MR imaging in the RT planning workflow is also related to the fact that CT is essential to achieve accurate radiation dose calculation for RT treatments. Several approaches have been developed and validated to generate a synthetic CT from MR imaging (MR for calculating attenuation [MRCAT]), particularly in the pelvis and brain.[38] Recently, Ahangari and colleagues[39] investigated the feasibility of a PET/MR imaging-only RT planning workflow for patients with cervical cancer. A dedicated RT set-up (coil holder and leg fixation) was used to perform the hybrid PET/MR imaging, with a logistic advantage for patients, no extradose exposure, and a scan time of less than 45 minutes, including the preparation time. Synthetic CT images were generated from a specific MR imaging sequence in less than 5 seconds. Dosimetric analysis of the MRCAT-based dose planning showed a mean absolute error of 0.17 Gy $\pm$ 0.12 Gy within the PTV.

SUMMARY

Integrated PET/MR imaging using different radiotracers can have several practical advantages in RT workflow.[40–44] The main advantage is that hybrid PET/MR imaging can provide a single acquisition for both PET and MR imaging, optimizing patient compliance. In addition, performing both images simultaneously would reduce tumor and organ movements caused by different scan times and setup changes, minimizing radiation exposure, and reducing coregistration discrepancies in CT simulation scanning.

PET/MR imaging can also play a role in improving target delineation for treatment planning, especially due to the higher soft tissue contrast. However, data in the literature are conflicting in demonstrating the superiority of hybrid PET/MR imaging over PET/CT and MR imaging performed separately.

Other interesting applications maybe in the field of treatment response assessment, and preliminary in adaptive RT.

Implementation of MR imaging set-up devices compatible with treatment planning systems would reduce image coregistration errors. Although in an early stage of development, another interesting application in the era of MR imaging-Linacs would be the development of hybrid PET/MR imaging for treatment planning with an MR imaging-only workflow.

Main limitations for reaching more robust conclusions are due to the relative low availability of hybrid PET/MR imaging devices, mainly limited to academic centers, with mostly single-center studies based on small sample sizes.

CLINICS CARE POINTS

- The main advantage in hybrid PET/MR imaging is based on the simultaneous acquisition of 2 modalities reducing the burden for the patient.
- Hybrid images show advantages in tumor delineation.
- PET/MR imaging performance is particularly good for the early evaluation of tumor response and allows better understanding intratumoral heterogeneity.

- Hybrid PET/MR imaging is still in early development for treatment planning.
- Evidence is based on monocentric experiences based on small patient samples.
- Availability and diffusion of PET/MR imaging is lower compared with PET/CT.

DISCLOSURE

The authors have nothing to disclose.

REFERENCES

1. Atun R, Jaffray DA, Barton MB, et al. Expanding global access to radiotherapy. Lancet Oncol 2015; 16(10):1153–86.
2. Decazes P, Hinault P, Veresezan O, et al. Trimodality PET/CT/MRI and radiotherapy: a mini-review. Front Oncol 2021;10:614008.
3. Créhange G, Soussan M, Gensanne D, et al. Interest of positron-emission tomography and magnetic resonance imaging for radiotherapy planning and control. Cancer Radiother 2020;24(5):398–402.
4. Zhu T, Das S, Wong TZ. Integration of PET/MR hybrid imaging into radiation therapy treatment. Magn Reson Imaging Clin N Am 2017;25(2): 377–430.
5. Thorwarth D, Henke G, Müller AC, et al. Simultaneous 68Ga-DOTATOC-PET/MRI for IMRT treatment planning for meningioma: First experience. Int J Radiat Oncol Biol Phys 2011;81(1):277–83.
6. Deantonio L, Beldì D, Gambaro G, et al. FDG-PET/CT imaging for staging and radiotherapy treatment planning of head and neck carcinoma. Radiat Oncol 2008;3:29.
7. Krengli M, Milia ME, Turri L, et al. FDG-PET/CT imaging for staging and target volume delineation in conformal radiotherapy of anal carcinoma. Radiat Oncol 2010;5:10.
8. Wang K, Mullins BT, Falchook AD, et al. Evaluation of PET/MRI for Tumor Volume Delineation for Head and Neck Cancer. Front Oncol 2017;7:8.
9. Samołyk-Kogaczewska N, Sierko E, Zuzda K, et al. PET/MRI-guided GTV delineation during radiotherapy planning in patients with squamous cell carcinoma of the tongue. Strahlenther Onkol 2019; 195(9):780–91.
10. Cao C, Xu Y, Huang S, et al. Locoregional extension patterns of nasopharyngeal carcinoma detected by FDG PET/MR. Front Oncol 2021;11:763114.
11. Graef J, Furth C, Kluge AK, et al. 68Ga-DOTATOC-PET/MRI-A secure one-stop shop imaging tool for robotic radiosurgery treatment planning in patients with optic nerve sheath meningioma. Cancers 2021;13(13):3305.

12. Zhang YN, Lu X, Lu ZG, et al. Evaluation of hybrid PET/MRI for gross tumor volume (GTV) delineation in colorectal cancer liver metastases radiotherapy. Cancer Manag Res 2021;13:5383–9.

13. Zhang S, Xin J, Guo Q, et al. Defining PET tumor volume in cervical cancer with hybrid PET/MRI: a comparative study. Nucl Med Commun 2014;35(7): 712–9.

14. Scharl S, Weidenbaecher CB, Hugo C, et al. First experiences with PET-MRI/CT in radiotherapy planning for cervical cancer. Arch Gynecol Obstet 2022; 306(5):1821–8.

15. Scobioala S, Kittel C, Wolters H, et al. Diagnostic efficiency of hybrid imaging using PSMA ligands, PET/CT, PET/MRI and MRI in identifying malignant prostate lesions. Ann Nucl Med 2021;35(5):628–38.

16. Daisne JF, Duprez T, Weynand B, et al. Tumor volume in pharyngolaryngeal squamous cell carcinoma: comparison at CT, MR imaging, and FDG PET and validation with surgical specimen [published correction appears in Radiology. Radiology 2004;233(1):93–100.

17. Terzidis E, Friborg J, Vogelius IR, et al. Tumor volume definitions in head and neck squamous cell carcinoma - Comparing PET/MRI and histopathology. Radiother Oncol 2023;180:109484.

18. Zhang YN, Lu ZG, Wang SD, et al. Gross tumor volume delineation in primary prostate cancer on [18F]-PSMA-1007 PET/MRI and [68Ga]-PSMA-11 PET/MRI. Cancer Imag 2022;22(1):36.

19. Bentzen SM, Gregoire V. Molecular imaging-based dose painting: A novel paradigm for radiation therapy prescription. Semin Radiat Oncol 2011;21:101–10.

20. Ma JT, Han CB, Zheng JH, et al. Hybrid PET/MRI-based delineation of gross tumor volume in head and neck cancer and tumor parameter analysis. Nucl Med Commun 2017;38(7):642–9.

21. Rasmussen JH, Nørgaard M, Hansen AE, et al. Feasibility of multiparametric imaging with PET/MR in head and neck squamous cell carcinoma. J Nucl Med 2017;58(1):69–74.

22. Witek ME, Kimple RJ, Avey GD, et al. Prospective study of PET/MRI tumor response during chemoradiotherapy for patients with low-risk and intermediate-risk p16-positive oropharynx cancer. Am J Clin Oncol 2022;45(5):202–7.

23. Mainta IC, Zilli T, Tille JC, et al. The Effect of Neoadjuvant Androgen Deprivation Therapy on Tumor Hypoxia in High-Grade Prostate Cancer: An [18F]-MISO PET-MRI Study. Int J Radiat Oncol Biol Phys 2018;102(4):1210–8.

24. Crimì F, Spolverato G, Lacognata C, et al. 18F-FDG PET/MRI for rectal cancer TNM restaging after preoperative chemoradiotherapy: Initial experience. Dis Colon Rectum 2020;63(3):310–8.

25. Freihat O, Tóth Z, Pintér T, et al. Pre-treatment PET/MRI based FDG and DWI imaging parameters for predicting HPV status and tumor response to chemoradiotherapy in primary oropharyngeal squamous cell carcinoma (OPSCC). Oral Oncol 2021; 116:105239.

26. Bosetti DG, Ruinelli L, Piliero MA, et al. Cone-beam computed tomography-based radiomics in prostate cancer: a mono-institutional study. Strahlenther Onkol 2020;196(10):943–51.

27. Capelli G, Campi C, Bao QR, et al. 18F-FDG-PET/MRI texture analysis in rectal cancer after neoadjuvant chemoradiotherapy. Nucl Med Commun 2022; 43(7):815–22.

28. Bertaux M, Berenbaum A, Di Stefano AL, et al. Hybrid [18F]-F-DOPA PET/MRI interpretation criteria and scores for glioma follow-up after radiotherapy. Clin Neuroradiol 2022;32(3):735–47.

29. Hojjati M, Badve C, Garg V, et al. Role of FDG-PET/MRI, FDG-PET/CT, and dynamic susceptibility contrast perfusion MRI in differentiating radiation necrosis from tumor recurrence in glioblastomas. J Neuroimaging 2018;28(1):118–25.

30. Fraioli F, Shankar A, Hyare H, et al. The use of multiparametric 18F-fluoro-L-3,4-dihydroxy-phenylalanine PET/MRI in post-therapy assessment of patients with gliomas. Nucl Med Commun 2020; 41(6):517–25.

31. Mongula JE, Bakers FCH, Vöö S, et al. Positron emission tomography-magnetic resonance imaging (PET-MRI) for response assessment after radiation therapy of cervical carcinoma: A pilot study. EJNMMI Res 2018;8(1):1.

32. Becker M, Varoquaux AD, Combescure C, et al. Local recurrence of squamous cell carcinoma of the head and neck after radio(chemo)therapy: Diagnostic performance of FDG-PET/MRI with diffusion-weighted sequences. Eur Radiol 2018;28(2): 651–63.

33. Lamanna G, Tabouret-Viaud C, Rager O, et al. Long-term Results of a Comparative PET/CT and PET/MRI Study of 11C-Acetate and 18F-Fluorocholine for Restaging of Early Recurrent Prostate Cancer. Clin Nucl Med 2017;42(5):e242–6.

34. Achard V, Lamanna G, Denis A, et al. Recurrent prostate cancer after radical prostatectomy: restaging performance of 18F-choline hybrid PET/MRI. Med Oncol 2019;36(8):67.

35. Evangelista L, Cassarino G, Lauro A, et al. Comparison of MRI, PET, and 18F-choline PET/MRI in patients with oligometastatic recurrent prostate cancer. Abdom Radiol (NY) 2021;46(9):4401–9.

36. Paulus DH, Oehmigen M, Grüneisen J, et al. Whole-body hybrid imaging concept for the integration of PET/MR into radiation therapy treatment planning. Phys Med Biol 2016;61(9):3504–20.

37. Brynolfsson P, Axelsson J, Holmberg A, et al. Technical Note: Adapting a GE SIGNA PET/MR scanner for radiotherapy. Med Phys 2018. https://doi.org/

10.1002/mp.13032. published online ahead of print, 2018 Jun 3.

38. O'Connor LM, Dowling JA, Choi JH, et al. Validation of an MRI-only planning workflow for definitive pelvic radiotherapy. Radiat Oncol 2022;17(1):55.

39. Ahangari S, Hansen NL, Olin AB, et al. Toward PET/MRI as one-stop shop for radiotherapy planning in cervical cancer patients. Acta Oncol 2021;60(8):1045–53.

40. Acker G, Kluge A, Lukas M, et al. Impact of 68Ga-DO-TATOC PET/MRI on robotic radiosurgery treatment planning in meningioma patients: First experiences in a single institution. Neurosurg Focus 2019;46(6):E9.

41. Vojtíšek R, Baxa J, Kovářová P, et al. Prediction of treatment response in patients with locally advanced cervical cancer using midtreatment PET/MRI during concurrent chemoradiotherapy. Strahlenther Onkol 2021;197(6):494–504.

42. Romeo V, Iorio B, Mesolella M, et al. Simultaneous PET/MRI in assessing the response to chemo/radiotherapy in head and neck carcinoma: Initial experience. Med Oncol 2018;35(7):112.

43. McDonald AM, Galgano SJ, McConathy JE, et al. Feasibility of dose escalating [18F]fluciclovine positron emission tomography positive pelvic lymph nodes during moderately hypofractionated radiation therapy for high-risk prostate cancer. Adv Radiat Oncol 2019;4(4):649–58.

44. Ivanidze J, Roytman M, Lin E, et al. Gallium-68 DO-TATATE PET in the evaluation of intracranial meningiomas. J Neuroimaging 2019;29(5):650–6.

Moving?

Make sure your subscription moves with you!

To notify us of your new address, find your **Clinics Account Number** (located on your mailing label above your name), and contact customer service at:

Email: journalscustomerservice-usa@elsevier.com

800-654-2452 (subscribers in the U.S. & Canada)
314-447-8871 (subscribers outside of the U.S. & Canada)

Fax number: 314-447-8029

Elsevier Health Sciences Division
Subscription Customer Service
3251 Riverport Lane
Maryland Heights, MO 63043

*To ensure uninterrupted delivery of your subscription, please notify us at least 4 weeks in advance of move.